Series Editors:
Steven F. Warren, Ph.D.
Marc E. Fey, Ph.D.

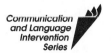

Communication
and Language
Intervention
Series

D0573183

Phonological Disorders in Children

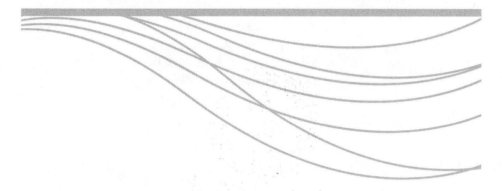

Also in the Communication
and Language Intervention Series:

Communication
and Language
Intervention
Series

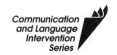

Phonological Disorders in Children

Clinical Decision Making in Assessment and Intervention

edited by

Alan G. Kamhi, Ph.D.
Northern Illinois University
DeKalb, Illinois

and

Karen E. Pollock, Ph.D.
University of Alberta
Edmonton, Alberta, Canada

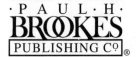

·P·A·U·L·H·
BROOKES
PUBLISHING CO.®

Baltimore • London • Sydney

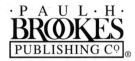

Paul H. Brookes Publishing Co.
Post Office Box 10624
Baltimore, Maryland 21285-0624

www.brookespublishing.com

Typeset by International Graphic Services, Newtown, Pennsylvania.
Manufactured in the United States of America
by Sheridan Books, Inc., Springfield, Virginia.

The individuals described in this book are composites or real people whose situations are masked and are based on the authors' experiences. Names and identifying details have been changed to protect confidentiality.

Library of Congress Cataloging-in-Publication Data

Phonological disorders in children : clinical decision making in assessment and intervention / edited by Alan G. Kamhi, and Karen E. Pollock.
    p.   cm.
  Includes bibliographical references and index.
  ISBN 1-55766-784-5 (pbk.)—(Communication and language intervention series)
  1. Articulation disorders in children. 2. Language disorders in children—Treatment. I. Kamhi, Alan G., 1950– II. Pollock, Karen E. III. Series.
RJ496.S7P464   2005
618.92'855—dc22   2005000733

British Library Cataloguing in Publication data are available from the British Library.

Contents

Series Preface

The purpose of the *Communication and Language Intervention Series* is to provide meaningful foundations for the application of sound intervention designs to enhance the development of communication skills across the life span. We are endeavoring to achieve this purpose by providing readers with presentations of state-of-the-art theory, research, and practice.

In selecting topics, editors, and authors, we are not attempting to limit the contents of this series to viewpoints with which we agree or that we find most promising. We are assisted in our efforts to develop the series by an editorial advisory board consisting of prominent scholars representative of the range of issues and perspectives to be incorporated in the series.

Well-conceived theory and research on development and intervention are vitally important for researchers, educators, and clinicians committed to the development of optimal approaches to communication and language intervention. The content of each volume reflects our view of the symbolic relationship between intervention and research: Demonstrations of what may work in intervention should lead to analysis of promising discoveries and insights from developmental work that may in turn fuel further refinement by intervention researchers. We trust that the careful reader will find much that is of great value in this volume.

An inherent goal of this series is to enhance the long-term development of the field by systematically furthering the dissemination of theoretically and empirically based scholarship and research. We promise the reader an opportunity to participate in the development of this field through debates and discussions that occur throughout the pages of the *Communication and Language Intervention Series.*

Editorial Advisory Board

About the Editors

Alan G. Kamhi, Ph.D., is Adjunct Professor in the Department of Communicative Disorders at Northern Illinois University. Since the mid-1970s, he has conducted research on many aspects of developmental speech, language, and reading disorders. He has written several books with Hugh Catts on the connections between language and reading disabilities as well as two books with Karen E. Pollock and Joyce Harris on communication development and disorders in African American speakers. His current research focuses on how to use research and reason to make clinical decisions in the treatment of children with speech, language, and literacy problems. He began a 3-year term as the Language Editor for the *Journal of Speech, Language, and Hearing Research* in January 2004 and served as Editor of *Language, Speech, and Hearing Services in Schools* from 1986 to 1992.

Karen E. Pollock, Ph.D., is Professor and Chair of the Department of Speech Pathology and Audiology at the University of Alberta. She has taught graduate courses, conducted research, and published in the area of child phonology for almost 20 years. In addition to co-editing two books with Alan G. Kamhi and Joyce Harris on communication development/disorders and literacy in African American children, she served as associate editor in the area of phonology for the *Journal of Speech, Language, and Hearing Research* from 1995 to 1997 and is currently an editorial consultant for several scholarly professional journals. Her recent research interests include vowel errors in children with phonological disorders, phonological variation in southern and African American English dialects, and speech-language development in internationally adopted children.

Contributors

Barbara Handford Bernhardt, Ph.D.
Associate Professor
School of Audiology and Speech Sciences
University of British Columbia
5804 Fairview Avenue
Vancouver, BC V6S 1A6, Canada

Barbara L. Davis, Ph.D.
Professor
Department of Communication Sciences
 and Disorders
The University of Texas at Austin
Jesse Jones Communication Complex
Austin, TX 78712

Judith A. Gierut, Ph.D.
Professor
Department of Speech and Hearing Sciences
Indiana University
200 South Jordan Avenue
Bloomington, IN 47405

Lisa Goffman, Ph.D.
Associate Professor
Department of Audiology and Speech Sciences
Purdue University
Heavilon Hall
West Lafayette, IN 47907

Paul R. Hoffman, Ph.D.
Professor
Department of Communication Sciences
 and Disorders
Louisiana State University
163 M&DA Building
Baton Rouge, LA 70803

Adele W. Miccio, Ph.D.
Associate Professor
Department of Communication Sciences
 and Disorders
The Pennsylvania State University
110 Moore Building
University Park, PA 16802

Janet A. Norris, Ph.D.
Professor
Department of Communication Sciences
 and Disorders
Louisiana State University
163 M&DA Building
Baton Rouge, LA 70803

Susan Rvachew, Ph.D.
Assistant Professor
School of Communications Sciences
 and Disorders
McGill University
1266 Pine Avenue West
Montreal, Quebec H3G 1A8, Canada

Ann A. Tyler, Ph.D.
Professor
Department of Speech Pathology &
 Audiology
University of Nevada School of
 Medicine
152 Nell J. Redfield Building
Reno, NV 89557

Shelley Velleman, Ph.D.
Associate Professor
Communication Disorders
 Department
University of Massachusetts at
 Amherst
715 N. Pleasant Street
Amherst, MA 01003

A. Lynn Williams, Ph.D.
Professor
Department of Communicative
 Disorders
East Tennessee State University
Post Office Box 70643
Johnson City, TN 37614

Foreword

Call me crazy, or boring, or both, but the truth is, when I go out for ice cream, I'm usually perfectly happy to shell out good money for *vanilla*. I think it was my grandmother who suggested to me that the best test of a great brand of ice cream is its vanilla, and for some reason that's always stuck with me. Despite my rather conservative taste in frozen confections, there are some days when vanilla just won't do. I need to spice things up a bit. On a wild day, I might throw caution to the wind and order up a fruit or nut flavor, or chocolate chunks, or a hot fudge–caramel sundae. Although I never lose my taste for vanilla, I rarely regret these explorations into the less common. Sometimes the adventure is extraordinary.

In many ways, Kamhi and Pollock's book, *Phonological Disorders in Children: Clinical Decision Making in Assessment and Intervention,* is like one of my more daring days at the ice cream store. There are plenty of vanilla options on the market. These texts follow a time-honored formula: a chapter or two on speech production, perception, and normal speech development; a chapter on characteristics of children with speech sound disorders; a couple of chapters on assessment; and then a couple more on intervention. These sorts of texts have served my students and me well for the past two decades. But sometimes, I'd like to be able to cut loose and try something different. That's what Kamhi and Pollock have now enabled me to do. Instead of following the typical formula, they enlisted a group of specialists on children's speech sound disorders. These individuals were known to have different perspectives on these problems: how to evaluate them, how to describe them, and how to treat them. Kamhi and Pollock then asked a subset of their cadre of authors to respond to a standard set of questions on assessment, goal selection, and intervention. Finally, they gave each author the freedom to address these issues from their own perspectives.

The result is anything but vanilla. Kamhi notes in his summary chapter that he finds it easier to agree with some authors than others, and all readers can expect to have the same experience. The views represented are too diverse to anticipate otherwise. Furthermore, some views have a firmer grounding in tradition and/or evidence than do others, making them more or less difficult to assimilate into existing clinical schemes. But clinicians who are interested in knowing *how* different experts address some of the clinical questions they routinely encounter and *why* these same individuals have selected their chosen paths will find this compelling reading. And instructors who like to use divergent clinical positions as the stimulus for classroom debates, for class projects, and for student explorations into the research literature will find this book a tasty resource. I invite you to dig in and urge you to use a big spoon.

Marc E. Fey, Ph.D.
University of Kansas

Preface

This book has an interesting history. We first started talking about doing a phonology book when we were still working together at the University of Memphis in the late 1990s. We had just finished editing a book for Paul H. Brookes Publishing Co. on communication development and disorders in African American children and enjoyed working with Elaine Niefeld and the excellent staff at Brookes Publishing. At that time there were not as many book choices in phonology as there were in other areas of speech pathology, and Brookes had yet to publish a book dealing exclusively with phonology.

We were interested in doing something a little different from the usual edited book that contains chapters from various authors. We don't remember exactly where the idea actually came from; it may have been from reading the commentaries in *Brain and Behavioral Sciences,* in which a lengthy article is followed by 10–15 commentaries. Our idea was to have chapters constructed around a set of related questions about assessment and intervention, followed by various contributors discussing their own approach.

Our next step was to identify the people we wanted to contribute. Barbara Hodson and Mary Louise Edwards had recently published an edited book containing chapters by the first generation of child phonologists such as David Ingram, Larry Shriberg, and Mary Elbert. The book was a remarkable collection of original writings, with contributors presenting their personal perspectives on the study of child phonology and how it has evolved over the past 20 years. For our book, we decided to seek out members of the "second generation," including some who had studied under one of the original leaders of the field, but who also had their own views shaped by clinical experience and/or new theoretical perspectives. Shelley Velleman, Adele W. Miccio, Barbara L. Davis, Mary Gordon-Brannan, Ann A. Tyler, Gregg Lof, and Lisa Goffman were our initial group of contributors. We set up a meeting at the American Speech-Language-Hearing Association convention to discuss the plan of the book. During that first meeting, we talked about the organization of the book, the kinds of questions contributors would be asked to address, and how authorship would be assigned. The initial plan was to have each of the eight authors contribute to each of the eight chapters, with authorship order rotating so that everyone would have one first-authored chapter. We planned to write an initial chapter in which we would set up the background and rationale for the questions being asked throughout the book. In the final chapter, we planned to summarize consistent or recurring themes from the book and identify and discuss apparent controversies.

After submitting a book proposal to Elaine Niefeld at Brookes, we both got distracted by other projects and major life changes, such as adopting a baby and moving across the country to Oregon. Without Elaine's encouragement, the book would have passed into that densely populated land of ideas that never see the light of day. In other words, Elaine would not let the book die. Prompted by her encouraging words and enthusiasm, the book was revived. The format was changed to accommodate concerns about overlapping contributions. Most importantly, instead of eight contributors writing a brief section for each chapter, only three to four contributors were assigned to each chapter. Many (but not all) of the initial contributors expressed continued interest in the project.

Ann A. Tyler and Shelley Velleman were our heroes. They both met the first deadline with time to spare. As the other chapters trickled in, it became clear that there was not uniformity in the contributions. Although we intended that the questions be used as the organizational framework for the chapter, some authors preferred writing a more traditional chapter in which the questions were addressed in a less explicit manner, whereas others used the questions as subheadings. Also, as often happens, some of the original authors were unable to contribute to the book because of unanticipated commitments. With fewer contributors to the original chapters, we were left with some gaps. Our first pinch hitters were Janet A. Norris, Paul R. Hoffman, and A. Lynn Williams. We asked Jan and Paul because their language-based perspective was very different from the phonologically oriented perspectives of the other contributors. We asked Lynn because she had written some excellent articles on goal selection. There was also another reason we wanted Lynn involved in the book.

When we got the August 2002 issue of the *American Journal of Speech-Language Pathology*, we were initially quite discouraged. Lynn had put together a special forum on phonology in which she had six authors (including some of ours) describe their assessment protocol for a sample case study. So much for the novelty of this book! But as we thought about it more, our book was not just about assessment; we also had sections on target selection and intervention.

The final change to the book occurred when we began to question the feasibility of merging contributions from three to four authors into one coherent chapter. The individual contributions were just too different. So, we modified the format once again. Instead of multiple-authored chapters, the questions were reassigned to three broad sections (assessment/diagnosis, goal selection, and treatment). Each section would contain five or more single-authored mini-chapters or "essays" offering different perspectives but still answering the same questions proposed initially. Elaine also encouraged us to add a few other contributors so that the book would represent an even broader range of perspectives. Barbara Handford Bernhardt, Judith A. Gierut, and Susan Rvachew were our second group of heroes. They submitted their chapters just 2 months after being asked. Lynn Williams also deserves a special word of mention for not only submitting her first chapter in a timely manner, but also volunteering to contribute a chapter to the intervention section. We would be remiss if we did not extend a special thank you to the original contributors to the book who were willing to make last-minute changes to their chapters. Our final thanks go to Denise Arend for proofing all of the chapters and to Janet Krejci and the staff at Brookes for helping to prepare the book for publication.

Alan G. Kamhi & Karen E. Pollock

Part I

Assessment and Classification

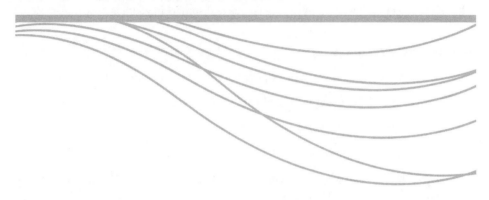

Many different classification systems have been proposed for differentiating subgroups of children with speech sound disorders. In addition, there is considerable variation among researchers and clinicians in the terms used to label these subgroups and the criteria used to define them. Therefore, the book begins with a series of questions about diagnostic classification systems.

We asked contributors to describe their typical approach to the assessment of articulation and phonology. We also asked how they coordinate the assessment of articulation and phonology with other components of language and whether they routinely assess phonological awareness or other literacy skills, which are now often seen as within the scope of practice for speech-language pathologists (SLPs).

With an increased emphasis on early intervention and inclusion practices, younger children and children with developmental disabilities and/or medical conditions are being seen by SLPs. The assessment of these children may be radically different from that of the typical preschooler. Today's clinicians are also faced with many new questions as a result of changing demographics. SLPs are seeing a rapidly increasing number of people who are bilingual, who speak English as a Second Language, or who speak a nonstandard dialect of English, and not all clinicians are equipped to provide a nonbiased assessment of such clients. Thus, we also asked contributors to address how they modify their assessment protocol for children of different ages, developmental levels, and linguistic backgrounds.

The specific questions posed to contributors were divided into three sections: diagnostic classification systems, assessment protocols, and special considerations.

Diagnostic Classification Systems

1. Which diagnostic classification system do you find useful?

2. Do you differentiate between articulation and phonological disorders, and if so, how?

3. What criteria do you use to identify children with developmental apraxia?

4. How do you deal with co-occurring language disorders in your classification system?

Assessment Protocols

5. Describe your typical assessment protocol for articulation/phonology.

6. Do you use standardized tests, and if so, which ones?

7. Do you use nonstandardized analyses, and if so, why?

8. Do you use computerized phonological analyses, and if so, which ones?

9. Does your protocol assess vowels, perception, prosody, or phonological awareness, and if so, which tests/measures do you use?

10. How would you coordinate the assessment of articulation/phonology with language assessment?

Special Considerations

11. How does your assessment protocol differ for children of different ages or developmental levels?

12. How do you assess a child who speaks a different language than you do or a nonstandard dialect at home?

Part I contains five chapters. The first chapter, by Barbara L. Davis, addresses all three sets of questions and provides a comprehensive overview of the assessment and diagnostic process. She nicely sets up many of the issues that arise in subsequent chapters. In Chapter 2, Shelley Velleman focuses on the first (Diagnostic Classification) and last (Special Considerations) sets of questions, paying particular attention to two difficult areas: the differential diagnosis of childhood apraxia of speech and the assessment of children who speak African American English (AAE). Adele W. Miccio (Chapter 3) and Ann A. Tyler (Chapter 4) focus on the second set of questions about typical assessment protocols. Along with the section in Chapter 1 describing Davis's typical assessment protocol, these chapters provide excellent illustrations of how well-versed researchers and clinicians integrate current theories and research findings into their own models of assessment. In the final chapter in Part I, Lisa Goffman considers the differential diagnosis of developmental apraxia and specific language impairment and the more general question of how approaches to classification affect assessment and treatment decisions.

Chapter 1

Clinical Diagnosis of Developmental Speech Disorders

Barbara L. Davis

The highest level of clinical interpretation relative to diagnostic classification is the decision of whether evaluation results (including assessment of spontaneous behaviors and formal test results) indicate that speech patterns should be considered the *primary* or the *secondary* category for differential diagnosis (see Table 1.1). If the observed speech patterns are considered as the primary diagnostic classification, the implication is that the clinician will be targeting these patterns as the major focus in intervention. In this case, the clinical prediction is that disorders related to developmental speech patterns are the primary diagnosis. After a period of intervention, speech patterns should normalize the child's communication delay or disorder relative to chronological age expectations. In children with conditions of known etiology (e.g., cerebral palsy), however, the primary developmental speech diagnosis may predict that these children's speech patterns will not normalize to age-appropriate expectations for intelligible speech based on the etiology classification.

If the disordered speech patterns observed are clinically judged as a secondary diagnosis, they are not considered to be the foundational classification for differential diagnosis but as clinical symptoms observed in addition to the primary diagnostic category assignment. This secondary level of differential diagnostic classification also has important implications for intervention. If the primary diagnostic category is not developmental speech disorder, intervention will be properly centered on other language and communication issues. Resolution of those symptoms should result in normalization of the child's

Table 1.1. Diagnostic classification for developmental speech disorders

Diagnostic evaluation		
Spontaneous behaviors		
Test results		

Primary diagnosis		Secondary diagnosis
Functional	Etiological	Primary clinical factor
Cause unknown	Mechanism	Speech production
	Perceptual	Fluency
	Motor	Voice
	Neural	Language
	General developmental	

clinically relevant speech production patterns related to chronological age expectations or severity level.

DEVELOPMENTAL SPEECH PATTERNS AS A PRIMARY DIAGNOSIS

When developmental speech patterns are considered the primary diagnostic category, two major classifications are available to the clinician. The first classification is termed *functional*. A functional developmental speech disorder or delay classification indicates that at the time of the clinical assessment, no known etiology can be pinpointed for clinically relevant behaviors observed. This functional category accounts for the largest group of children with developmental speech disorders when speech is the primary diagnostic classification (Bernthal & Bankson, 2002). In this category, the clinician may implement intervention based on either phonological or phonetic principles, but the underlying cause of the clinical speech patterning is simply not available based on contemporary techniques for diagnosis in communication sciences and disorders.

The second classification in which developmental speech patterns are designated as the primary diagnostic category is termed *etiological* classification. Etiological classification related to differential diagnosis falls into two areas related to *peripheral mechanism* considerations: production system causes and perception system causes. *Neural* control for speech production or perception may also be implicated as an etiological factor. Finally, *general developmental* issues may be the etiological basis for a diagnosis of primary developmental speech impairment.

In the case of peripheral mechanism etiology, the respiratory, phonatory, or articulatory subsystems of the speech production system can be implicated in a variety of ways directly related to observed speech pattern impairments. For example, respiratory insufficiency is implicated in cerebral palsy, in which energy to support speech production may be insufficient or uncoordinated. In addition, intensity and voicing may be directly involved as well as problems with control of the speech articulation subsystem. Phonation characteristics may underlie speech production impairment associated with injured vocal folds. Here, voicing and fundamental frequency aspects of speech production patterns may be implicated. The articulatory subsystem may be the major etiological factor in a variety of conditions as diverse as velar insufficiency, cleft palate, or tongue muscle weakness (e.g., dysarthria). These differences in articulatory subsystem structures and functions relate to both articulatory shaping of the sound source and to resonance properties underlying speech production patterns.

Perceptual subsystem factors relevant to etiology for developmental speech disorders relate primarily to characteristics of the auditory system, although other sensory systems, including vision and kinesthetic systems, can also be implicated. Level of hearing acuity has been studied for many years relative to predictions for development of intelligible oral speech production, even when children receive intensive therapeutic intervention. Recent instantiation of universal newborn hearing screening programs adds very young children or toddlers to the category of auditory perceptual etiology that may be a part of the scope of practice in assessment and intervention for the contemporary speech-language pathologist. At this time, relationships between sensory factors other than the auditory perceptual status have not been well documented by data-based research.

In addition to peripheral mechanism considerations, neural factors may be implicated as an etiological consideration for observed patterns in developmental speech impairments. The advent of more sophisticated instrumentation such as positron emission tomography (PET) scanning and functional magnetic resonance imaging (fMRI) technologies may signal the beginning of an era in which more straightforward links can be made between neurological structure and function and etiology for developmental speech disorders. At present, the proposed diagnostic classification of developmental apraxia of speech is, in some theoretical perspectives, considered as a difference in speech motor planning based on proposed neurological differences (e.g., Hall, Jordan, & Robin, 1993). Instrumentation currently available is not capable of establishing the validity of this proposal, however. Clearly, some severe categories of developmental speech disorder such as dysarthria are based on underlying neurological damage that can be documented with present instrumentation.

General developmental considerations can also lead to a diagnosis of primary speech delay or disorder. For example, "general motor clumsiness" is a DSM-V (American Psychiatric Association, 2000) category that may also be accompanied by primary developmental speech production impairment (e.g., Hodge, 1998). Profound cognitive delays may stem from a diversity of etiological factors, which result in a primary developmental speech impairment. (This speech impairment may co-occur with primary impairment in language or other areas of communication.) Birth-related risk factors can also constitute a general developmental consideration in which infants experience pre-, peri-, or postnatal birth traumas (Bleile, 1995). These general developmental factors can result in a primary communication disorder affecting typical speech acquisition along with general developmental delays and, potentially, co-occurring primary disorders in other areas of language and communication development.

DEVELOPMENTAL SPEECH PATTERNS AS A SECONDARY DIAGNOSIS

Developmental speech impairment that is clinically relevant based on expectations for a child's chronological age may be a secondary diagnostic classification related to a number of factors (see Table 1.1). In these children, the speech production impairment may either be functional or derive from a known etiological base. In either case, however, clinician judgment will implicate another area as the primary basis for the child's communication or language disorder. In this regard, the developmental speech disorder would likely be at the mild to moderate level relative to age-related expectations for intelligibility. A severe to profound level of developmental speech disorder would more likely, although not always, be considered as the primary clinical classification, even with a co-occurrence of other clinical diagnoses, if the child's intelligibility were extremely low overall.

Developmental speech disorder or delay may be secondary to clinical involvement in other areas of the speech production system. Stuttering or voice disorders, considered aspects of speech production (Kent, 2004), would fit within this category. For example, a child may exhibit stuttering, which is a speech rhythm disorder. The diagnosis of stuttering may be considered the highest priority for clinical classification and planning remediation, even if developmental speech production impairments coexist. A voice disorder affecting the areas of pitch, loudness, rate, or resonance characteristics could also be considered a primary diagnostic category even in the presence of a developmental speech disorder. If the child's voice characteristics are based on etiological factors (e.g., paralyzed vocal fold), a primary diagnostic classification of voice disorder is more likely. As with stuttering, however, the severity of the child's speech production impairment would be important for the clinician in determining the primary area of clinical diagnosis.

Developmental speech delay may also be secondary to *language* delay or disorder. Differential diagnosis of speech versus language disorder as the primary diagnostic category is based on typical speech and language expectations for a child's chronological age. For example, a 5-year-old child who uses primarily open syllables with some consonant-vowel-consonant (CVC) forms (e.g., "cat") and most consonants expected for his age but who demonstrates a mean length of utterance (MLU) of only one to two words might more likely be classified with primary expressive language delay even though his speech production patterns are not considered age appropriate. A 6-year-old with receptive language impairment who does not produce complex word shapes consistently and leaves off some final consonants would receive a primary diagnosis of receptive language delay despite the lack of age appropriate speech production patterns.

A variety of other clinical diagnoses may also include developmental speech production impairment as a secondary diagnostic component for intervention classification. *Socially* based language disorders, such as an autism spectrum disorder, may likely contain a speech production component in children who are considered low functioning, but they would be primarily classified with reference to socially motivated language issues. Children with *cognitively* based language disorders related to intellectual capacity may also exhibit a developmental speech component. The speech patterns would not necessarily be a primary diagnostic focus if the child's language function were significantly impaired.

PHONETIC OR PHONOLOGICAL CLASSIFICATION OF DEVELOPMENTAL SPEECH DISORDERS

One contemporary issue related to classification of developmental speech disorders relates to the dichotomy between phonetic and phonological designations for patterns observed in children who are evaluated clinically. Briefly, *phonetic* perspectives relate to the operation of the motor and sensory processes used to support speech production as well as to neurally instantiated brain–behavior relationships known to support speech production and perception. This dimension of description has been termed the *performance* aspect of speech production (Chomsky & Halle, 1968). In short, an example of performance is what a child does with her body to learn to speak and what the child or adult speaker does to produce speech. In contrast, *phonological* designations relate to what a child or adult speaker *knows* about the phonemic categories and sequence restrictions in the ambient language that allow construction of linguistic messages. Phonological *competence* underlies coding of meanings in a language community.

At present, systems of clinical assessment and intervention in speech-language pathology fall into either phonetic or phonological categories, depending on the background and orientation of the clinician/researcher. Cases in which the etiology is clearly known have been described using the type of classification that is prominent in the professional community, regardless of whether the implication of a phonetic or phonological basis is well founded. For example, the phonological process classification (Stampe, 1979) was used in the 1980s for all types of etiologies, including children with hearing impairment, dysarthria, or cleft palate, despite the clear basis for natural phonological processes within phonological theory. In short, the descriptive utility of clinical speech patterns using phonological descriptors dominated, even in cases in which a clear phonetic or peripheral mechanism etiology was present.

In general, the history of diagnostic classification has represented a pendulum swinging back and forth from predominantly motor-based classifications to primarily phonological classifications for developmental speech involvement. One prominent early classification system for developmental speech disorder or delay was based on Van Riper and Irwin's (1958) original "substitution," "distortion," and "omission" descriptors related to a proposed motor basis for observed speech symptoms. Succeeding that classification system were the linear distinctive feature systems of the 1970s, largely based on the Chomsky and Halle (1968) feature descriptions for underlying phonological competence. Some competence-based feature classifications are still available to contemporary therapists (e.g., Lowe, 2003; Yavas, 1998). In the 1980s and early 1990s, phonological processes (e.g., Hodson & Paden, 1994) were used as the predominant classification system for clinical diagnosis and treatment of developmental speech disorders. As new phonological theories became increasingly predominant in linguistics to replace some of the inadequacies of linear distinctive feature systems, new applications of these theories have emerged in systems of classification available within communication sciences and disorders. Two prominent representatives of these theoretical orientations can be found in nonlinear phonology (e.g., Bernhardt & Stoel-Gammon, 1994) and optimality theory (Pater, 1999). In contrast, contemporary systems of classification based on motor speech theoretical orientations (e.g., Yorkston, Beukelman, Strand, & Bell, 1999) suggest classification based on principles of motor learning with the implication that many developmental speech disorders can be appropriately understood with respect to motor programming and motor planning designations for observed impairments.

The variety of classification systems employed since the 1970s in speech pathology for description of developmental speech disorders reflects a "borrowing" process. Researchers and therapists borrow from available theories in linguistics or motor learning to describe patterned regularities in children diagnosed with developmental speech impairments relative to expectations for their chronological ages. At present, no consensus exists on how to make principled decisions about the proposed phonetic or phonological basis for children's observed clinical impairments. Combined with the situation in which the largest category of children is designated with functional bases for clinical patterns observed, the state of contemporary speech pathology practice in this area of communication sciences and disorders is founded on the clinician's or researcher's theoretical orientation rather than on any objective basis for classification of speech patterns as phonetic or phonological. This "noisy" status of classification relative to the possibility of performance or competence bases for observed clinical symptoms remains a challenge to precision in clinical classification in our speech-language pathology.

ASSESSMENT FRAMEWORK FOR CLINICAL DIAGNOSIS

An overall assessment framework for articulation/phonology has three areas of focus. The first area of focus is related to the primary phonetic/phonological patterns. In this area, the single-word articulation test and the connected speech and language sample are the two tools of choice for assessment. The classic single-word articulation test can be given either in a screening form or as a full test of consonants or syllable structure phonological processes. The connected sample of a child's communication within a developmentally appropriate communication context is another necessary component of valid assessment in this area.

The second major area of assessment focus relates to the child's overall language system and potential relationships between phonetic/phonological delay or disorder and more general language abilities. In this case, the connected speech and language sample is the most important tool for assessing the interface between phonetic/phonological variables and language variables. General language testing may be appropriate to note areas of impairment that may be contributing to the child's clinically relevant phonetic/phonological patterns as well as areas of strength in language abilities that may support therapeutic intervention.

The third, most general, area of assessment focus is related to the larger context of each child's communication profile, as these issues relate to understanding of the phonetic/phonological delay or disorder related to issues of etiology, functional intelligibility or communication ability, and family or cultural factors.

Phonetic/Phonological Assessment

Single-Word Articulation Tests

The single-word articulation test gives a quick picture of a child's ability to produce the consonant phonemes of English in initial, medial, and final position. Some single-word tests also afford analysis of syllable-level phonological processes. These tests are very helpful for children from mainstream American culture who are between the chronological ages of $2^{1}/_{2}$ to 20 years. Single-word articulation tests are helpful for a quick look at consonant patterns and, in the case of phonological process analyses, syllable and word-level patterns as well. If the child's speech is unintelligible, a single-word test format allows an avenue to understand production patterns when the clinician knows the lexical target. The language targets for children whose speech is unintelligible may be difficult to discern in spontaneous utterances, particularly on topics introduced by the child without much contextual support.

Because many single-word tests have normative data available (at least normative data on Anglo-American children), they can also be used to qualify children for services in some intervention contexts, such as public school settings, in which a qualification score for intervention services is needed. Many articulation tests are available giving clinicians the ability to complete this quick measure of a child's speech patterns in single-word citation forms; a visual picture or toy can also be used as support for formulating the needed word. The response format is consistent, allowing task variable comparison across children relative to their ability to relate to familiar and developmentally appropriate materials.

The content of the single-word articulation test misses some very important aspects of assessment of the primary phonetic/phonological delay or disorder. Missing aspects include consistent testing of vowels, stress and intonation patterns, variations related to word- or utterance-level complexity (Pollock, 1991), and the potential and varied relationships of phonetic/phonological delay or disorder to other aspects of the language system such as pragmatic, semantic, syntactic, or discourse variables. These variables are crucial to understanding the status of the child's phonetic/phonological impairments as they relate to overall intelligibility. In addition, each of these aspects missing from the data gained from a single-word articulation test may be a focus for therapeutic goals that cannot be accessed successfully using this testing format alone.

Connected Speech and Language Sample

In contrast, the connected speech and language sample neutralizes many of the drawbacks related to the single-word test for comprehensive clinical assessment. The flexibility available in the connected sample enables assessment of differences between familiar and unfamiliar communication partners, as well as differences in intelligibility in initiated versus response utterances from the child, and differences related to task structure (e.g., novel topics versus familiar topics; structured sentences versus spontaneous speech). Each of these variables is critically important in order to evaluate the client's functional communication abilities as well as to assess the diversity of clinically relevant patterns for intervention that may be observed across contexts.

Because the connected speech sample is based on topics familiar to the child, it is less likely that words outside of the child's semantic capacity will be required. Primary phonetic/phonological variables such as vowels, stress and intonation patterns, and variations related to word- or utterance-level complexity can be observed in the child's connected speech. Finally, the clinician can build into the sampling procedure stimulability testing as well as dynamic assessment (see Peña & Gillam, 2000, for a review of these issues) of the client's ability to make changes on a short-term basis. These aspects can support fuller understanding of clinically relevant speech patterns as well as helping to build appropriate clinical goals based on the assessment process. In addition, the connected sample allows the clinician to assess the child's abilities across all language and communication systems, including visual, gestural, and other nonverbal supports for communication intelligibility.

Despite these benefits, however, some drawbacks for full assessment are inherent in the use of a connected sampling procedure. The child may not be willing to cooperate in the communication context, even with developmentally appropriate materials. As a result, not enough language or communicative vocalizations may be available to get a valid sample of clinically relevant patterns for planning intervention. If the child is unwilling to participate in a variety of activities, the language or vocalizations obtained in the sample may be very restricted and not supportive of understanding the child's speech patterns within the context of overall language abilities. If the child becomes intensely focused on one activity, the distribution of language observed may be severely reduced relative to systematic patterns the child is capable of producing. In addition, analysis of a connected speech and language sample is vastly more time consuming than the single-word articulation test both in collecting a sample and analyzing the patterns that may result.

Table 1.2 lists components that should be incorporated into assessment of each child's phonetic/phonological abilities based on the connected sample. These components include

Table 1.2. Assessment areas for phonetic/phonological analysis

---

Phonetic independent analysis

1. Consonant phones × word position × place × manner × voicing × adult phonology frequency of occurrence
2. Vowel phones × word position × place × manner × voicing × adult phonology frequency of occurrence
3. Syllable and word shapes (CV patterns × syllable and word shapes)
4. Sequential constraints on occurrence
   a. Initial, medial, final
   b. Intrasyllabic CV patterns
5. Prosodic characteristics
   a. Pitch
   b. Loudness
   c. Duration (syllables)
   d. Rate (words and sentences)
   e. Expressive jargon
   f. Stress
   g. Intonation

Phonological/phonetic relational analysis

1. Phonological processes
   a. Syllabic
   b. Assimilatory
   c. Substitution
2. Error analysis
   a. Consonants
   b. Vowels
   c. Clusters
3. Word and syllable matching
   a. Syllable shapes
   b. Word shapes
   c. Word-based patterns
4. Sequential accuracy patterns
   a. Initial, medial, final
   b. Intrasyllabic CV patterns
5. Prosodic accuracy
   a. Stress
   b. Intonation

Key: CV, consonant–vowel.

an *independent* and a *relational* analysis of each client's production patterns. The independent analysis looks at production patterns for consonants, vowels, syllable and word shapes, and prosodic capacities regardless of their accuracy in relationship to language targets. This type of analysis is generally related to a phonetic level of description of speech production patterns. A relational analysis relates to the accuracy a child achieves in producing meaning-based language targets. Relational analysis can be used to describe either phonetic patterns based on motor-based descriptions of the child's patterns or phonological analysis based on phonological descriptions of the individual's patterns. In the case of both independent and relational analyses, the clinician will need to judge the need for the types of analysis employed to describe clinically relevant patterns. These analysis types should be considered to be tools that the clinician selects as needed for valid clinical description. For example, an 8-year-old with residual errors on [s] and [r] does not need an independent/phonetic analysis. In contrast, it is clear that a 3-year-old who does not produce any consonants but [b] and [d] with neutral vowels does not need a relational or error analysis.

Independent Analyses

For the independent analysis of consonants, occurrences should be described by word position relative to place, manner, and voicing characteristics and related to frequency of occurrence values for the child's primary language. For independent analysis of vowels, occurrences should be documented by syllable position relative to height, front–back, and rounding dimensions and should be related to frequency of occurrence values for the child's primary language. Syllable shapes used in the sample should be enumerated (i.e., in English, the range of potential syllable shapes is [CC]CV[CCCC]). Frequency of occurrence of word shapes should also be counted (i.e., monosyllables, disyllables, and polysyllables). Intrasyllabic constraints on occurrence (i.e., reduplication or variegation patterns or initial, medial, or final patterns) should be described. In addition, within-syllable consonant–vowel patterns can also be described to provide a foundation for intervention where there are CV phonetic constraints in the child's production system. Prosodic characteristics related to use of pitch, loudness, duration, and rate parameters should be described. In addition, use of stress (if disyllables are present) and intonation should be observed and described, regardless of accuracy. For stress analysis, the child's ability to produce asymmetric stress in disyllables should be observed. For intonation, the child's ability to change pitch within a word or sentence should be observed, again regardless of accuracy. In the child operating at the single-word level, co-occurrence of expressive jargon should be described, as this type of vocalization potentially indicates an ability to produce longer strings of vocalization with language-like stress and intonation even if the child is only employing single words for meaningful communication.

Relational analysis can be pursued from a variety of theoretical vantage points, including phonological processes (Hodson & Paden, 1991) or nonlinear phonology (Bernhardt & Stemberger, 1998), or "least" rather than the more traditional "most" knowledge (Gierut, 1986). In addition, traditional substitution, distortion, and omission analysis can be employed from a motor-based perspective in describing error patterns (Strand, 2003). From this perspective, matching of language targets for words and syllables is also beneficial for observing the client's achievement of complexity relative to the target language. Analysis of accuracy by word position as well as within-syllable accuracy can help to plan intervention targets. Accuracy analysis in the area of prosody should include description of patterns of error for stress and intonation to estimate the nature of these patterns relative to supporting intelligibility of sound and structure-based patterns.

Language Assessment

Pragmatic, semantic, syntactic, or discourse variables can also be assessed as they relate to the client's ability to manage communication in the connected speech sample. Clinically relevant phonetic/phonological patterns that form the primary focus of intervention must be evaluated as they relate to diverse aspects of communication or language abilities. In the case of the child who is producing meaning-based verbal output, other formal aspects of language may be affected in addition to phonetic/phonological abilities. If syntax, semantic, pragmatic, or discourse aspects of language are impaired, as well as the child's intelligibility, intervention programming will need to appropriately incorporate these issues relative to goal setting and prioritization of clinical goals. Alternatively, if the child's phonetic/phonological patterns of delay or disorder are found to exist in isolation from clinical level of involvement in other language areas, these areas need to be explored and described to provide supportive scaffolding in intervention for the primary goal of achieving age-appropriate intelligibility.

General language testing to establish the client's developmental level is needed at both of these levels of clinical involvement. In addition to structured language testing, the connected sample can double as a language sample for examination of the client's general communication and/or language abilities and the ways in which they affect intelligibility. Concurrent assessment of this more general context of communication and/or language abilities is crucial for adequate intervention planning, either to detect strengths to support intervention or to document concurrent areas of clinical relevance for intervention. Table 1.3 gives examples of potential interfaces between speech and language variables that should be considered in assessment of the connected sample.

General Profile

The general level of clinical assessment is related to the larger context of each child's communication profile. Each of these issues is appropriately included as they relate to understanding of the focal referral issue of phonetic/phonological delay or disorder. These issues are diverse and are properly related to potential etiology for the observed clinical patterns, to issues of functional intelligibility and/or communication competence, and to family and cultural expectations for the child.

The most general statement of these types of issues in assessment is found in the World Health Organization (WHO) Chronic Disabilities Model (Wood, 1980). This model provides a framework for the background considerations that should be incorporated into the assessment to understand each child at the broadest level (see Table 1.4 for an overview of the WHO levels of analysis). Each of the levels of the model will be appropriately related to the chronological and developmental level of the child as well as to family and cultural expectations for the child. The *pathophysiology level* is related to considerations

Table 1.3. Interactions of phonetic/phonological patterns and language variables

Area	Example
Syntax	Mean length of utterance Syntactic complexity of sentences (question forms, negations) Length of sentences
Morphology	Final position grammatical morphemes Auxiliary verbs Stress on morphemes
Pragmatic/discourse	Pragmatic intentions coded Topic familiarity Initiation versus response Novel versus familiar material; communication partner
Semantic	Function versus content words Familiarity and relevance of lexical items Syllable and word complexity of lexical items Other sounds in lexical items that may influence target sound

Table 1.4. World Health Organization levels of disability

Pathophysiology level
Cellular or tissue level of a disorder. Focuses on the anatomical or neurological basis of a disorder.

Impairment level
Anatomical or physiological deficits in structure and function associated with subsystems. Language function can be divided into several subsystems such as semantics, syntax, and phonology. Speech can be divided into four subsystems including respiration, phonation, velopharyngeal function, and articulation.

Functional limitation level
Extent to which an individual is restricted or unable to perform an action in a manner or range considered normal as a result of his or her impairment. In speech the focus is on overall measures such as intelligibility, speaking rate, or naturalness.

Disability level
Extent to which an individual successfully performs socially defined communicative activities within natural communicative contexts. This level involves an additional layer of information that approximates functional communication more readily than intelligibility measures alone.

Societal limitation level
Extent to which an individual is able to succeed in communication roles within social situations. Specifically, how effective is the speaker in special communication situations such as speaking with a stranger or a friend, speaking in groups, and speaking in adverse environments such as those involving noise, interpersonal conflicts, and emotion.

of etiology which are accessed in the assessment through the case history and medical records as well as by referrals to appropriate medical professionals (i.e., audiologists, neurologists, occupational or physical therapists) as needed. In addition, examination of the client's sensory acuity would fall into the pathophysiological category. The *impairment level* relates to structural and functional impairments associated with subsystems describing speech and language. In the case of phonetic levels of assessment, these subsystems relate to the status of respiratory, phonatory, resonance, and articulation structures and their function for speech production. This type of analysis is often based on observation and, in the case of phonatory and articulatory subsystems, on oral-peripheral mechanism examination. Occupational or physical therapy evaluation would also provide understanding of the impairment level as well as the pathophysiological level. Relative to phonological variables, the impairment level would describe the language systems detailed in the previous section. The *functional limitation level* describes the extent to which an individual is restricted or unable to perform an action in a manner or range considered typical as a result of his or her impairment. In phonetic/phonological assessment, the focus is on overall measures such as speech intelligibility, speaking rate, or naturalness. The *disability level* relates to description of the extent to which an individual can successfully perform socially defined communicative activities within natural communicative contexts. This level involves an additional layer of information that approximates functional communication more readily than intelligibility measures alone. The *societal limitation level* focuses on the extent to which an individual is able to succeed in communication roles within social situations. Specifically, this aspect relates to the child's effectiveness in special communication situations such as speaking with a stranger or a friend, speaking in groups, and speaking in adverse environments such as those involving noise, interpersonal conflicts, and emotion. These WHO levels assess appropriately the individual at the most specific to the most general level of overall function relative to the impact of his or her clinical speech disorder.

Special Considerations

A clinical assessment protocol differs for children of differing chronological and developmental age levels. The types of analyses and inferences the clinician draws from data gathered during the assessment process are related to the child's developmental level. Based on results of clinical assessment, clients are properly designated by their developmental level of function in designing therapeutic intervention goals. Mismatches between developmental level in the primary area of phonetic/phonological delay or disorder and the child's chronological age form crucial parts of the decision matrix related to both interpreting behaviors observed during assessment and formulating goals for intervention. In addition, other aspects of functional communication surrounding the primary clinical diagnosis will need to be accounted for in designing an intervention plan that utilizes each client's individualized profile of strengths and areas of clinical involvement.

Table 1.5 describes an assessment framework for individuals at differing developmental levels. The basis for comparison of the client's level of function in the assessment process is relative to information on the typical course of development of phonetic/phonological patterns. Types of assessment across the stages of typical development fall in two areas, listed on the left side of Table 1.5. The first area is termed *developmental* and relates to areas of analysis appropriate for describing the client's phonetic/phonological system. The second area is termed *functional* and relates to the individual's general abilities in communication and language (i.e., semantic, pragmatic, and discourse variables). These areas are seen as supporting or background issues for consideration in planning intervention and in understanding the client's overall communicative and language profile relative to the primary clinical diagnosis.

Typical Speech Development

Developmental age expectations are generated based on the clinician's understanding of the client's behaviors in relationship to typical phonological development milestones. In

Table 1.5. Developmental levels in typical phonological development

	Vocal (phonetic)		Verbal (phonological)	
	8–14 months (pre-speech)	14–20 months (emerging system)	20–30 months (establishing system)	30+ months (completing system)
Developmental (System)	Independent	Independent (Relational)	Relational (Independent)	Relational
Segmental/ complexity	Consonants Vowels Phonotactics	Consonants Vowels Phonotactics	Consonants Vowels Phonotactics Utterance level	Consonants Vowels Phonotactics Utterance level
Prosody	Pitch Duration Intensity Resonance	Stress Intonation Rate/pause Expressive jargon	Stress Intonation Rate/pause	Stress Intonation Rate/pause
Functional (Communication/language)	Gestures/signs Nonverbal Semantic Pragmatic Discourse	Gestures/signs Nonverbal Semantic Pragmatic Discourse	Self-monitoring	Self-monitoring

the typical developmental process, children develop vocal ability for use of the voice before they begin to use it for communicating meaning at the onset of first meaningful words. Stages of prelinguistic vocal development have been described in detail by a number of researchers (e.g., Davis & MacNeilage, 1995; Oller, 1980; Stark, 1980). Early development of phonetic and phonological abilities as a part of language development have also been described over a number of years from both phonetic (e.g., Davis, MacNeilage, & Matyear, 2002) and phonological (e.g., Bernhardt & Stoel-Gammon, 1994; Gierut, 1986) perspectives. As a result, a rich matrix of information is available to clinicians for evaluating the relationship between expectations for speech production based on a client's chronological age and developmental level described as a part of the assessment process. For purposes of clinical assessment and intervention, two major phases are noted in Table 1.5 across the top of the page. The first, termed *vocal*, relates to vocalizations that are not meaning based, occurring before the onset of word use. The second overall category, *verbal*, relates to the period of acquisition of a meaning-based phonological system in which the individual is using verbal means to code language-based communication. Under these two major designations, four categories of development are labeled. They are related to the developmental status of the child on a typical developmental continuum. Although any stage-based description is arbitrary, these categories are meant to provide a helpful guide to assessment and intervention planning by relating to important aspects of development to this process.

Use of Developmental Periods in Assessment

The *pre-speech* period is consistent with vocal development between 8 and 14 months, roughly the period from the onset of speech-like and syllable-based vocalization of canonical babbling until the appearance of first meaningful words. In this period, an independent analysis of vocalizations is appropriate, as the child may not yet produce enough language-based communication to allow an accuracy or relational analysis related to precise lexical targets. In the developmental area, the clinician will want to note what segmental/complexity and prosodic characteristics the child has available to produce speech (i.e., what raw materials are within the child's capacity to build a language-based system). The expectation is that the child will present with a limited range of behaviors characteristic of typically developing children during babbling. In the area of functional communication, use of gestures or signs, use of nonverbal means of communication, and precursors to language-based semantic, pragmatic, and discourse variables in the client's communication system should be assessed appropriately. These areas should be considered as independent analyses, as they do not yet clearly relate to language targets (except in the case of lexical signs that may have been taught by parents). These areas of assessment relate to the behaviors available to the client for interacting with communication partners, whereas the phonological system is the primary focus in intervention.

Use of a single-word articulation test implies that the child is able to perform the response task in looking at a picture or toy and producing a focused response to name it. Children who are functioning at a prelinguistic developmental level or who have multiple disabilities or motor, sensory, or cognitive impairments, thus functioning at the severe-to-profound level of vocal ability, and are developmentally delayed, may not be able to successfully participate in a single-word articulation test. An additional challenge is faced in testing children with significant concurrent language issues who may have difficulty naming the test items consistently, complicating assessment of phonetic/phonological patterns.

Because the single-word articulation test is not appropriate, the connected sample can be used for assessment of developmentally young children or children with severe to profound impairment through observation of vocalizations and other patterns of communication with appropriate materials and diverse communication partners. These partners can include caregivers who may be able to elicit more sophisticated communication than the clinician. The clinician can take into account the child's individualized deficits in the areas of motor, cognitive, or sensory impairment in designing the communication environment during the sampling. In the case of children who are still operating at a prelinguistic level of vocal communication, auxiliary areas such as nonverbal, gestural, or even visual regard abilities for communication need to be explored. These areas are intrinsically related to the child's ability to communicate within his or her environment, as the clinician is building vocal competence toward use of consistent meaning-based communication. In addition, crucial prelinguistic behaviors such as joint attention, turn-taking, and imitation will need to be explored to understand fully the child's ability to participate actively in intervention.

The *emerging system* period relates to the early phonetic and phonological behaviors observed in the single-word period of acquisition in typical development, approximately 14–20 months of age. In assessment, the clinician may also perform an independent analysis of segmental/complexity characteristics and prosody, but a relational analysis may also be appropriate if there are enough word forms available to allow a preliminary look at the child's accuracy patterns. In the area of prosody, the clinician may wish to begin to assess language-related areas of stress, intonation, speech rate, and use of pause. Expressive jargon may be present and can be diagnostically helpful in discerning whether a child who is producing mostly single-word communication is capable of producing longer strings of vocalization.

Functional assessment will still focus on use of gestures or signs, nonverbal means of communication, and semantic, pragmatic, and discourse variables related to language. However, in these areas, the expectation is different if the child is functioning in the emerging system period. The child would be expected to be mostly communicating verbally, with gesture and sign taking a supplementary role rather than forming the main centerpiece of the child's communication system (Thal & Tobias, 1991). Semantic and pragmatic variables would be coded in language-based forms and interactions. Discourse variables such as eye contact, turn-taking, and initiation response would be expected to be intact and supportive of communication intelligibility at this developmental stage.

The *establishing system* period sees the child developmentally using many, if not all, of the phonemes of the ambient language, although complexity of individual words may continue to be reduced. This period is roughly equivalent to a typically developing 20–30-month-old child, regardless of chronological age. A typically developing child at this stage is developing multiword utterances and beginning to achieve intelligible speech with most listeners. A child at this stage can usually be expected to complete a single-word articulation test successfully. The expectation for connected sample assessment of a child operating developmentally in the establishing system period is that the relational analysis for accuracy of sounds and word complexity relative to attempted targets will be the most relevant aspect of clinical analysis. Independent analysis of raw materials available (either sounds or word/syllable complexity) is less likely to provide important information at the establishing system level of development. However, categories of sounds (i.e., dorsals or fricatives) or complexity issues (i.e., deletion of final consonants or cluster reduction) may remain outside the child's production inventory. Most vowels should be produced accurately, at least in single words, although vowel accuracy may diminish with longer utterances. Accuracy in use of stress, intonation, and pause or juncture for support of intelligibility will also be an important aspect of some children's assessment, related to severity of clinical involvement. It may be relevant to assess the relationship between accuracy patterns and utterance level considerations for a child who is functioning in the establishing system period because the child may loose accuracy when producing multiword utterances when both accuracy and inventory can be maintained at a higher level in single words. At the functional level, the child's ability to display awareness of clinically relevant error patterns may form an important part of assessment of readiness for therapeutic intervention.

The *completing system* period is related to developmental expectations for a typically developing child who is 30+ months of age. In this period, most phonemes and aspects of complexity may be accurate and only a few residual errors remain on late-developing sounds such as [r], [l], [s], and voiced or voiceless "th." Complexity issues that remain will often relate to late-developing constructs such as clusters. Maintaining intelligibility related to increase in length of utterance might also continue to be a clinically relevant pattern. The relational analysis of sounds and phonotactic complexity (e.g., cluster use) will be the predominant type of analysis. If only a few sounds remain in error, the single-word articulation test can capture most irregularities; however, the connected sample can be used to ascertain variations potentially related to language complexity. Prosody should be intact at this developmental stage and should be expected to be a support for intelligibility. The client's awareness of error patterns should also be assessed at a functional level relative to intervention.

Severity Level

Clinicians also need to make qualitative judgments about the severity level of each client's phonetic/phonological delay or disorder as a part of assessment (Davis & Bedore, 2003). Terms frequently used to qualitatively describe the degree of involvement include *mild*, *moderate*, and *severe*. Many factors are considered when making valid judgments about severity level. These include overall intelligibility, etiological factors, potential impact on the child's social and communicative functioning in daily living, as well as family and cultural expectations about speech development. Mismatch between the child's chronological and developmental age and observed phonetic/phonological characteristics is the primary factor, however. Mismatches between developmental expectations and chronological age are indicative of speech *delay*. However, information about the course of typical development can also inform the clinician about those error patterns that are not seen typically and are indicative of speech *disorder*. Some examples of disorder include substitution of a glottal stop for all oral consonants or pervasive nasality. As the child's chronological age increases, the gap or mismatch between the observed speech characteristics and expectations for the child's chronological age gradually increases.

Judgments of severity in assessment are important for several reasons. Predictions of prognosis and length of therapeutic intervention are often based on judgments of severity, as well as on other factors. Information about severity is important when communicating with families. Quantification of severity may be a part of qualifying clients for services in both educational and medical settings. These judgments also affect decisions about the frequency and intensity of intervention. Statements of severity do not, however, link to decisions about the type of intervention that is most beneficial for a client. Such statements also do not allow for differential diagnosis of functional versus etiological bases for observed clinical symptoms. However, assessment of severity can provide general guidelines across individuals at different chronological ages.

In a client with a mild speech impairment, phonetic inventory and segmental error patterns are delayed relative to the child's chronological age. Most consonant and vowel phonemes and word and syllable shapes are present and produced correctly. Errors are more likely to be distortions (e.g., /r/) or substitutions (e.g., d/s) that are considered immature for the child's chronological age. The youngest children may show some stereotypical word-based patterns (e.g., reduplication in two-syllable words) or may use patterns typical of the single-word period. In addition, the use of only a few meaning-based spontaneous vocalizations for communication may signal mild vocal delay in a very young child (i.e., a 30-month-old toddler). Prosody and vowels are not usually impaired. In an older child, intelligibility may be close to 100%, but the child's speech calls attention to itself in spontaneously produced utterances. The impact on expressive language is minimal with a mild level of speech delay (e.g., marking of final morpheme inflections). These clients are delayed relative to typically developing peers rather than children who present with patterns not observed in typical development. For their chronological age, production patterns are like those of a somewhat younger child.

In children with moderate delay, the phonetic inventory of consonants and syllable/word shapes may be incomplete (i.e., dorsals may be missing or final consonants may be deleted). The inventory of vowels is likely to be complete. Even if the child's inventory of consonants, vowels, and syllable/word shapes is complete, it may not be used accurately. Intelligibility is further reduced by inconsistent accuracy for the complexity of word targets attempted (i.e., cluster reduction or final consonant deletion). Intelligibility is influenced by the amount of contextual support available for the listener and the complexity of language produced by the client. When prosodic aspects of speech production are not intact, intelligibility is affected further. Very young children may not be using vocalization consistently to communicate, accompanied by speech characteristics appropriate to the onset of first-word production. The impact on expressive language is more pronounced. For example, the child may omit function words (e.g., "the") and there may be an accompanying reduction in morphosyntactic complexity. Volubility may also be lower than expected for the child's chronological age (although this varies across differing cultural contexts). These children show a larger delay relative to their typically developing peers than do children rated as having mild involvement. They may also show some atypical patterns indicative of disorder in addition to delay.

In children with severe delay or disorder, the phonetic inventory of consonants, vowels, and syllable/word shapes is likely to be incomplete (i.e., only low vowels may be produced). In addition, accuracy of those elements in the child's inventory may be very low, with the exception of single words in short utterances. Intelligibility is severely compromised in all communicative contexts. Clients of all chronological ages may use communicative gestures and eye contact to supplement communication. If contextual support is available, communication with a familiar listener is more likely to be successful. Prosody is frequently impaired. Youngest children may not be using vocalization consistently to communicate. In these infants and toddlers, the mismatch between observed vocal behaviors and chronological age may not be so large. However, etiological considerations leading to early identification may indicate a poor prognosis for development of oral communication and contribute to a rating of severe impairment. Older children may have developed avoidance strategies for oral communication such as poor eye contact or alternative word choices. Oral expressive language is severely compromised. Children may be unable to generate multiword utterances. These children show a very large delay relative to their typically developing peers. Disordered or atypical patterns usually occur in conjunction with these delayed speech production patterns.

Culturally and Linguistically Diverse Children

The United States is increasingly diverse culturally and linguistically. Children for whom English is not a first language may present difficulties related to use of assessment focused on English phonology for a child whose primary target phonology may be very different from English. There are many drawbacks to the use of single-word articulation tests for assessment and formulation of goals for clinical intervention with these children. First, a child from a nonmainstream culture may not be familiar with the task required in responding to the test stimuli because that type of response format is not usual within his or her cultural background. Tests of English phoneme articulation have been normed primarily on Anglo-American children. As a result, phonemes in other languages may not be tested. All aspects of the child's phonological system may potentially be different from English, including prosody, consonant and vowel patterns, and word and syllable complexity. In addition, children who are bilingual may produce forms that are intermediate to either of the monolingual systems involved. Consequently, most published articulation tests are not valid for use on children who are from nonmainstream cultures and/or who are linguistically diverse. Use of this test type in assessment may lead to overdiagnosis of speech delay or disorder and inappropriate choice of intervention targets.

In addition, in a connected speech and language sample, ideally the communication partner should be proficient in the child's primary language. Obviously, not all clinicians are presently equipped to deal with the varied language backgrounds of the children they serve. However, the connected sample potentially can include interactions with parents or other familiar communication partners who can understand the child's phonetic/phonological patterns and the relationship of these patterns to English phonology. Including individuals who speak the child's primary language in the assessment environment can assist the clinician in assessing the child's intelligibility. In addition, differences in the child's performance with familiar cultural partners and within familiar communication patterns versus communication with the clinician can be integrated into assessment findings.

SUMMARY

Considerations for clinical diagnosis of developmental speech disorders have been reviewed. Major aspects of this process include the issue of primary diagnostic category relative to differential diagnosis of expressive language versus phonetic or phonological delay or disorder. The issue of how to characterize the nature of speech disorder relative to phonetic or phonological theoretical perspectives and terminology is another major facet of clinical diagnosis as well as in intervention in contemporary clinical practice. This diversity in theoretical perspectives leads directly to the types of assessment frameworks proposed as being comprehensive for differential diagnosis. Finally, a number of special considerations must be accounted for in valid clinical diagnosis, including consideration of developmental level and severity level relative to expectations for the child's chronological age. Cultural and linguistic diversity, with the diverse expectations created from different languages and cultural backgrounds in the United States, is another complex aspect of clinical diagnosis faced by contemporary speech-language practitioners in diagnosis of clinical speech disorders.

REFERENCES

American Psychiatric Association. (2000). *Diagnostic and statistical manual of mental disorders* (DSM-V) (5th ed.). Washington, DC: Publisher.

Bernhardt, B., & Stemberger, J. (1998). *Handbook of phonological development from the perspective of non-linear phonology.* New York: Elsevier.

Bernhardt, B., & Stoel-Gammon, C. (1994). Non-linear phonology: Introduction and clinical application. *Journal of Speech, Language, and Hearing Research, 37,* 123–143.

Bernthal, J.E., & Bankson, N.W. (2002). *Articulation and phonological disorders.* Boston: Allyn & Bacon.

Bleile, K.M. (1995). *Manual of articulation and phonological disorders: Infancy through adulthood.* Clifton Park, NY: Delmar Learning.

Chomsky, N., & Halle, M. (1968). *The sound pattern of English.* New York: Harper & Row.

Davis, B.L., & Bedore, L. (2003). *The speech disorders clinical archive.* The University of Texas at Austin, unpublished CD-ROM.

Davis, B.L., & MacNeilage, P.F. (1995). The articulatory basis of babbling. *Journal of Speech and Hearing Research, 38,* 1199–1211.

Davis, B., MacNeilage P., & Matyear, C. (2002). Acquisition of serial complexity in speech production: A comparison of phonetic and phonological approaches to first word production. *Phonetica, 59,* 75–107.

Gierut, J. (1986). *On the relationship between phonological knowledge and learning in misarticulating children.* Bloomington, IN: IULC Publications.

Hall, P.K., Jordan, L.S., & Robin, D.A. (1993). *Developmental apraxia of speech: Theory and clinical practice.* Austin, TX: PRO-ED.

Hodge, M. (1998). Developmental coordination disorder: A diagnosis with theoretical and clinical implications for developmental apraxia of speech. *American Speech, Language, and Hearing Association Special Interest Division 1 Newsletter: Language Learning and Education, 5,* 8–12.

Hodson, B., & Paden, E. (1991). *A phonological approach to remediation: Targeting intelligible speech* (2nd ed.). Austin, TX: PRO-ED.

Kent, R.D. (2004). *The MIT encyclopedia of communication disorders.* Cambridge, MA: MIT Press.

Lowe, R. (2003). *Workbook for the identification of phonological processes and distinctive features* (3rd ed.). Austin, TX: PRO-ED.

Oller, D.K. (1980). The emergence of the sounds of speech in infancy. In G. Yeni-Komshian, J. Kavanagh, & C. Ferguson (Eds.), *Child phonology: Vol. 1. Production* (pp. 93–112). New York: Elsevier.

Pater, J. (1999). Minimal violation and language development. *Language Acquisition, 6,* 201–253.

Peña, E.D., & Gillam, R.B. (2000). Dynamic assessment of children referred for speech and language evaluations. In C. Lidz & J. Elliott (Eds.), *Dynamic assessment: Prevailing models and applications* (Vol. 6). Oxford, UK: Elsevier Science.

Pollock, K. (1991). The identification of vowel errors using traditional articulation or phonological process test stimuli. *Language, Speech, and Hearing Services in Schools, 22,* 39–50.

Stampe, D. (1979). *A dissertation on natural phonology.* New York: Garland.

Stark, R. (1980). *Stages of speech development in the first year of life.* In G. Yeni-Komshian, J. Kavanagh, & C. Ferguson (Eds.), *Child phonology: Vol. 1. Production* (pp. 113–142). New York: Elsevier.

Strand, E. (2003). Childhood apraxia of speech: Suggested diagnostic markers for the younger child. In L.D. Shriberg & T.F. Campbell (Eds.), *Proceedings of the 2002 childhood apraxia of speech symposium* (pp. 75–79). Carlsbad, CA: Hendrix Foundation.

Thal, D., & Tobias, S. (1991). Communicative gestures in children with delayed onset of oral expressive vocabulary. *Journal of Speech and Hearing Research, 35,* 1281–1289.

Van Riper, C., & Irwin, J. (1958). *Voice and articulation.* Englewood Cliffs, NJ: Prentice Hall.

Wood, P. (1980). Appreciating the consequences of disease: The classification of impairments, disabilities, and handicaps. *The World Health Organization Chronicles, 34,* 376–380.

Yavas, M. (1998). *Phonology: Development and disorders.* San Diego: Singular Publishing.

Yorkston, K.M., Beukelman, D.R., Strand, E.A., & Bell, K.R. (1999). *Management of motor speech disorders in children and adults.* Austin, TX: PRO-ED.

Chapter 2

Perspectives on Assessment

Shelley Velleman

For me, phonology encompasses a wide range of phonetic and cognitive elements, from the motoric/articulatory level to much higher levels of processing such as phonemic awareness. This includes interactions with other linguistic systems (e.g., morphology). More generic organizational foundations, such as sequencing and pattern recognition skills, must also be considered.

Most of the children that I see clinically are fairly young (i.e., younger than 5 years of age) and/or they have severe impairments (i.e., less than 75% intelligible). I take a very pragmatic, eclectic, and individual-focused approach. When thinking about a child's phonology, my first question has to do with function: What is not working here? That is, what aspects of this child's phonology are interfering the most with successful communication? Some of the most common answers are:

- **Too much homonymy:** The child's substitutions yield phoneme collapses that obscure important contrasts in the language. The most extreme examples I've seen are in children who produce essentially one consonant sound, typically [d]. In other extreme cases, all vowels may be neutralized to an undifferentiable group of mid-low central vowels. The children with the most severe impairments produce no consonants at all.

- **Too much variability:** The child produces a given word or a given phoneme so inconsistently that listeners cannot learn to recognize the intended target. Children who fall within this category range from those with quite varied phonetic repertoires that are nonfunctional despite their variety (but because of their variability), to those with very limited, yet inconsistent, phonetic repertoires.

- **Unexpected patterns:** Adults who spend time with young children come to expect certain substitution patterns, such as [w] for /r/, and are able to accommodate these fairly automatically, even when they are produced by a child who is already beyond the age at which such patterns are expected. Children whose substitution patterns are atypical or whose patterns change frequently are far less intelligible to those who have not had the chance to become accustomed to their speech.

I begin the process by carrying out several independent analyses: phonotactic repertoire (word and syllable shapes; reduplication and harmony), phonetic repertoire (consonant and vowel repertoires), and, where appropriate, consonant–vowel interactions (syllable restrictions based on consonants and vowels that share similar articulatory configurations, e.g., [ba], [di], [gu]). These independent analyses give me a picture of the phonological elements and structures that are available to the child, which may include (but are not limited to) two-syllable words, vowels from all corners of the vowel triangle, a variety of consonant manners and places, syllables that incorporate significant articulatory changes, and words that include two different consonant manners or places of articulation. Furthermore, independent analyses make it possible to compare the capabilities of this system with the requirements of the language that the child is trying to learn. For example, a lack of consonant clusters is of no concern in a child who is learning Hawaiian, because no clusters occur in that language. When a child is learning English, however, clusters must eventually be mastered.

Next, relational analyses are performed: phonemic repertoire (consonants and vowels used contrastively), processes (substitution, omission, harmony, and movement patterns), and constraints (avoidance of certain structures or elements; consistent production of other structures and elements, perhaps at some cost to other aspects of the target word). Percent consonants correct (PCC), a calculation of the proportion of consonants that the child attempted that were pronounced correctly, is a useful summary measure of the severity level of the child's impairment (Shriberg & Kwiatkowski, 1982; Shriberg, Kwiatkowski, Best, Hengst, & Terselic-Weber, 1986). These are the basic questions that are answered by relational analyses: 1) How accurate are the child's productions of words, and in what ways are they inaccurate? 2) Are minimal pairs produced in such a way that a listener can tell the difference between the two words? and 3) When the target word includes a consonant cluster or a fricative or an iambic stress pattern (unstressed + stressed, as in giRAFFE), does the child produce it as such? If not, what is produced instead?

Not until I have established what is going on in the child's phonological system do I ask, "Why?" That is, what is the source of the homonymy, variability, or unexpected patterns? Why are the child's phonotactic, phonetic, or phonemic repertoires limited? What is the reason for the child's frequent use of stopping, gliding, or cluster reduction? Why is he or she avoiding production of initial clusters (via deletion, epenthesis, or metathesis) yet producing final clusters where they are not even called for? This is where I begin to try to distinguish between more phonetically based versus more cognitively based phonological disorders and consider deeper sources such as pattern recognition, auditory processing, motor sequencing/planning, muscle tone, and training.

PHONETICS VERSUS PHONOLOGY

Some children show clear signs of motoric deficits.

- Droopy face, protruding tongue, slow movements, and a quiet, breathy voice may indicate low muscle tone, which may or may not be present in other parts of the body (usually demonstrated by poor posture, w-sitting, and so forth). Phonetic characteristics of low tone may include frication of stops; frequent omissions, especially of final consonants and of elements of consonant clusters; and articulatory inaccuracy, for example, centralized vowels (indicating undershoot). This is a type of dysarthria.

- Muscle tension, overactive reflexes (e.g., bite, gag), and hard glottal attack may indicate high muscle tone, which may or may not be present in other parts of the body (e.g., as seen in spasticity). Phonetic characteristics may include poor grading of movements, for example, stopping of fricatives or even glides, and overshoot of vowels (i.e., tendency to substitute corner vowels [i], [a], [u] for less peripheral ones, to tense lax vowels, or to diphthongize simple vowels); this is another type of dysarthria.

- Groping for articulatory positions (e.g., articulatory false starts, inability to imitate articulatory postures or sequences); signs of effort with no payoff (e.g., mouth wide open with no sound coming out); inability to combine elements into a larger whole (e.g., to combine a consonant and a vowel into a syllable, two syllables into a word, two words into a phrase); mis-sequencing of sounds within a word (metathesis, e.g., [bost] for *boats*), morphemes within a phrase (e.g., "it's don't float" or "it don't floats" for "it doesn't float"; "mow lawner" for "lawn mower"), or words within a sentence (e.g., "Pick-up trucks beep don't") may be signs of a motor planning disorder, typically referred to as *childhood apraxia of speech* (CAS; also called *developmental apraxia of speech, developmental verbal dyspraxia,* and several other terms).

Others' symptoms appear to be completely within the realm of the cognitive phonological system, with symptoms depending on the age of the child.

- Phonetic and phonotactic repertoires are appropriately varied for age, but sounds are not used properly within target phonological structures (i.e., many phonological processes are observed) or are used very inconsistently (e.g., the same phoneme may be substituted with several different phones in different, yet phonologically similar, words or on different occasions).

- The child does not spontaneously use sounds that can be produced in imitation. Poor phonological discrimination is noted; that is, the child does not appear to attend to phonemic contrasts within the language receptively or expressively.

- Poor phonological awareness; that is, reading readiness skills such as rhyming, segmentation, blending, and phoneme–grapheme correspondences are delayed or deficient.

- Poor phonological storage or retrieval; that is, the child performs poorly on phonological fluency tasks (e.g., "Tell me all the words you can think of that start with the [s] sound") or makes phonemic word finding errors (e.g., "house" for *horse*).

In some cases, these deficits may be mirrored by parallel language deficits (especially with respect to learning morphological patterns and other lexical storage and retrieval difficulties) or parallel learning deficits (difficulties with pattern recognition, concept generalization, abstract concept formation, or information storage and retrieval).

Because children with CAS may exhibit symptoms from both of these lists, CAS is considered by this author to span the entire range of phonology. It has been noted by various researchers (e.g., K. Strand, personal communication; A. Meredith, personal communication) that children's symptoms may appear to be very motoric when they are quite young (e.g., 24–36 months) yet gradually become more and more phonological, to the point where a speech-language pathologist (SLP) evaluating a child for the first time at age 7 or 8 might be surprised to hear that the child has a history of motor planning deficits as well as a more organizational/cognitive phonological disorder.

The phonological deficits of children with CAS tend to be more phonotactic than phonetic; that is, their syllable and word structures (e.g., final consonants, clusters, multisyllabic words, varied stress patterns) are less mature than one would expect given their phonetic repertoires. Therefore, measures that rely on segmental accuracy alone, such as PCC, may give an inappropriate view of the child's progress in therapy. For example, one child assessed over time by this author was included in the Shriberg, Aram, and Kwiatkowski (1997) study. At age 5, he was profoundly unintelligible and heavily reliant on mime and gestures to communicate. His typical word was one syllable long, usually either a vowel alone or a consonant–vowel (CV) syllable. Sentences consisted of two to three words separated by vocalizations of "uh" used to mark missing function words. Most of his word attempts could not be used to calculate PCC because they were unintelligible; one cannot judge whether a consonant is correct unless one knows what the target consonant is. At age 8, this child was vastly more intelligible. He was able to produce multisyllabic words with final consonants and consonant clusters. Many of his consonants remained inaccurate but in more predictable ways (e.g., gliding, deaffrication). However, his PCC had not changed. Therefore, the authors concluded that, "Child 7/14 made virtually no gains in his speech development during a 3-year period" (Shriberg et al., p. 316)! Fortunately, the child's insurance company was not using PCC as its measure of progress.

IATROGENIC (TREATMENT-INDUCED) PHONOLOGICAL DEFICITS

Because of my clinical interest in autism spectrum disorders, I have often evaluated children "on the spectrum." Many times, such children's phonological systems are characterized by both too much homonymy and too much variability, for reasons that I attribute to the children's training. In particular, many practitioners of the applied behavioral analysis (ABA) approach address phonology in a very arbitrary way, choosing target words based on preschool vocabulary categories (e.g., vegetables) without consideration of function (What does this child want/need to be able to say?) or of the child's phonological/phonetic capabilities (What is this child likely to be able to pronounce distinctively?). The result is that, during ABA picture-naming drills, any gross approximation to the word target is accepted. The child is rewarded (in a manner that is unrelated to the meaning of the word) for vocalizing in response to the picture stimulus or to the modeled phonetic form. The adult may make some attempt to shape the vocalization to yield a slightly more accurate phonetic form, but this is typically not based on systematic, phonologically based objectives. Such children usually exhibit significant cognitive, pragmatic, and behavioral difficulties as well, but in many cases their unintelligibility has been exacerbated by treatment that is not based on any sort of phonological assessment. Sometimes, attempts at oral communication are abandoned after a time, despite the fact that no systematic phonological analysis of their capabilities has taken place.

NONSTANDARDIZED ASSESSMENT PROCEDURES

For children such as those described previously (very young children, those with severe impairments, or those on the autistic spectrum), standardized testing is often inappropriate or even impossible and therefore it is vital to perform independent phonological analysis. Independent analysis consists of collecting data from a language sample regarding the sounds and sound structures (e.g., syllable and word shapes) that the child produces, regardless of the adult target. Children who do not yet have identifiable adult-based words, who speak a language or dialect unknown to the evaluator, or who are not cooperative for word elicitation (e.g., using a picture-based articulation test) can still be assessed quite thoroughly in this way. The results can be used to determine the severity of the disorder with respect to the extent of the child's impairment. For example, a child who only produces a single syllable shape (e.g., CV), one consonant type (e.g., a stop), or one vowel type (e.g., a low central vowel) clearly has quite a significant disorder. Furthermore, the child's repertoires can be compared with typical repertoires in development (e.g., stops are typically acquired before fricatives) and with phonological universals (e.g., stops are more prevalent in the languages in the world than fricatives) in order to estimate the severity of the disorder. For example, a child who only produces three different vowels that also are all low vowels has a more deviant phonological system than a child who produces only the three corner vowels ([i], [a], [u]). The impact of these limitations on a learner of a particular language can be assessed without fluency in the language, using only book knowledge. For example, on the one hand, if the child is learning Hawaiian as a native language, the lack of final consonants or of consonant clusters is not of concern; these are not used in this language. The communicative success of a child learning English, on the other hand, would be significantly affected by such limitations.

Of course, it is highly preferable to be able to perform relational analysis as well as independent analysis, comparing the child's forms with the words that he or she is attempting to say, if the child does have identifiable word targets. In addition, an SLP who speaks the child's language fluently is unquestionably the best professional to carry out any type of evaluation on the child (Goldstein, 2000). However, it is not appropriate to do no phonological analysis at all simply because the child speaks another language or is too young, has too severe an impairment, or is too uncooperative to be given a standardized test.

A further option for children who have identifiable word targets in a different language or dialect from that of the SLP is to have a family member who speaks both languages repeat the child's target word or utterance after the child has spoken. In this way, the evaluator can compare the child's production with the adult target in order to identify substitutions, simplifications, and structural alterations (e.g., metathesis) that have occurred. Finally, it is vital to interview family members and others who interact with the child on a regular basis to determine the degree of functionality of the child's phonology. That is, how often do the client's attempts at oral communication succeed without the support of manual, gestural, or pictorial communication?

That said, it certainly does behoove all SLPs to learn as much as they possibly can about phonological universals as well as particular languages and dialects spoken in their geographical area. In addition, it is important to become consciously aware of one's own assumptions about phonology and phonological development. For example, initial consonant deletion is seen as a bright red flag for phonological disorder in children learning English. Yet, this is a very common, normal pattern among young learners of Finnish. Similarly, /v/ is considered to be a late, difficult phoneme for children learning English, but it is learned quite early among children learning Swedish.

Differences such as these do not occur only in languages that are completely different from Mainstream American English (MAE). The phonological development of children speaking other American dialects, such as African American English (AAE), have been shown to differ in important ways and may differ in even more ways that have not yet been verified through longitudinal research. These differences will be described in detail in the subsequent section because AAE is the nonmainstream dialect that is most prevalent across the United States. Although the recent development of the Developmental Evaluation of Language Variance (DELV; Seymour, Roeper, & DeVilliers, 2003) has filled a gap in our field with respect to our ability to assess the phonology (as well as syntax, morphology, semantics, and pragmatics) of children who are learning AAE in an unbiased manner, many aspects of AAE phonology remain that have not yet been explored fully. Furthermore, the DELV is not appropriate for children younger than age 4 years.

PHONOLOGICAL ASSESSMENT
OF SPEAKERS OF AFRICAN AMERICAN ENGLISH

As with other dialects, AAE is a systematic, rule-governed linguistic system (Labov, 1972; Linguistic Society of America, 1997; Wolfram & Fasold, 1974) and children should not be viewed as having a speech and language problem because they speak AAE (American Speech-Language-Hearing Association, 1987). AAE is spoken by many African Americans, who represented 12.3% of the U.S. population as of the 2000 census (U.S. Census Bureau, 2002). Coda constraints, resulting in absence of final stops and nasals (with selective preservation before onsetless words), absence or reduction of final clusters, and metathesis of final /s/ + stop, are typical of the dialect. Metrical differences, especially absence of initial weak syllables from iambic words, stress shift onto initial weak syllables ("trochaicization") in iambic words, and absence of medial weak syllables particularly in reduplicated contexts (e.g., *Mississippi*) have also been widely reported. Vocalization or absence of /r/ intersyllabically, in syllabic contexts, postvocalically, and after consonants (after *th* and in unstressed syllables) are also typical of AAE (Pollock et al., 1998; Pollock & Meredith, 2001; Stockman, 1996; Wolfram, 1994), although some speakers of AAE seem instead to hyperarticulate postvocalic /r/ (Pollock & Berni, 1996). Some of these patterns occur in other dialects of American English, but more frequently in AAE, whereas others are unique to AAE (Bailey & Thomas, 1998).

Most of the information available about AAE has been gleaned from adult speakers of the dialect, although an increasing number of studies have been conducted on the development of syntax and morphology in young speakers of AAE. However, Stockman (1996) reports that even the studies that have been performed to investigate AAE phonological development have been limited. Most studies have either proposed to describe the differences between the performance of children who speak AAE versus MAE on standardized tests normed on mainly white speakers of MAE (Haynes & Moran, 1989; Ratusnik & Koenigsknecht, 1976; Seymour & Seymour, 1981) or have focused on the development of a specific phoneme (or set of phonemes) or on phonological process frequencies (Haynes & Moran, 1989; Moran, 1993; Seymour, Green, & Huntley, 1991; Stockman, 1993). Seymour and Seymour (1981) found that 4- and 5-year-old children learning AAE omitted word-final stops more frequently than did MAE speakers and also made more errors on all consonants except /r/, /l/, /ʧ/, and /ʤ/. Interestingly, although the characteristics of AAE should result in children exposed to this dialect hearing fewer tokens of the phoneme

/r/ overall, these children acquired prevocalic singleton /r/ ahead of children learning MAE. Stockman (1993) found that 36–96-month-old AAE-speaking children had difficulty with medial clusters that violated English initial cluster constraints (e.g., –ts–). Moran (1993) reported that AAE-speaking children 4–9 years of age deleted final stop consonants at least 20% of the time in conversational speech. They compensated for these deletions with vowel lengthening before target voiced stops.

Velleman, Bryant, Abdulkarim, and Seymour (2004) investigated resyllabification, sonority, and voicing as potential factors in the maintenance versus reduction of coda consonant clusters in ten 5-year-old AAE speakers. Sonority differences were found to account for the majority of the variance in the data, with voicing contributing to a lesser extent. Charko and Velleman (2003) investigated metrical versus segmental factors in children ages 4–6 years learning AAE versus MAE and classified as typically developing versus language disordered. They found that, whereas AAE and MAE speakers did not differ in their overall percent correct on these items, all AAE speakers were more likely to exhibit phonotactic differences (e.g., absence, movement, or epenthesis of syllables or segments), and MAE speakers exhibited more phonetic differences on the phonology subtest of the DELV (Seymour, Roeper, & DeVilliers, 2003). This contrast was especially evident in children age 6 years and older (Charko & Velleman, 2003).

Stockman (1996) pointed out that although these studies provide valuable information on a number of very specific aspects of AAE phonology in children, a large gap still exists in the literature on the process of phonological development of young African American children. Very little has been written about phonological development in AAE learners who are younger than 4 years of age.

Metrical phonological development is an area with potentially important diagnostic implications. Although Stoel-Gammon (1987) found that 27 of 34 (79%) MAE-speaking 24-month-olds used CVCV words sometimes, several studies have shown that English-learning children up to the age of 3 tend to omit weak syllables, especially from initial position in iambic words (Allen & Hawkins, 1980; Demuth, 1996; Fikkert, 1994; Gerken, 1991, 1994; Gerken & McIntosh, 1993; Kehoe, 1997; Kehoe & Stoel-Gammon, 1997a, 1997b; Schwartz & Goffman, 1995), yielding a word that fits the primary trochaic (strong–weak) template of English nouns. Syllables in final position are far less vulnerable to omission. Much less commonly, stress shifts result in iambic words being pronounced trochaically (e.g., *giRAFFE* shifts to *GIraffe*). Velleman and Shriberg (1999) reported that children with phonological delays and disorders exhibit patterns of metrical errors that are very similar to children developing typically, but some with phonological delays persist in weak syllable deletion up to the age of 6 and some with a diagnosis of suspected CAS continue to exhibit weak syllable deletion, as well as stress shifts and excess equal stress, up to the age of 14. Aguilar-Mediavilla, Sanz-Torrent, and Serra-Raventos (2002) recently reported a similar finding for children with specific language impairment in contrast to children with language delay or normal acquisition. Thus, persistence of weak syllable deletion and stress shifts is a red flag for phonological delay or disorder in MAE. However, stress shifts (e.g., *police* pronounced with primary stress on the first syllable), absence of weak syllables in initial and medial positions (e.g., "member" for *remember,* "sectary" for *secretary*), and haplology (e.g., "Missippi" for *Mississippi*) result in decreased frequencies of iambic words in adult AAE (Stockman, 1996; Wolfram, 1994). Thus, it may be normal for children exposed to AAE to demonstrate more frequent stress shifts/trochaiciza-tion and more persistent and pervasive patterns of weak syllable omission even in words that are pronounced iambically in MAE. This question remains to be investigated systemati-cally, but this possibility should be kept in mind by SLPs evaluating children who speak AAE.

Phonotactic frequency differences between MAE and AAE can also be expected to have an impact on learners of these two dialects. In AAE, alveolar stops in coda position and various coda morphemes (–t, –d, –s, –z) are frequently omitted. Thus, AAE learners are exposed to far fewer codas. Moran (1993) noted that AAE speakers between 4 and 9 years old deleted final stop consonants, although they compensated for these deletions with a vowel length contrast before target voiced versus voiceless stops. The occurrence of such compensations in child-directed speech and the developmental process of this variable in younger children learning AAE are unknown, although evidence has been found of similar compensatory lengthening in Japanese spoken in early childhood (Ota, 2001). It has been proposed (Demuth & Fee, 1995) that children's early words are constrained to contain at least two weight units; a monosyllabic word must include at least two moras (a long vowel, a diphthong, or a vowel–consonant sequence). Kehoe and Stoel-Gammon (2001) have recently confirmed that children do produce codas more often after lax vowels than after tense vowels, possibly due to the need for extra syllable weight following a lax vowel. It is not known whether vowel length influences coda retention in adults or children speaking AAE, but again the frequency of final consonant deletion in children learning AAE may normally remain higher longer than in children learning MAE.

Another important phonotactic difference between MAE and AAE is the occurrence of coda clusters. About 50% of typically developing MAE-learning 2-year-olds produce some combinations of consonants (Stoel-Gammon, 1987); 3¹/₂-year-olds produce full clusters 75% of the time or more (Roberts, Burchinal, & Footo, 1990). The range, diversity, and accuracy of clusters develop over time (McLeod, van Doorn, & Reed, 2001), pro-gressing from complete deletion of the cluster (rare for onset clusters in English-learning children), to deletion of one element of the cluster, to substitution of one element, to correct production (Greenlee, 1974). Coda clusters typically emerge earlier than onset clusters in children learning MAE (Kirk & Demuth, 2002). Due to coda cluster reduction in addition to morphological absences, however, AAE learners are exposed to far fewer coda clusters than are MAE learners, and the types of clusters to which they are exposed differ. It is not known whether young children learning AAE therefore acquire initial consonant clusters before final consonant clusters (the opposite order from that of children learning MAE), or exactly what the developmental course of coda cluster acquisition is in this group.

SUMMARY

The frequencies of occurrence of certain structures or sounds in a particular dialect or language can often have an impact on the child's order and thoroughness of acquisition of that structure or sound. Errors that may serve as red flags of disorder in one language or dialect may be quite normal in another. Therefore, SLPs evaluating children from different linguistic backgrounds must learn as much as possible about that language or dialect; question their own assumptions about the typical course of phonological develop-ment; carry out thorough, independent analyses of such clients' phonologies; and rely heavily on reports or observations of the child's oral communicative function in a variety of communicative contexts.

Independent phonological analyses are also critical for very young children, children with severe phonological disorders, and those with disorders on the autism spectrum. For such children, the SLP's task is first to identify the overall source of the unintelligibility (homonymy, variability, unexpected patterns, or some combination of these three) and the general nature of the disorder (phonetic, phonological, or some combination of the two). Once these determinations have been made, then more detailed independent as well as relational analyses will reveal the child's specific error patterns and possibly shed light on underlying causes.

REFERENCES

Aguilar-Mediavilla, E.M., Sanz-Torrent, M., & Serra-Raventos, M. (2002). A comparative study of the phonology of preschool children with specific language impairment (SLI), language delay (LD), and normal acquisition. *Clinical Linguistics and Phonetics, 16,* 573–596.

Allen, G.D., & Hawkins, S. (1980). Phonological rhythm: Definition and development. In G.H. Yeni-Komshian, J.F. Kavanagh, & C.A. Ferguson (Eds.), *Child phonology* (pp. 227–256). New York: Academic Press.

American Speech-Language-Hearing Association. (1987). Social dialects: Position paper. *ASHA, 19*(1), 45.

Bailey, G., & Thomas, E. (1998). Some aspects of African-American Vernacular English phonology. In S. Mufwene, J.R. Rickford, G. Bailey, & J. Baugh (Eds.), *African-American English: Structure, history, and use* (pp. 85–109). New York: Routledge.

Charko, T.A., & Velleman, S.L. (2003, November). *Dialectal influence on disordered children's phonotactic constraint rankings.* Paper presented at the American Speech-Language-Hearing Association, Chicago, IL.

Demuth, K. (1996). The prosodic structure of early words. In J. Morgan & K. Demuth (Eds.), *Signal to syntax: Bootstrapping from speech to grammar in early acquisition* (pp. 171–184). Hillsdale, NJ: Lawrence Erlbaum Associates.

Demuth, K., & Fee, E.J. (1995). *Minimal words in early phonological development.* Unpublished manuscript, Brown University and Dalhousie University.

Fikkert, P. (1994). *On the acquisition of prosodic structure.* Dordrecht: Holland Institute of Generative Linguistics.

Gerken, L. (1991). The metrical basis for children's subjectless sentences. *Journal of Memory and Language, 30,* 431–451.

Gerken, L. (1994). A metrical template account of children's weak syllable omissions from multisyllabic words. *Journal of Child Language, 21,* 565–584.

Gerken, L., & McIntosh, B.J. (1993). The interplay of function morphemes and prosody in early language. *Developmental Psychology, 29,* 448–457.

Goldstein, B. (2000). *Cultural and linguistic diversity resource guide for speech-language pathologists.* San Diego: Singular Publishing Group.

Greenlee, M. (1974). Interacting processes in the child's acquisition of stop-liquid clusters. *Papers and Reports in Child Language Development, 7,* 85–100.

Haynes, W., & Moran, M. (1989). A cross-sectional developmental study of final consonant production in southern black children from preschool through third grade. *Language, Speech, and Hearing Services in Schools, 20,* 400–406.

Kehoe, M. (1997). Stress error patterns in English-speaking children's word productions. *Clinical Linguistics & Phonetics, 11,* 389–409.

Kehoe, M., & Stoel-Gammon, C. (1997a). The acquisition of prosodic structure: An investigation of current accounts of children's prosodic development. *Language, 73,* 113–144.

Kehoe, M., & Stoel-Gammon, C. (1997b). Truncation patterns in English-speaking children's word productions. *Journal of Speech Language and Hearing Research, 40,* 526–541.

Kehoe, M.M., & Stoel-Gammon, C. (2001). Development of syllable structure in English-speaking children with particular reference to rhymes. *Journal of Child Language, 28,* 393–432.

Kirk, C., & Demuth, K. (2002, November). *Coda/onset asymmetries in the acquisition of clusters.* Paper presented at the 30th Boston University conference on language development, Boston.

Labov, W. (1972). *Language in the inner city: Studies in the Black English vernacular.* Philadelphia: University of Pennsylvania Press.

Linguistic Society of America. (1997). *LSA resolution on the Oakland "Ebonics" issue.* Washington, DC: Author.

McLeod, S., van Doorn, J., & Reed, V.A. (2001). Normal acquisition of consonant clusters. *American Journal of Speech-Language Pathology, 10,* 99–110.

Moran, M. (1993). Final consonant deletion in African American children speaking Black English: A closer look. *Language, Speech, and Hearing Services in Schools, 24,* 161–166.

Ota, M. (2001). Phonological theory and the development of prosodic structure: Evidence from child Japanese. *Annual Review of Language Acquisition, 1,* 65–118.

Pollock, K.E., Bailey, G., Berni, M.C., Fletcher, G., Hinton, L.N., Johnson, I., et al. (1998). *Phonological features of African American Vernacular English (AAVE).* Retrieved September 23, 2004, from the University of Alberta Web site: http://www.rehabmed.ualberta.ca/spa/phonology/features.htm

Pollock, K., & Berni, M.C. (1996, October). *Vocalic and postvocalic /r/ in African American Memphians.* Paper presented at New Ways of Analyzing Variation in English (NWAVE), Las Vegas, NV.

Pollock, K.E., & Meredith, L.H. (2001). Phonetic transcription of African American Vernacular English. *Communication Disorders Quarterly, 23*(1), 47–54.

Ratusnik, D., & Koenigsknecht, R. (1976). Influence of age on black preschooler's non-standard performance of certain phonological and grammatical forms. *Perceptual and Motor Skills, 42,* 199–206.

Roberts, J.E., Burchinal, M., & Footo, M.M. (1990). Phonological process decline from 2;6 to 8 years. *Journal of Communication Disorders, 23,* 205–217.

Schwartz, R.G., & Goffman, L. (1995). Metrical patterns of words and production accuracy. *Journal of Speech and Hearing Research, 38,* 876–888.

Seymour, H., Green, L., & Huntley, R. (1991, November). *Phonological patterns in the conversational speech of African-American children.* Poster presented at the national convention of the American Speech-Language-Hearing Association, Atlanta, GA.

Seymour, H.N., Roeper, T., & de Villiers, J. (2003). *Diagnostic evaluation of language variation.* San Antonio, TX: Harcourt Assessment.

Seymour, H., & Seymour, C. (1981). Black English and Standard American English contrasts in consonantal development of four- and five-year-old children. *Journal of Speech and Hearing Disorders, 46,* 276–280.

Shriberg, L.D., Aram, D.M., & Kwiatkowski, J. (1997). Developmental apraxia of speech III: A subtype marked by inappropriate stress. *Journal of Speech, Language, and Hearing Research, 40*(2), 313–337.

Shriberg, L.D., & Kwiatkowski, J. (1982). Phonological disorders I: A diagnostic classification system. *Journal of Speech and Hearing Disorders, 47,* 226–241.

Shriberg, L.D., Kwiatkowski, J., Best, S., Hengst, J., & Terselic-Weber, B. (1986). Characteristics of children with phonologic disorders of unknown origin. *Journal of Speech and Hearing Disorders, 51,* 140–161.

Stockman, I. (1993). Variable word initial and medial consonant relationships in children's speech sound articulation. *Perceptual and Motor Skills, 76,* 675–689.

Stockman, I.J. (1996). Phonological development and disorders in African American children. In A.G. Kamhi, K.E. Pollock, & J.L. Harris (Eds.), *Communication development and disorders in African American children: Research, assessment, and intervention* (pp. 117–153). Baltimore: Paul H. Brookes Publishing Co.

Stoel-Gammon, C. (1987). Phonological skills of 2-year-olds. *Language, Speech, and Hearing Services in Schools, 18,* 323–329.

U.S. Census Bureau. (2002). *United States census 2000.* Washington, DC: Author.

Velleman, S.L., Bryant, T., Abdulkarim, L., & Seymour, H. (2004). *Predictors of coda consonant cluster reduction in African American English.* University of Massachusetts, Amherst. Manuscript in preparation.

Velleman, S.L., & Shriberg, L.D. (1999). Metrical analysis of the speech of children with suspected developmental apraxia of speech and inappropriate stress. *Journal of Speech, Language, and Hearing Research, 42,* 1444–1460.

Wolfram, W. (1994). The phonology of a sociocultural variety: The case of African American Vernacular English. In J.E. Bernthal & N.W. Bankson (Eds.), *Child phonology: Characteristics, assessment, and intervention with special populations* (pp. 227–244). New York: Thieme Medical Publishers.

Wolfram, W., & Fasold, R.W. (1974). *The study of social dialects in American English.* Englewood Cliffs, NJ: Prentice Hall.

Chapter 3

Components
of Phonological Assessment

ADELE W. MICCIO

B y the time a typically developing child is 3 years of age, he or she is likely to be intelligible to any listener most of the time (Vihman & Greenlee, 1987). Even 2-year-olds produce speech sounds from a range of manner classes and syllable structures (Stoel-Gammon, 1985). Consequently, when parents or caregivers are very concerned about their child's inability to be understood by others and seek a professional assessment, it is likely that a problem exists. Although phonological disorders are relatively easy to identify in preschool children with unintelligible speech, determining the nature of the disordered sound system and the severity of the problem is a challenge to the speech-language pathologist (SLP).

A PROTOCOL FOR ARTICULATION/PHONOLOGY ASSESSMENT

A typical assessment must gather enough information to determine whether the prerequisite behaviors for spoken language are present, including the status of the hearing and speech mechanisms and the status of speech and language skills. Any underlying cause or contributing factors must also be determined before recommendations can be made regarding treatment or prognosis for change (Miccio, 2002).

Background Questionnaire and Interview

To save assessment time, caregivers may complete a background questionnaire before a child's speech production is assessed (Miccio, 1995). The purpose of the questionnaire is to gain information on general development and to call attention to factors that may need further exploration at the time of the assessment, such as a history of middle ear infections, the use of more than one language in the home, and so forth. In addition, it is important to identify any cultural differences that may indicate different child-rearing practices or other factors that may influence the outcome of an assessment. The family's responses to the questionnaire alert the SLP to incomplete or inconsistent information that can be clarified during the assessment. This process also allows a clinician to better understand a family's attitudes toward communication disorders. The parents' responses and reactions are also a window into the potential success of intervention.

Even when much information has been obtained, it is important to remember that an assessment is dynamic. Tasks that are undertaken will vary depending on a child's responses or on additional information obtained from parents during the course of the assessment. Any phonological assessment, however, must include a screening for related factors, including other aspects of communication that may be of concern but may not have been recognized by the parents. This is important to ensure that clinicians can identify any associated behaviors that may contribute to speech production problems (Shriberg & Kwiatkowski, 1982a).

Receptive Language Test

Although a phonological impairment may be part of a more general problem or a problem with multiple aspects of language development, I plan an assessment around the suspected problem (Miccio, 2002). Even so, testing for receptive and expressive language difficulties is a crucial part of any phonological assessment because of the high incidence of co-occurring language problems (Shriberg & Austin, 1998; Shriberg, Kwiatkowski, Best, Hengst, & Terselic-Weber, 1986).

It is important to determine whether other components of the linguistic system and phonological development are in sync with each other or whether lexical and syntactic development have continued to grow at a rapid pace in the absence of a strong phonetic base. A rapidly expanding vocabulary in a child who produces only a few phonemes will inevitably result in widespread homonymy and may also trigger atypical speech production as the child struggles to produce phonemic contrasts with a severely limited sound system.

In a typical assessment, receptive language tests such as the Preschool Language Scale–3 (PLS-3; Zimmerman, Steiner, & Pond, 1992), Test of Early Language Development–3 (TELD-3; Hresko, Reid, & Hammill, 1999), or a similar test that yields a standard score are convenient initial tasks because they do not require verbal responses from the child. Small children, especially those with speech intelligibility problems, are often hesitant to speak with strangers. Receptive tests primarily require the child to point at pictures and allow the clinician and child to become comfortable with each before engaging in tasks that require the extensive speech production that is needed to complete a phonological assessment.

Later in the assessment, when the child is comfortable with the clinician and the process, a connected speech sample can be obtained to facilitate sampling of expressive language. This can be done through conversational tasks during play, through narrative tasks during a book-reading task, or both. In addition to more extensive phonological analyses, the language sample will provide data for syntactic, morphological, and pragmatic analyses at a later date, if needed.

Standardized Articulation or Phonology Test

A standardized picture-naming test is completed to provide a quick snapshot of a child's speech production abilities and to provide a comparison to other children's performance on the same instrument (e.g., Bankson–Bernthal Test of Phonology [BBTOP]; Bankson & Bernthal, 1990). The test also identifies children with only a few errors or error patterns and alerts a clinician to a child with multiple or atypical errors and the sounds or structures that will need to be probed more extensively to adequately describe a child's phonological system. If a child produces only a few errors, the sample provided by the articulation test in addition to any information gained from conversation or a language sample are adequate for making intervention decisions (Kamhi, 1992).

Results of a standardized test in comparison with a normative sample, however, do not reveal whether errors are typical or atypical in development or whether substitutions for particular sounds or patterns are consistent. If a child has multiple sounds in error, the standardized test results alone do not provide adequate information to characterize the child's phonological system because of the limitations in the size of the speech sample as well as limitations of the method for obtaining the responses. Standardized tests do, however, provide helpful information because the intended target words are identifiable through the picture-naming task. Consequently, whole-word transcriptions of the test items provide valuable initial information about a child's phonological system and its relation to the adult system. Transcriptions can be scanned for place, voice, and manner problems. The BBTOP, for example, allows the clinician to visually scan the error grid to identify basic error patterns (Tyler & Tolbert, 2002). The information gained from a standardized test alerts a clinician to the sounds or structures that need to be probed more extensively.

If an error pattern is not identifiable from the test, it is likely that the child's phonology does not correspond directly to the target sound system in a sound-by-sound manner. Rather, it is likely that problems are due to reduplication, consonant-vowel dependencies, or problems with vowel or consonant harmony. These suspicions can then be assessed later with a supplementary probe. It is important to note that all standardized tests are culturally biased to some degree, because test items may not be representative of items in a child's home environment or dialect. Names of items differ in various parts of the country, as does the way in which a word is pronounced. In such instances, a supplementary probe should be used.

Audiological and Oral Mechanism Screenings

Screening for the existence of any causal factors such as a craniofacial deficit or hearing problem is important. Attention must be given to any problems in this domain because remediation of the problems (e.g., hearing aids or prostheses) could assist in more efficient and effective treatment of the phonological problem. Consequently, a pure-tone audiometric screening, immittance audiometry, and a brief oral mechanism screening are included. Because these tasks may remind a child of a visit to the doctor's office, they are purposely left toward the middle of an assessment so that some speech production and receptive language data have already been obtained. If a hearing problem is suspected, an audiological referral is made. If middle ear pathology, nonspeech motor problems, or possible structural abnormality is noted, a medical referral is made. Only a brief oral mechanism screening is necessary, because little pharyngeal function is observable during an oral mechanism screening and nonspeech tasks do not reflect a child's ability to produce speech (Lof, 2002, 2003; Moore & Ruark, 1996; Moore, Smith, & Ringel, 1988). Miccio (2002) provided an example of an oral mechanism screening protocol that takes these factors into account.

Nonstandardized Supplementary Phonological Probe

Despite their usefulness in providing a comparison to a normative sample, standardized test results may not be representative of a child's true abilities or provide adequate information on the systematic nature of a child's phonology from which to make judgments of severity or prognosis for change. A supplementary picture-naming probe allows the clinician to obtain multiple tokens of sounds and syllabic structures found to be in error on the initial test so that a child's phonology may be described more fully (Miccio, 2002).

Multiple probes provide the opportunity to elicit a target sound in a variety of contexts. From this information, the consistency of an error pattern can be observed. Probes typically provide the opportunity to produce each English consonant a minimum of five times (Miccio, 1995). More extensive probes also provide multiple opportunities for children to produce each sound in each possible word or syllable position (Elbert & Gierut, 1986; Williams, 2003). If time is a concern, however, only items related to the suspected error pattern or later developing sounds are probed because eliciting later developing sounds will result in the production of early developing sounds.

If a child is either too young or too active to respond reliably to a picture probe, the supplementary information can be obtained from a play routine by strategically selecting toys that will elicit the sounds, syllable structures, or word structures of interest. This information facilitates independent analysis of a child's consonant and vowel inventories and the distribution of sounds across word positions as well as analysis of a child's syllable system and use of word-level stress. Because the targets are known, a relational analysis of a child's phonological system is also possible and a preliminary judgment of severity can be made.

Speech and Language Sampling

Although picture or object naming tasks allow the clinician to know the intended target, single-word responses have other limitations. Single words provide limited information on intelligibility and no information on phrase-level phonological patterns. Consequently, the phonological assessment includes a connected speech sample that optimizes the opportunity for further language analysis. A connected speech sample allows the clinician to observe a large number of speech skills in a relatively short time (e.g., prosody, intelligibility, phrase-level phonological patterns). The same sample can also be used to assess expressive language abilities, fluency, and voice quality.

Speech samples can be gathered in many ways, and the clinician has to be prepared to resort to different methods of obtaining a representative sample. Some preschoolers will talk about activities and people not present, such as a family trip or their preschool friends. Other children are reluctant participants in pretend play or casual conversation and are more comfortable talking during an activity of daily living such as preparing food. Alternatively, children may enjoy a table-top game or activity. Broken toys or missing game pieces may elicit conversation. For example, an action figure may have a leg missing or a game may have the wrong pieces. Children are likely to notice if something is wrong and will comment on it. It is important to use simple tasks that require minimal concentration so that a child is not too preoccupied with a game to talk. Family members may also be invited to participate in this task so that a family's communicative interaction can be observed. It is important to keep in mind that communicative interactions may be different in the home, where many other distractions are present.

Another option is to elicit a speech sample while reading a wordless picture book using tell or retell strategies. If the phonological deficit appears to be part of a larger language problem, a book-reading sample can also be used for narrative analysis at a later date. A language sample provides information about the complexity of a child's grammatical system and the extent of his or her vocabulary as well as speech production. A videotaped sample provides an opportunity to examine the phonological system in more detail at a later date and to observe use of eye contact, facial expression, and gestures to communicate.

Information gained from the supplementary probe or language sample is used to complete independent analyses of a child's consonant and vowel inventories as well as information on stress and intonation and phrase-level phonology (Bernhardt & Holdgrafer, 2001; Velleman, 1998). The sample also illuminates occurrences of lexical selection and homonymy. These factors contribute to unintelligibility and are not examined easily in a single-word probe. Information from the connected speech sample can also be used to determine percent consonants correct (PCC) or another appropriate quantitative measure of severity (Shriberg, Austin, Lewis, McSweeny & Wilson, 1997; Shriberg & Kwiatkowski, 1982b).

Stimulability Testing

A stimulability probe is administered for consonants that appear to be absent from a child's phonetic inventory (Bernthal & Bankson, 2004; Miccio, 2002). *Stimulability,* that is, a child's ability to imitate a sound that is absent from his or her phonetic inventory immediately following an examiner's model, can be determined easily (Powell & Miccio, 1996). This task provides useful information for treatment planning and for determining the prognosis for change. A typical stimulability probe elicits production of a speech sound missing from a child's phonetic repertoire in isolation and in three contexts: CV (prevocalic), VCV (intervocalic), and VC (postvocalic). The sounds that a child imitates without the benefit of specific phonetic placement cues are presumed stimulable and are most likely to be learned in the absence of treatment (Miccio, Elbert, & Forrest, 1999). Thus, stimulability testing illuminates the difference between performance of a speech production task under a typical condition (e.g., spontaneous speech) and a highly supportive condition such as imitation of a syllable (Bain, 1994).

Other Supplemental Assessments: Vowels, Speech Perception, and Phonological Awareness

If a child's responses to a standardized test suggest a possible vowel disorder, this may be probed further at a later date using the protocol developed by Pollock and Keiser (1990). I do not assess perception formally, nor do I evaluate phonological awareness if the referral is for speech production problems. Phonological awareness problems are most likely to occur in children with severe phonological disorders and concomitant language problems (Bird, Bishop, & Freeman, 1995). If I suspect difficulties with speech perception as intervention progresses, goals can easily be adjusted to address speech perception and phonological awareness problems concomitantly with speech production goals (Tyler & Tolbert, 2002). Most interventions for phonological disorders inherently involve activities that require a child to perceive phonological contrasts and to segment words into smaller units.

PROGNOSIS AND RECOMMENDATIONS

The information gathered in the steps described above is used to analyze a child's phonological system both independent of the adult form and in relation to the adult form. Independent analysis of the speech sample provides information on the size of a child's phonetic system, how the sounds a child produces are distributed across word positions, and whether the child's phonetic development is typical when viewed independently from the adult phonological system. The relational analysis identifies patterns of correspondence between a child's system and an adult's system.

The prognosis is determined based on a holistic view of all the information gathered during the assessment. Any causal factors, the nature of the error pattern, severity, stimulability, motivation, and family support are all taken into account. In general, a consistent error pattern with easily identified relationships between a child's productions and the adult phonology would predict rapid change and generalization across the sound system in response to treatment. Multiple substitutions for the same sound, however, are more likely to be a poor prognostic indicator (Forrest, Elbert, & Dinnsen, 2000). A child who is highly stimulable for production of sounds that are absent from the phonetic inventory also has a more positive prognosis than a child who is not stimulable (Miccio et al., 1999; Powell & Miccio, 1996). If a child is not stimulable for production of sounds that are absent from the inventory, rapid gains are unlikely (Miccio et al., 1999; Powell, Elbert, & Dinnsen, 1991; Rvachew, Rafaat, & Martin, 1999). This information is also valuable for planning intervention.

If a child's phonology does not appear to be changing positively in the absence of treatment, treatment is recommended. Based on the information gathered in the assessment, a tentative treatment plan is designed and probes are developed to observe change as intervention progresses. As a problem is more fully understood, goals may be changed and refined.

Because assessment is dynamic, intervention not only addresses problems that were identified during an initial assessment but also serves as an extended longitudinal assessment. Carefully planned treatment and attention to a child's responses during intervention and during production probes provides data for ongoing analysis and continuous refinement of treatment goals.

REFERENCES

Bain, B.A. (1994). A framework for dynamic assessment in phonology: Stimulability revisited. *Clinics in Communication Disorders, 4,* 12–22.

Bankson, N., & Bernthal, J. (1990). *Bankson–Bernthal Test of Phonology.* Austin, TX: PRO-ED.

Bernhardt, B.H., & Holdgrafer, G. (2001). Beyond the basics I: The need for strategic sampling for in-depth phonological analysis. *Language, Speech, and Hearing Services in Schools, 32,* 18–27.

Bernthal, J.E., & Bankson, N.W. (2004). *Articulation and phonological disorders* (5th ed., p. 214). Boston: Pearson Allyn & Bacon.

Bird, J., Bishop, D.V.M., & Freeman, N.H. (1995). Phonological awareness and literacy development in children with expressive phonological impairments. *Journal of Speech and Hearing Research, 38,* 446–462.

Elbert, M., & Gierut, J.A. (1986). *Handbook of clinical phonology: Approaches to assessment and treatment* (pp. 54–55). San Diego: Singular Publishing Group.

Forrest, K., Elbert, M., & Dinnsen, D.A. (2000). The effect of substitution patterns on phonological treatment outcomes. *Clinical Linguistics & Phonetics, 14,* 519–532.

Hresko, W.P., Reid, D.K., & Hammill, D.D. (1999). *Test of Early Language Development–3.* Austin, TX: PRO-ED.

Kamhi, A.G. (1992). The need for a broad-based model of phonological disorders. *Language, Speech, and Hearing Services in Schools, 23,* 261–268.

Lof, G.L. (2002). Two comments on this assessment series. *American Journal of Speech-Language Pathology, 11,* 255–256.

Lof, G.L. (2003). Oral motor exercises and treatment outcomes. *Perspectives on Language Learning and Education, 10,* 7–11.

Miccio, A.W. (1995). *A spectral moments analysis of the acquisition of word-initial voiceless fricatives in children with normal and disordered phonologies.* Unpublished doctoral dissertation, Indiana University, Bloomington.

Miccio, A.W. (2002). Clinical problem solving: Assessment of phonological disorders. *American Journal of Speech-Language Pathology, 11,* 221–229.

Miccio, A.W., Elbert, M., & Forrest, K. (1999). The relationship between stimulability and phonological acquisition in children with normally developing and disordered phonologies. *American Journal of Speech-Language Pathology, 8,* 347–363.

Moore, C.A., & Ruark, J.L. (1996). Does speech emerge from earlier appearing oval motor behaviors? *Journal of Speech and Hearing Research, 39,* 1034–1047.

Moore, C.A., Smith, A., & Ringel, R. (1988). Task-specific organization of activity in human jaw muscles. *Journal of Speech and Hearing Research, 31,* 670–680.

Pollock, K.E., & Keiser, N.J. (1990). An examination of vowel errors in phonologically disordered children. *Clinical Linguistics & Phonetics, 4,* 161–178.

Powell, T.W., Elbert, M., & Dinnsen, D.A. (1991). Stimulability as a factor in the phonological generalization of misarticulating preschool children. *Journal of Speech and Hearing Research, 34,* 1318–1328.

Powell, T.W., & Miccio, A.W. (1996). Stimulability: A useful clinical tool. *Journal of Communication Disorders, 29,* 237–254.

Rvachew, S., Rafaat, S., & Martin, M. (1999). Stimulability, speech perception skills, and the treatment of phonological disorders. *American Journal of Speech-Language Pathology, 8,* 33–43.

Shriberg, L.D., & Austin, D. (1998). Comorbidity of speech-language disorders: Implications for a phenotype marker for speech delay. In R. Paul (Ed.), *The speech-language connection* (pp. 73–117). Baltimore: Paul H. Brookes Publishing Co.

Shriberg, L.D., Austin, D., Lewis, B.A., McSweeny, J.L., & Wilson, D.L. (1997). The Percentage of Consonants Correct (PCC) metric: Extensions and reliability data. *Journal of Speech, Language and Hearing Research, 40,* 708–722.

Shriberg, L.D., & Kwiatkowski, J. (1982a). Phonological disorders I: A diagnostic classification system. *Journal of Speech and Hearing Disorders, 47,* 236–241.

Shriberg, L.D., & Kwiatkowski, J. (1982b). Phonological disorders III: A procedure for assessing severity of involvement. *Journal of Speech and Hearing Disorders, 47,* 256–270.

Shriberg, L.D., Kwiatkowski, J., Best, S., Hengst, J., & Terselic-Weber, B. (1986). Characteristics of children with phonologic disorders of unknown origin. *Journal of Speech and Hearing Disorders, 51,* 130–161.

Stoel-Gammon, C. (1985). Phonetic inventories, 15–24 months: A longitudinal study. *Journal of Speech and Hearing Research, 28,* 505–512.

Tyler, A.A., & Tolbert, L.C. (2002). Speech-language assessment in the clinical setting. *American Journal of Speech-Language Pathology, 11,* 215–220.

Velleman, S.L. (1998). *Making phonology functional: What do I do first?* (pp. 24–25). Woburn, MA: Butterworth-Heinemann.

Vihman, M.M., & Greenlee, M. (1987). Individual differences in phonological development: Ages one and three years. *Journal of Speech and Hearing Research, 30,* 503–521.

Williams, A.L. (2003). *Speech disorders resource guide for preschool children* (pp. 163–167). Clifton Park, NY: Thomas Delmar Learning.

Zimmerman, I., Steiner, V., & Pond, R. (1992). *Preschool Language Scale–3.* San Antonio, TX: Harcourt Assessment.

Chapter 4

Assessment for Determining a Communication Profile

Ann A. Tyler

My assessment protocol for articulation/phonology consists of both standardized tests and nonstandardized analyses. Standardized tests are important for identifying whether a disorder exists because they allow for comparison to a normative sample. Scores provided by standardized tests are especially useful for helping parents to understand how their child is performing in relation to his or her same-age peers, certifying children for services through school districts and public service agencies, and securing payment from third-party payers. Whereas standardized measures help in the identification of the presence or absence of a problem, nonstandardized analyses are useful for describing the problem in detail and designing an intervention program. In this regard, computerized phonological analyses are particularly useful because of the wide array of analysis procedures they employ.

My typical assessment protocol includes the following:

1. Case history

2. Standardized test for articulation/phonology and, if necessary, phonological awareness

3. Collection of a conversational speech-language sample and nonstandardized analyses of various components

4. Standardized language test

5. Stimulability testing

6. A cursory oral-peripheral examination

7. Hearing screening

Language assessment is an integral part of the evaluation because research indicates that approximately 60% of children with phonological disorders have co-occurring language impairment (Bishop & Edmundson, 1987; Paul & Shriberg, 1982; Shriberg & Austin, 1998; Shriberg & Kwiatkowski, 1994; Shriberg, Kwiatkowski, Best, Hengst, & Terselic-Weber, 1986; Tallal, Ross, & Curtiss, 1989). Although our assessment protocol may be designed primarily for diagnosing articulation/phonology disorders, as communication specialists it is our job to evaluate the range of behaviors involved in communication and those particularly relevant to articulation/phonology, such as language and fluency.

CASE HISTORY

To obtain a case history, we send a questionnaire approximately a week before the scheduled evaluation and ask that the family or caregivers complete it and bring it with them to the evaluation session. This questionnaire contains items designed to elicit information regarding the child's birth history, speech-language development, motor development, social-emotional development, medical history, and familial history concerning speech and language delays and other learning difficulties. We review the completed questionnaire at the beginning of the evaluation, and in a short interview we ask questions about topics that we wish to have clarified or expanded. Frequently, these topics are related to the reason for referral, the history and course of ear infections, or the child's speech and language development. We also ask the family for their expected outcome from the evaluation so that we may address their questions and concerns adequately in the recommendation session.

ARTICULATION/PHONOLOGY TEST

For a standardized articulation/phonology instrument we use the Goldman–Fristoe Test of Articulation–3 (GFTA-3; Goldman & Fristoe, 2000), which provides the option of also applying the Khan–Lewis Phonological Analysis (KLPA-2; Khan & Lewis, 2002). Both of these tools have been revised to include standard scores as well as percentile ranks and accompanying confidence intervals. If one has a phonological process approach and is interested in comparing phonological error patterns with developmental norms, the KLPA-2 is quite useful and is now easier to score. Prior to these revisions, few standardized articulation/phonology instruments provided true standard scores; one exception is the Bankson–Bernthal Test of Phonology (BBTOP; Bankson & Bernthal, 1990). Although the BBTOP provides a moderately large sample of 80 words in comparison with the GFTA's 53 words, the time required for scoring is a major drawback. We often found it necessary to "eyeball" the error patterns and score the test after the evaluation session.

The purpose of using a standardized test is to be able to quickly compare a child's performance with that of a normative sample so that parents can be given this information at the time of the evaluation in order to know how their child is doing in relation to other children. With the revisions of the GFTA-3 and the KLPA-2, this has become a reasonable expectation.

CONVERSATIONAL SAMPLE

Conversational samples are used as a context from which to make clinical judgments about voice, fluency, and grammatical errors. I use a play session between the examiner and child, sometimes also including the parents, to elicit a conversational speech-language sample. Playmobil houses and related accessories are useful for these sessions because they provide familiar contexts for young children (e.g., furniture, cars, animals, people). We provide a wordless picture book from the *Carl* series by Alexandra Day to elicit a narrative sample as well. For older children, I focus more on narratives and elicit a variety of these using the procedures described by Hadley (1998). My goal is to elicit a 100–200 utterance sample, which should take about 15 minutes. From this sample, information can be obtained about articulation/phonology, expressive language skills, fluency, and voice.

Although I make an audio recording of the conversational sample, I transcribe on-line 50 utterances from which I tabulate a preliminary mean length of utterance (MLU) for comparison with Miller and Chapman's (1981, 2000) reference data. In this sample, I also note the presence or absence of finite morphemes (e.g., past tense –ed, third person singular regular, auxiliary and copula be), because these have been shown to be especially problematic for children with speech and language disorders (Bedore & Leonard, 1998; Rice, Wexler, & Cleave, 1995). With respect to fluency, I would expect a disfluency frequency no greater than approximately 2%, comprising normal nonfluencies (Conture, 1990). These are characterized by between-word types of disfluencies, such as phrase repetitions, as opposed to "core" disfluencies, such as sound repetitions or prolongations. I also judge pitch, resonance, loudness, and overall quality of voice, but I could do so more systematically using Shriberg, Kwiatkowski, and Rasmussen's (1990) Prosody-Voice Screening Profile, if necessary.

When time permits, I prefer to complete a phonological analysis of a 100-word sample. I select approximately 47 words from the spontaneous sample to augment the citation sample obtained from administration of the GFTA-3 and analyze this 100-word sample using the computer program module PROPH (Computerized Profiling; Long, Fey, & Channell, 2000). A nonstandardized analysis such as this one includes both independent and relational components (Stoel-Gammon, 1985). An independent analysis provides information about a child's phonological system regardless of how it compares with the ambient system the child is learning. Thus, parts of an independent analysis, such as a phonetic inventory, simply provide summary data regarding which phones the child produces, whether or not they are accurate. In contrast, a relational analysis compares the child's productions with targets in the ambient system. Phonological processes, substitution patterns, and quantitative measures such as percentage of consonants correct (PCC; Shriberg & Kwiatkowski, 1982) are all pieces of information that result from relational analyses. PROPH provides comprehensive independent and relational analyses including phonetic inventory, syllable structure inventory and match, phonemic inventory, substitution analysis, phonological process analysis, PCC, and phonological mean length of utterance (PMLU; Ingram & Ingram, 2001). PMLU is a measure of phonological complexity of words that represents both the accuracy of consonant production and the number of segments in the word. PMLU has been found to be highly correlated with PCC (Nelson, 2002). Not only is PROPH generally user-friendly, it is downloadable shareware that is as comprehensive as any other marketed analysis program. I highlight inventory constraints, syllable structure limitations, positional constraints, overall severity as indicated by PCC, and primary error patterns with reference to Grunwell's (1982) data used in PROPH. All of these pieces of information are crucial in describing the child's phonological system and designing an intervention plan.

If cursory analysis of 50 utterances from the conversational speech-language sample indicates the presence of expressive language difficulties, I submit the sample to analysis using Systematic Analysis of Language Transcripts (SALT; Miller & Chapman, 2000) to obtain more in-depth data regarding grammatical morpheme usage, number of different words used, type-token ratio, and use of mazes. Again, this computerized nonstandardized analysis provides information that describes the specific characteristics of the child's system and aids in intervention planning.

LANGUAGE TEST

I administer a standardized language test to make norm-referenced comparisons for specific aspects of both expressive and receptive language. It is particularly important to assess receptive language because I can obtain expressive language information from the conversational sample and because receptive skills are often overestimated by parents. For preschoolers, I often choose the Preschool Language Scale–3 (PLS-3; Zimmerman, Steiner, & Pond, 1992) because 1) it provides an auditory comprehension, expressive communication, and total communication scores without administration of numerous subtests; 2) it can be administered in a reasonable time period; 3) it is not too difficult for children in the 4-year-old range; and 4) it appears to have an acceptable level of concurrent validity. It can also be scored quickly at the time of an evaluation so that results can be reported for parents. For older school-age children I would select from the Test of Language Development-Primary-3 (TOLD-P3; Newcomer & Hammill, 1997), the Oral and Written Language Scales (OWLS; Carrow-Woolfolk, 1995), the Clinical Evaluation of Language Fundamentals–3 (CELF-3; Semel, Wiig, & Secord, 1995), or the Comprehensive Assessment of Spoken Language (CASL; Carrow-Woolfolk, 1999). I would not expect to be able to administer one of these instruments in its entirety; that would make for an unreasonably lengthy evaluation session given the other necessary standardized and nonstandardized measures. Instead, I would focus on the different types of receptive skills that are assessed, their task requirements, and the types of receptive quotients that are provided in selecting from among the instruments. For example, a receptive quotient on the CASL is obtained from a subtest requiring the identification of synonyms and a paragraph comprehension subtest. In comparison, the receptive language score on the CELF-3 is obtained from three subtests: 1) a sentence comprehension task requiring picture identification to match the spoken sentence; 2) a concepts and directions task involving pointing to shapes specified by an increasing number of referents; and 3) a word classes task involving the identification of words that go together from a group of three.

ADDITIONAL ARTICULATION/PHONOLOGY TESTING

Stimulability testing, which can also be thought of as dynamic assessment of articulation change, is crucial for making a prognosis for response to intervention. Sounds that are not present in the inventory but that are found to be stimulable are likely to enter the child's phonological system without direct intervention; however, children in whom those sounds are nonstimulable are likely to need treatment (Miccio, Elbert, & Forrest, 1999; Powell, Elbert, & Dinnsen, 1991). The numbers of sounds that fall into these two categories, as well as the relative effort the child displays in the stimulability task, help the speech-language pathologist provide some gauge of the therapy time required. I first check for stimulability on sounds that are not present in the child's inventory—in isolation first, and, if correct, in CV and VC syllables. Next, stimulability for positional constraints is checked in the target position of syllables and words. Finally, sounds that are inconsistent at the word level can be checked in words and sentences.

I conduct a cursory oral-peripheral examination that involves rating of structures and function as normal, marginal/emerging, or abnormal, following the framework used in many published protocols. In general, we are interested in whether structures and function of the oral mechanism are within the required range to support normal speech production. The oral examination is presented as an exploratory game in which examiner and child get to look in each other's mouths. Observations are made of the size and symmetry of structures, the child is required to imitate speech and nonspeech movements, and diadochokinetic rates for the production of syllabic sequences are evaluated. If I wish to have a more comprehensive oral-peripheral examination, I use that found in Robbins and Klee (1987), which includes both a structural and a functional protocol. The structural protocol provides a score based on normal (1) or abnormal (0) ratings across structures. The functional protocol results in a total functional score based on a rating scale where 2 = adult-like function, 1 = emerging skill, and 0 = absent function. Robbins and Klee (1987) provide normative data on their functional and structural protocols for certain ages.

Cumulative research about the relationship of phonological awareness skills to early reading performance and successful interventions to promote those skills suggests that phonological awareness is an important area to evaluate, particularly for children in kindergarten and first grade. Not only are measures of phonological awareness powerful predictors of early reading success but also phonological awareness training has been shown to improve phoneme awareness, word decoding, and word encoding skills of 6-year-old children with language impairment who had early signs of reading delay (Gillon, 2000). Children with phonological disorders are a heterogeneous group and, as such, experience varying degrees of phonological awareness difficulties. The presence of impairment in phonological awareness and the extent of that impairment appear to be influenced by two factors: 1) the overall severity of the phonological disorder and 2) the diagnosis of co-occurring language impairment. The likelihood of phonological awareness difficulties is greater when there is co-occurring language impairment (Bishop & Adams, 1990; Catts, 1993). As the severity of the phonological disorder increases, a greater likelihood exists of impairment in phonological awareness (Bird, Bishop, & Freeman, 1995; Catts, 1993; Larrivee & Catts, 1999). Thus, for 5- to 6-year-old children presenting with either of these influencing characteristics, it is important to assess their level of functioning in phonological awareness, particularly in the skill area of segmentation, because this is the most robust predictor of reading success.

Ideally, both standardized and nonstandardized assessments should be completed, but because I am interested in determining how a child performs in comparison with his or her peer group, I would administer a standardized test at the evaluation and follow up with specific nonstandardized assessments in initial therapy sessions. The Comprehensive Test of Phonological Processing (CTOPP; Wagner, Torgeson, & Rashotte, 1999), the Test of Phonological Awareness (TOPA; Torgesen & Bryant, 1994), or the Phonological Awareness Test (Robertson & Salter, 1997) is good for the identification of a problem. The CTOPP is well-normed on ages 5;0 to 24;11, with seven core subtests for kindergartners and first graders and one supplemental test. It is designed to identify impairment in phonological awareness skills as well as impairment in related rapid automatized naming skills and phonological memory, with quotients provided for all of these domains. The TOPA is normed for ages 5–8 and is a shorter test designed more specifically for assessment of phonological awareness skills related to early reading. The Phonological Awareness Test is also normed for a similar age group (5–9 years old) and has subtests arranged developmentally by skill level from rhyming and segmentation to graphemes and decoding, although it has a smaller normative sample. Follow-up with criterion-referenced tasks from Swank and Catts (1994), Catts (1993), and Ball (1993) can be adjusted to specific age-level expectations so that, for example, rhyming and syllable segmentation tasks can be given to younger children and phoneme blending and elision tasks can be given to older children.

My assessment protocol does not typically include evaluation of perceptual skills. If these are in question, particularly as they relate to specific sound errors, Locke's (1980) Speech Production-Perception Task (SPPT) remains one of the best formats for assessing a child's perception for specific target-error contrasts. Although perceptual skills are complex to assess, internal discrimination tasks, such as the SPPT, have been considered better measures of a child's perception with respect to specific sound errors than external discrimination tasks. In the SPPT, the child discriminates his or her own spoken form with target forms of the same words. For example, if the child produces "fumb" for "thumb," he or she is required to judge whether the clinician said the right word as both pictures are pointed to alternately. Flipsen (2002) advocated using the SPPT in a decision tree designed to help determine types of errors (phonetic or phonemic) and intervention approaches and whether auditory training should be incorporated in the intervention. Although it may not be necessary to determine the type of error, there may be instances in which a child's error is affected by perceptual factors, particularly in the case of residual errors, and when perceptual assessment and training may be appropriate.

REFERENCES

Ball, E.W. (1993). Assessing phoneme awareness. *Language, Speech, and Hearing Services in Schools, 24,* 130–139.

Bankson, N., & Bernthal, J.E. (1990). *Bankson–Bernthal Test of Phonology.* Austin, TX: PRO-ED.

Bedore, L.M., & Leonard, L.B. (1998). Specific language impairment and grammatical morphology: A discriminant function analysis. *Journal of Speech and Hearing Research, 41,* 1185–1192.

Bird, J., Bishop, D.V.M., & Freeman, N.H. (1995). Phonological awareness and literacy development in children with expressive phonological impairments. *Journal of Speech and Hearing Research, 38,* 446–462.

Bishop, D.V.M., & Adams, C. (1990). A prospective study of the relationship between specific language impairment, phonological disorders, and reading retardation. *Journal of Child Psychology and Psychiatry, 21,* 1027–1050.

Bishop, D.V.M., & Edmundson, A. (1987). Language-impaired 4-year-olds: Distinguishing transient from persistent impairments. *Journal of Speech and Hearing Disorders, 52,* 156–173.

Carrow-Woolfolk, E. (1995). *Oral and Written Language Scales.* Circle Pines, MN: American Guidance Service.

Carrow-Woolfolk, E. (1999). *Comprehensive Assessment of Spoken Language.* Circle Pines, MN: American Guidance Service.

Catts, H.W. (1993). The relationship between speech-language impairments and reading disabilities. *Journal of Speech and Hearing Research, 36,* 948–958.

Conture, E. (1990). *Stuttering* (2nd ed.). Englewood Cliffs, NJ: Prentice Hall.

Flipsen, P., Jr. (2002, November). *Articulatory or phonological intervention: Which one?* Seminar presented at the annual meeting of the American Speech-Language-Hearing Association. Atlanta, GA.

Gillon, G.T. (2000). The efficacy of phonological awareness intervention for children with spoken language impairment. *Language, Speech, and Hearing Services in Schools, 31,* 126–141.

Goldman, R., & Fristoe, M. (2000). *Goldman-Fristoe Test of Articulation–3.* Circle Pines, MN: American Guidance Service.

Grunwell, P. (1982). *Clinical phonology.* Rockville, MD: Aspen Publishers.

Hadley, P.A. (1998). Language sampling protocols for eliciting text-level discourse. *Language, Speech, and Hearing Services in Schools, 29,* 132–147.

Ingram, D., & Ingram, K.D. (2001). A whole-word approach to phonological analysis and intervention. *Language, Speech, and Hearing Services in Schools, 32,* 271–283.

Khan, L.L., & Lewis, N. (2002). *Khan-Lewis Phonological Assessment–2.* Circle Pines, MN: American Guidance Service.

Larrivee, L.S., & Catts, H.W. (1999). Early reading achievement in children with expressive phonological disorders. *American Journal of Speech-Language Pathology, 8,* 118–128.

Locke, J.L. (1980). The inference of speech perception in the phonologically disordered child: Part II. Some clinically novel procedures, their use, some findings. *Journal of Speech and Hearing Disorders, 45*(4), 445–468.

Long, S.H., Fey, M.E., & Channell, R.W. (2000) Computerized profiling (Version 9.27) [Computer software]. Retrieved August, 2004, from http://www.computerizedprofiling.org

Miccio, A.W., Elbert, M., & Forrest, K. (1999). The relationship between stimulability and phonological acquisition in children with normally developing and disordered phonologies. *American Journal of Speech-Language Pathology, 8,* 347–363.

Miller, J., & Chapman, R. (1981). Research note: The relation between age and mean length of utterance in morphemes. *Journal of Speech and Hearing Research, 24,* 154–161.

Miller, J., & Chapman, R. (2000). *Systematic analysis of language transcripts.* Madison, WI: Language Analysis Laboratory, Waisman Research Center.

Nelson, L. (2002). *The relationship among four phonological measures.* Unpublished master's thesis, University of Nevada, Reno.

Newcomer, P.L., & Hammill, D.D. (1997). *Test of Language Development-Primary–3.* Austin, TX: PRO-ED.

Paul, R., & Shriberg, L.D. (1982). Associations between phonology and syntax in speech-delayed children. *Journal of Speech and Hearing Research, 25,* 536–547.

Powell, T.W., Elbert, M., & Dinnsen, D.A. (1991). Stimulability as a factor in the phonological generalization of misarticulating preschool children. *Journal of Speech and Hearing Research, 14,* 1318–1328.

Rice, M., Wexler, K., & Cleave, P. (1995). Specific language impairment as a period of extended optional infinitive. *Journal of Speech and Hearing Research, 38,* 850–863.

Robbins, J., & Klee, T. (1987). Clinical assessment of oropharyngeal motor development in young children. *Journal of Speech and Hearing Disorders, 52,* 271–277.

Robertson, C., & Salter, W. (1997). *Phonological Awareness Test.* East Moline, IL: LinguiSystems.

Semel, E., Wiig, E.H., & Secord, W. (1995). *Clinical Evaluation of Language Fundamentals–3.* San Antonio, TX: Harcourt Assessment.

Shriberg, L.D., & Austin, D. (1998). Comorbidity of speech-language disorders: Implications for a phenotype marker for speech delay. In R. Paul (Ed.), *The speech-language connection* (pp. 73–117). Baltimore: Paul H. Brookes Publishing Co.

Shriberg, L.D., & Kwiatkowski, J. (1982). Phonological disorders III: A procedure for assessing severity of involvement. *Journal of Speech and Hearing Disorders, 17,* 256–270.

Shriberg, L.D., & Kwiatkowski, J. (1994). Developmental phonological disorders I: A clinical profile. *Journal of Speech and Hearing Research, 37,* 1100–1126.

Shriberg, L.D., Kwiatkowski, J., Best, S., Hengst, J., & Terselic-Weber, B. (1986). Characteristics of children with phonologic disorders of unknown origin. *Journal of Speech and Hearing Disorders, 51,* 140–161.

Shriberg, L.D., Kwiatkowski, J., & Rasmussen, C. (1990). *Prosody-Voice Screening Profile (PVSP).* Tucson, AZ: Communication Skill Builders.

Stoel-Gammon, C. (1985). Phonetic inventories, 15–24 months: A longitudinal study. *Journal of Speech and Hearing Research, 28,* 505–512.

Swank, L.K., & Catts, H.W. (1994). Phonological awareness and written word decoding. *Language, Speech, and Hearing Services in Schools, 25,* 9–14.

Tallal, P., Ross, R., & Curtiss, S. (1989). Familial aggregation in specific language impairment. *Journal of Speech and Hearing Disorders, 54,* 167–173.

Torgesen, J., & Bryant, P. (1994). *Test of Phonological Awareness.* Austin, TX: PRO-ED.

Wagner, R., Torgesen, J.K., & Rashotte, C. (1999). *Comprehensive Test of Phonological Processing.* Austin, TX: PRO-ED.

Zimmerman, I., Steiner, V., & Pond, R. (1992). *Preschool Language Scale–3.* San Antonio, TX: Harcourt Assessment.

Chapter 5

Assessment and Classification

An Integrative Model of Language and Motor Contributions to Phonological Development

LISA GOFFMAN

C lassification schemes strive to subgroup children with phonological impairments on the basis of language and motor contributions to their observed impairments. Language-based approaches consider how children learn the phonological rules of the language, including, for example, contrasts, patterns or processes, constraints, and interactions with morphosyntax (e.g., Barlow & Gierut, 1999; Bernhardt & Stemberger, 1998). Conversely, motor approaches emphasize the development of feeding, oral-motor, and motor programming capacities that are presumed to support speech production (e.g., Hall, Jordan, & Robin, 1993; Morris & Klein, 1987). An assumption of these principles of classification is that language and motor systems are encapsulated. However, neurophysiological and behavioral evidence demonstrates mutual dependencies between motor and language development, leading to a reconsideration of traditional models of speech sound disorders in which language and motor domains are viewed as modular. In this section, I first review some of the evidence that language and motor development are highly interactive. If the developmental process is not dissociable across these broad domains, then it follows that particular diagnostic classifications that rely on relatively discrete characterizations of motor processes (e.g., childhood apraxia of speech [CAS]) or language processes (e.g., specific language impairment [SLI] with concomitant speech sound disorders) may be problematic. Finally, clinical case studies illustrate why traditional categories need to be rethought and a more integrative developmental model of speech production disorders generated.

Neurophysiologically, during infancy, localization of language functions to the left hemisphere is protracted (Bates, 1999; Mills, Coffey-Corina, & Neville, 1993; Molfese, 1990). In general, as demonstrated by imaging studies as well as recovery profiles of infants with focal lesions, great neural plasticity can be seen early in the process; language

I am grateful to Bill Saxton and Christine Weber-Fox for their assistance with this project. This work was supported by Grant DC04826 from the National Institutes of Health, National Institute on Deafness and Other Communicative Disorders.

functions are not tied to specific areas of the brain. Bates (2004) makes a strong case for looking beyond the language system when considering language development and disorders. She suggested that multiple domain general capacities—such as social, cross-modal perceptual, sensorimotor, and computational—underlie language. As an example, Bates suggested that "by intersecting cross-modal perception with sensorimotor precision, human infants develop an ability to associate sounds with their meanings" (2004, p. 251). Thus, little evidence may be seen early on for domain-specific classification.

Even as functions become more localized, Greenfield (1991) argued that general computational capacities, such as those associated with the acquisition of hierarchical structure, similarly influence both language and motor behaviors. Much of her evidence is behavioral, based on observations of 2- to 3-year-old children's engagement in complex motor and language tasks such as sentence formation and assembly of nesting blocks. She suggested that these complex motor and language functions are related as a consequence of a shared neural substrate roughly corresponding with Broca's area. Diamond (2000) also made the case that cognitive and motor development are closely interconnected, citing evidence that the cerebellum and prefrontal cortex are both involved in complex cognitive (including linguistic) and motor tasks. Overlapping impairments in cognitive and motor domains in clinical populations, such as dyslexia, attention-deficit/hyperactivity disorder, and specific language impairment, provide further evidence that cognitive-linguistic and motor development are closely intertwined, rather than independent and modular (Diamond, 2000).

Turning to observations of speech behaviors, canonical babbling in infants perhaps provides the most thoroughly investigated example of the co-development of language and motor behavior (MacNeilage & Davis, 1990, 2000; Oller, 2001; Stark, 1980). Babbling is defined as the phase of infant vocal development in which the timing characteristics of speech production begin to resemble mature consonants and vowels; yet, babbling also is thought to be comprised of rhythmic, or reduplicated, oscillations of the jaw (MacNeilage & Davis, 1990, 2000; Oller, 2001; Stark, 1980). The rhythmic properties of canonical babbling have been hypothesized to provide a biological substrate for the production of speech. Such rhythmicity is pervasive and is seen across multiple behaviors during development, such as chewing (MacNeilage & Davis, 1990, 2000), kicking (Thelen, 1981), and object banging (Ejiri, 1998). Thus, babbling is seen as a movement primitive for speech that is also closely related to many other motor behaviors.

According to this biologically based view, the rhythmic oscillatory movements of the jaw observed during canonical babbling evolve to accomplish language-specific goals such as the production of differentiated segments (MacNeilage & Davis, 1990, 2000) and prosodic structures (Goffman, 1999; Goffman & Malin, 1999). Early segmental differentiation is reliant on the natural position of the tongue during jaw oscillation; a child is not yet independently controlling movements of the tongue (MacNeilage & Davis, 1999, 2000). Thus, the segments produced by the infant and toddler are driven by propensities of the motor system. In the prosodic domain, even 4-year-old children produce movement patterns associated with early developing strong–weak (or trochaic; e.g., "BAby") stress sequences with undifferentiated movements of the lips and jaw that do not distinguish strong from weak syllables (Goffman, 1999; Goffman & Malin, 1999). It is only in later developing weak–strong (or iambic; e.g., "balLOON") sequences that speech movements associated with weak syllables are small and well-controlled. Overall, there is substantial evidence that, early in development, observed segmental and prosodic distinctions are intricately tied to motor biases.

In the preschool and early school years, Kent (1992) argued that segmental development relies on changes in motor control as well as linguistic processing. For example, early stop consonants are less complex in terms of motor processes than are later fricatives. These stop consonants rely on simple ballistic movements, whereas fricatives require fine force regulation (also see Green, Moore, & Reilly, 2002, for empirical data supporting this developmental shift). Kent (1992) also described an error pattern that is familiar to speech-language pathologists; namely that for children acquiring English, [r] is particularly problematic. Yet [r] is perceptually salient and also occurs frequently in English. Therefore, it seems that movement complexity explains why [r] is so difficult for some children to acquire.

Physiological recording methods have only recently been used to evaluate directly how motor and language capacities interact over the course of development of speech production. In these studies, articulatory movements of the upper lip, lower lip, and jaw are recorded. Multiple productions of the same form are compared to determine how similarly the movement trajectories are produced on each replication. Such direct recordings of oral articulatory movements demonstrate that even when children produce words and sentences that are segmentally accurate, they do so with more variable movement patterns than do adults (e.g., Sharkey & Folkins, 1985; Smith, 1994; Smith & Goffman, 1998; Smith & Zelaznik, 2004; Walsh & Smith, 2002). Increased variability in speech movement patterns shows a protracted developmental time course and persists in adolescence (Smith & Zelaznik, 2004; Walsh & Smith, 2002).

Interestingly, children diagnosed with SLI show movement patterns that are particularly variable (Goffman, 1999, 2004). Perhaps even more striking, however, these children show a reduced capacity to produce small and short movements associated with weak, or unstressed, syllables, even in cases that are perceptually judged as accurate. Thus, even in a disorder that is defined by language variables (usually those associated with impairments in grammatical morphology), speech motor output is immature relative to age-matched peers. These data provide a direct example of how language and motor aspects of development interact. Impairments are observed both in the production of movements associated with prosodic structure and in the capacity to produce patterned, stable, and replicated speech movements. As described in the text that follows, variable movements and difficulty with prosody are associated with CAS. However, direct recordings of movement reveal these characteristics even in young normally developing children and in children with SLI.

Language and motor aspects of speech development continue to change across a very long time scale, from infancy through adolescence. Moreover, language and motor processes are intimately tied to the production of speech. With this backdrop, it should not be surprising that differential diagnosis of speech sound disorders is so difficult. In discussing disorders, I first review two major diagnostic categories, one motor (CAS) and one linguistic (SLI with concomitant speech production impairments). A basic description of these categories is included, followed by evidence that even an extremely motor-based speech production impairment (CAS) almost always involves language impairments and even the most language-based impairment (SLI) also involves motor impairments. It is then important to consider how approaches to classification influence the actual implementation of assessment and intervention, which is the topic of the final section.

CHILDHOOD APRAXIA OF SPEECH

CAS is classically described as an impairment in motor planning (Hall et al., 1993; Strand, 2002). This diagnostic category has been controversial. As discussed at a 2002 symposium on CAS (Shriberg & Campbell, 2002), several characteristics of speech production have been proposed as central to differential diagnosis. Many investigators consider motor impairments to be the hallmark of the disorder (e.g., Hall et al., 1993; Strand, 2002). Others are a bit broader in their conceptualization, suggesting, for example, that impairments in hierarchical organization (e.g., of speech, language, and even play) underlie the disorder (e.g., Velleman & Strand, 1994). When turning to specific characteristics of CAS, the following speech behaviors are cited frequently: inappropriate stress/abnormal word and sentence stress (e.g., Shriberg, Aram, & Kwiatkowski, 1997); variability/inconsistent error patterns (e.g., Hall et al., 1993); difficulty with initial articulatory configurations (e.g., Strand, 2002; Velleman, 2002); reduced phonemic repertoire (e.g., Campbell, 2002); increased errors with increased word length and phonetic complexity (e.g., Strand, 2002; Velleman, 2002); groping and/or trial and error behaviors (e.g., Hall et al., 1993; although Davis, 2002, suggested that these groping errors do not persist and, thus, are not consistent behavioral markers); vowel distortions (e.g., Davis, 2002; Pollock & Hall, 1991); reduced speech rate (e.g., Campbell, 2002); receptive–expressive gap (e.g., Hall et al., 1993); and automatic–volitional gap (e.g., Hall et al., 1993).

One problem has been that no single or subset of characteristics provides a differential diagnosis in children with CAS (Davis, 2002). This is illustrated in a study by Shriberg and colleagues (1997) that carefully examined the speech behaviors of 53 children with this diagnosis. Misplaced stress was the only characteristic that showed up in a significant number of children (52%, in contrast to 10% of children with speech production impairments of unknown origin). It is problematic that no small set of criteria can be used to distinguish children with CAS. Without stable behavioral characteristics, a genetic marker will be difficult to identify (Vargha-Khadem, 2002).

In addition, children who fit into other diagnostic categories (or even very young children who are developing typically) often show most of the characteristics associated with CAS. For example, as noted, misplaced stress is one of the most frequently cited differentiating attributes of CAS. However, children with SLI have also been found to produce stress errors in their speech (Del Duca et al., 1998; Goffman, 1999). Another identifying characteristic, slowed speech rate, is also seen in young typically developing children as well as in those with other speech and language disorders (e.g., Goffman & Smith, 1999; Smith, 1994; Smith & Zelaznik, 2004). It is well established that error rates increase as a function of length and complexity demands (e.g., Kamhi, Catts, & Davis, 1984; Paul & Shriberg, 1982). Variability is another oft-cited feature of CAS that also is evident in young children who are typically developing and in those with phonological impairments (Ferguson & Farwell, 1975; Leonard, Rowan, Morris, & Fey, 1980; Vihman, 1996). At the level of movement, less mature speakers, whether they are typically developing (Sharkey & Folkins, 1985; Smith & Goffman, 1998) or have disordered language

(Goffman, 1999; Goffman, 2004), show more variability in lip and jaw movement than do older children and adults. It is clear that a gap between receptive and expressive language occurs in many other diagnostic categories, above all in SLI (Leonard, 1998). This gap leaves few characteristics remaining, most notably vowel errors and articulatory groping. These characteristics are typically not measured in early development or in other speech and language disorders. It is unclear whether they are specific to CAS.

Overall, CAS does not appear to form a coherent diagnostic category. Given the interactive nature of speech and motor development, it seems unlikely that a disorder exists that encapsulates only motor variables. The research in CAS has led to some essential analytical approaches that incorporate motor control into the developmental model (e.g., Caruso & Strand, 1999; Crary, 1993; Hall et al., 1993; Square, 1994). I hypothesize that for some children with speech production disorders, these motor variables are more heavily weighted. To date, however, these analyses have not revealed a differenti-able category. Furthermore, as discussed later, most of these characteristics also apply to the assessment and treatment of language-based phonological disorders such as SLI.

SPECIFIC LANGUAGE IMPAIRMENT

At the other extreme from CAS, SLI has been identified as the hallmark type of proprietary language impairment. Children with SLI are diagnosed in relation to their language abilities, with specific impairments in either receptive or expressive language that are not explained by psychosocial, cognitive, auditory, or overt motor impairments (Leonard, 1998; Stark & Tallal, 1981). A primary focus of research and of clinical assessment and treatment has been on grammatical morphology. Specifically, these children show particular vulnerabilities in the production of grammatical inflections, most notably those applied to verbs. Indeed, probably the most sensitive diagnostic marker to date is the finite verb morphology composite, which is obtained from percent correct usage of verb inflections (i.e., regular past tense, regular third person singular, copula, and auxiliary) in spontaneous language (Goffman & Leonard, 2000; Leonard, Miller, & Gerber, 1999; Rice, Wexler, & Hershberger, 1998). Children with SLI may or may not show phonological impairments. However, at least in the preschool years, phonological disorders often co-occur with language impairments. SLI is theoretically the strongest example of a language-based speech production impairment.

Although children with SLI demonstrate language impairment, interestingly they also perform below expected levels on many motor tasks. For example, fine motor skills requiring spatiotemporal precision (e.g., copying shapes) are correlated with receptive language abilities (Schwartz & Regan, 1996). Children with SLI also perform more slowly on a task involving the movement of pegs (Bishop & Edmundson, 1987). They show difficulties with imitating gestures such as saluting and brushing teeth (Hill, Bishop, & Nimmo-Smith, 1998). There is evidence that gross and fine motor skills are also impaired for many of these children (for a review, see Hill, 2001).

In the motor domain for speech, group findings have revealed that children diagnosed with SLI show oral movements that are more variable than those of their age-mates (Goffman, 1999, 2004). Furthermore, these children are poorer at producing the contiguous small and large movements required for the production of differentiated stress patterns.

Overall, at least as a group, children with SLI show impairments in gross motor, fine motor, and speech motor areas, thus providing evidence that motor and language domains do not develop in isolation. At least in some cases, motor development should also be considered even in children whose diagnostic classification is defined by their language impairment. Although a less severe example than CAS (i.e., some individual children's impairments are likely dominated by language variables), the case of SLI once again supports a far more interactive view than do typical classification schemes.

CLINICAL IMPLICATIONS

It is crucial to consider how diagnostic classification relates to clinical treatment. Presumably, the importance of classification is that it leads to differential interventions. As stated at the outset, intervention approaches are generally linked to traditional classification categories such as CAS, phonological impairments, and SLI with concomitant speech impairment. Some of these approaches are illustrated in a special issue of the journal *Seminars in Speech and Language* devoted to the topic of phonological intervention. Several major researchers contributed chapters on treatment approaches, including, for example, oral-motor (Forrest, 2002), pattern based (Stoel-Gammon, Stone-Goldman, & Glaspey, 2002), minimal contrasts (Barlow & Gierut, 2002), and language based (Tyler, 2002). All of these approaches are likely to be effective in some cases, although empirical data are limited for the oral-motor approach. A more interesting question for the present purposes is "How should the appropriate approach be selected for a given child?" In the case studies included in these articles, much overlap was seen in the developmental descriptions of the children, even though different approaches were recommended.

The case studies reported in the context of the phonological patterning (Stoel-Gammon et al., 2002) and language-based (Tyler, 2002) approaches were very similar with regard to the children's developmental profiles. Critically, both 4-year-old children who participated in the studies had typical intelligence, normal hearing, and impaired expressive language and phonology. Both of these children had multiple errors leading to unintelligibility. In the pattern-based approach, intervention consisted of using cycles (Hodson & Paden, 1991) in which treatment is rotated across a group of phonological patterns such as final consonant deletion, velar fronting, and stopping of fricatives. In the language-based approach, treatment focused on the production of phonemes associated with grammatical morphemes. The child described in the minimal pairs approach, also a 4-year-old, differed in that he showed no language impairments. His speech sound repertoire was extremely reduced and treatment consisted of teaching how minimal pair distinctions would contribute to effective communication. Although the interventions are distinct in each of these published cases, much overlap was observed in the developmental qualities of the children themselves. The intervention approach focuses on a particular aspect of the child's profile but does not appear to link closely to diagnostic classification. This does not seem surprising when considering a more interactive framework of language and motor contributions to phonological development.

The oral-motor approach (Forrest, 2002) did not include a case study. Perhaps an explanation for this is that, in general, oral-motor approaches have grown out of clinically based observation rather than controlled experimental research; models such as neurodevelopmental treatment (NDT) hold great promise but beg for careful investigation regarding efficacy. Approaches that are motor based, including NDT, along with models based on principles of motor control (e.g., Hall et al., 1993), have far less empirical backing than do language-based approaches. More study is required in treatments associated with motor contributions to speech development and disorders.

Three clinical case studies, along with data from a typically developing child, will be used to further explicate how an interactive, rather than a modular, view provides a more accurate model of development. The three children participating in these studies fit a classic profile associated with SLI. Although the children fit the same general criteria that appropriately lead to this diagnosis, the relative weighting of motor factors on their speech production differs markedly. Individual and rather detailed analyses of motor, speech, and language behaviors—not general diagnostic category—lead to treatment choices. Also interesting to note is that these children have profiles that are similar to those reported by Stoel-Gammon and colleagues (2002) and Tyler (2002).

General assessment data leading to a diagnosis of SLI are first reported. Assessment data reported from T were collected from age 5;1 to 6;0. T has a history of speech and language impairments. He was diagnosed with SLI, for which he clearly fit the exclusionary criteria. His auditory status was normal, and his score on a nonverbal intelligence test, the Columbia Mental Maturity Scale (Burgemeister, Blum, & Lorge, 1972), was well within the expected range. His receptive language skills were also appropriate for his age. Expressively, however, T exhibited significant deficits. His finite verb morphology composite (i.e., grammatical morphemes associated with tense and agreement; regular past tense –ed, regular third person singular, copula, and auxiliary) was 28%, which is well below expected levels of 85%–100% (Goffman & Leonard, 2000). Significantly, T's grammatical errors were not all explainable by phonological factors. For example, he was able to mark final [d] and [z] in monomorphemic contexts (e.g., "nose") and he produced frequent pronoun errors. This finding suggests that not all of his production impairment can be seen as articulatory or even phonological. Some language-specific aspects are also implicated.

T's speech production was also below expected levels. His standard score on the Bankson–Bernthal Test of Phonology (BBTOP; Bankson & Bernthal, 1990) was 77 for consonant inventory. His speech production was characterized by typically observed processes, similar to one of the children in the study presented by Stoel-Gammon and colleagues (2002). For example, T frequently stopped fricatives, fronted velars, omitted weak syllables, and reduced clusters.

J, age 4;7, also fits the classification of SLI, again with concomitant phonological impairments. His profile is similar to T's. J's nonverbal cognitive skills were normal (score of 113 on the Columbia Mental Maturity Scale [Burgemeister et al., 1972]), as were his auditory and oral-motor functioning. However, J demonstrated a significant language impairment, as indicated by a score of less than the first percentile on the Structured Photographic Expressive Language Test–Preschool (SPELT-P; Werner & Kresheck, 1983) and a finite verb morphology composite of 15%. J also showed a phonological impairment. His standard score on the consonant inventory analysis of the BBTOP (Bankson & Bernthal, 1990) was 76. Patterns observed included fronting, cluster reduction, gliding, and weak syllable omission.

M is a child who, as with J and T, shows a classic profile associated with SLI. At age 4;11, his nonverbal cognitive skills (standard score of 113) and receptive language skills were normal. However, on the SPELT-P (Werner & Kresheck, 1983) he scored at the 3rd percentile and his finite verb morphology composite score was 34%. He also showed concomitant speech production impairments, as indicated by a score of less than 65 on the BBTOP (Bankson & Bernthal, 1990).

All three boys clearly fit a diagnosis of SLI. They showed particular impairments in grammatical morphology but normal hearing, oral-motor, and receptive language status. In addition, they each had a concomitant speech production disorder, which is consistent with the diagnosis of SLI (e.g., Leonard, 1998). T, J, and M also participated in group studies of speech motor development in children with SLI (e.g., Goffman, 1999; Goffman, 2004; Goffman, Heisler, & Chakraborty, in press). Examples of their movement data are shown in Figure 5.1. These plots show lower lip movements recorded for the repeated production of the utterance "Bobby's pə'pʌp is falling." (Goffman, Heisler, & Chakraborty, in press). The top plot for each child shows lower lip movements for 10 repeated productions of this sentence. The middle plot shows the same 10 productions, now normalized for time and amplitude to remove the effects of changes in rate or loudness. The bottom panel is an index of variability, the spatiotemporal index (Smith, Goffman, & Zelaznik, et al., 1995), in which standard deviations of the normalized records are obtained at 2% intervals and are summed. This sum is an index of variability and is displayed in the bottom panel of data for each child. The higher numbers shown for T and J reflect more variability, as can also be seen in the movement trajectories in the top and middle panels. Also notable is that T and J produce movements that are larger in amplitude than those of their peers. Interestingly, many aspects of T's and J's speech production may be viewed as consistent with CAS rather than SLI, most notably direct observations of variability in the movement domain. In fact, in another clinical context, T may easily have been diagnosed as having CAS. He fits many of the diagnostic criteria, including inappropriate stress, variability, reduced phonemic inventory, increased errors with increased complexity, slowed rate, and receptive-expressive gap. Direct observation of the motor evidence, although not clinically feasible to incorporate at this time, provides substantiation that these clinical categories of CAS and SLI overlap, at least in some cases, in that the implementation of stable and well-planned oral movements is impaired in some children who fall squarely into the category of SLI.

The purpose of these case studies is to illustrate that even when children appear to be well matched according to the basic criteria for a diagnosis, enriched assessment data show that very different treatment approaches should follow. T, J, and M displayed normal auditory, gross oral-motor, and nonverbal cognitive status. Each child also had impairment in expressive language, with a receptive-expressive gap. Finite verb morphology and morphosyntax, signature characteristics of SLI, are implicated strongly for all of these children. However, for two children, T and J, intervention should also be weighted toward including motor planning and implementation. For M, however, although speech production impairment was most severe, motor factors were less heavily weighted. Traditional classification systems do not allow for the incorporation of language, phonological, and motor variables in the assessment of every developing child.

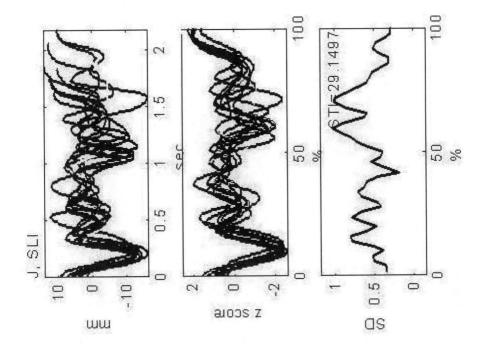

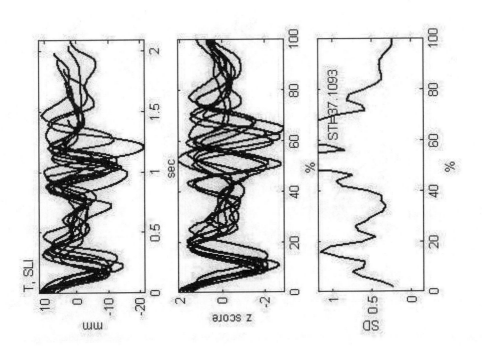

Figure 5.1. Spatiotemporal stability of three children with SLI compared with a typical age-matched control (ND). All three children are producing the utterance "Bobby's pɔ pʌp is falling." Note that two of these children (T and J) produced movements that were more variable and of larger amplitude than another child (M) with SLI and than a typically developing age-matched control (ND). A detailed description of this figure is included in the text.

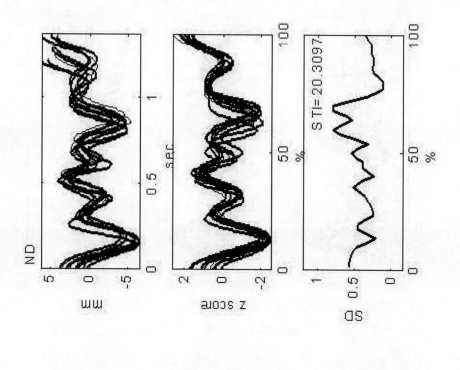

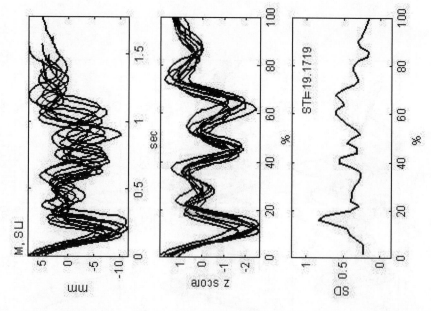

FUTURE DIRECTIONS AND IMPLICATIONS
FOR ASSESSMENT AND TREATMENT MODELS

The contributions of theoretical constructs from linguistics and from motor control provide strong and crucial bases for considering how speech production impairments are assessed and treated. However, with new evidence, it becomes important to develop new models of speech disorders that explicitly integrate the acquisition of language and motor representations in concert with one another. Such an approach modifies how each child is examined in the assessment and treatment process. Traditional diagnostic categories only minimally guide treatment decisions. The assessment process needs to go beyond existing measures of segmental repertoires, syllable shapes, and error patterns to include more elaborated and integrative measures of language and motor development and how they interact for the production of speech. Morphosyntactic, semantic, phonological, and motor contributors to a child's speech production impairment should be evaluated to determine the appropriate course of intervention.

A NOTE ON ASSESSMENT

As a clinician working in early intervention, I became aware early on that, dependent on perspective, therapists had two general repertoires on which to base their assessment and treatment: language or motor skills. Clinicians who had been trained in a language-based model typically assessed children by obtaining a speech sample (either single-word naming or, ideally, continuous speech) and completing an independent (e.g., sound and syllable shape inventory) and a relational (e.g., processes and substitution patterns) analysis (e.g., Stoel-Gammon & Dunn, 1985). Within this same general approach fall perceptual judgments of prosody and, in older children, acquisition of phonological awareness. Also, for these clinicians, phonological skills were always evaluated in the context of semantic, syntactic, and pragmatic domains, with, for example, careful consideration of relations to lexical and morphological development.

Conversely, another group of clinicians analyzed oral-motor and general motor skills, including, for example, feeding, respiration, positioning, and speech. Generally, these assessments were derived from neurodevelopmental treatment approaches (e.g., Morris & Klein, 1987). The only commonality across approaches was an audiological assessment. I believe, however, that assessing the child from either side of the dichotomy only looks at "part of the elephant." Clearly, speech production is a motor and a linguistic process. Models of normal and disordered development need to be broadened to consider the interactive nature and interdependent components of speech production.

REFERENCES

Bankson, N.W., & Bernthal, J.E. (1990). *Bankson–Bernthal Test of Phonology.* Chicago: Riverside.

Barlow, J.A., & Gierut, J.A. (1999). Optimality theory in phonological acquisition. *Journal of Speech, Language, and Hearing Research, 42,* 1482–1498.

Barlow, J.A., & Gierut, J.A. (2002). Minimal pair approaches to phonological remediation. *Seminars in Speech and Language, 23,* 57–67.

Bates, E.A. (1999). Language and the infant brain. *Journal of Communication Disorders, 32,* 195–205.

Bates, E.A. (2004). Explaining and interpreting deficits in language development across clinical groups: Where do we go from here? *Brain and Language, 88,* 248–253.

Bernhardt, B.H., & Stemberger, J.P. (1998). *Handbook of phonological development from the perspective of constraint-based nonlinear phonology.* San Diego: Academic Press.

Bishop, D.V.M., & Edmundson, A. (1987). Specific language impairment as a maturational lag: Evidence from longitudinal data on language and motor development. *Developmental Medicine and Child Neurology, 29,* 442–459.

Burgemeister, B., Blum, L., & Lorge, I. (1972). *Columbia Mental Maturity Scale* (3rd ed.). San Antonio, TX: Harcourt Assessment.

Campbell, T.F. (2002). Childhood apraxia of speech: Clinical symptoms and speech characteristics. In L.D. Shriberg & T.F. Campbell (Eds.), *Proceedings of the 2002 childhood apraxia of speech research symposium.* Carlsbad, CA: The Hendrix Foundation.

Caruso, A.J., & Strand, E.A. (1999). *Clinical management of motor speech disorders in children.* New York: Thieme.

Crary, M.A. (1993). *Developmental motor speech disorders.* San Diego: Singular.

Davis, B.L. (2002). Patterns of vowel production in childhood apraxia of speech. In L.D. Shriberg & T.F. Campbell (Eds.), *Proceedings of the 2002 childhood apraxia of speech research symposium.* Carlsbad, CA: The Hendrix Foundation.

Del Duca, G., Petrille, L., Bourne, P., Leavy, H., McMillin, A., Wieting, S., Dollaghan, C., Davis, D., Liddell, M., & Metzler, R. (1998, June). *Prosodic features of children with language impairments.* Paper presented at the symposium for research in child language disorders, Madison, WI.

Diamond, A. (2000). Close interrelation of motor development and cognitive development and of the cerebellum and prefrontal cortex. *Child Development, 71,* 44–56.

Ejiri, K. (1998). Relationship between rhythmic behavior and canonical babbling in infant vocal development. *Phonetica, 55,* 226–237.

Ferguson, C.A., & Farwell, C.B. (1975). Words and sounds in early language acquisition: English initial consonants in the first fifty words. *Language, 51,* 419–439.

Forrest, K. (2002). Are oral-motor exercises useful in the treatment of phonological/articulatory disorders? *Seminars in Speech and Language, 23,* 15–25.

Goffman, L. (1999). Prosodic influences on speech production in children with specific language impairment: Kinematic, acoustic, and transcription evidence. *Journal of Speech, Language, and Hearing Research, 42,* 1499–1517.

Goffman, L. (2004). Kinematic differentiation of prosodic categories in normal and disordered language development. *Journal of Speech, Language, and Hearing Research, 47,* 1088–1102.

Goffman, L., Heisler, L., & Chakraborty, R. (in press). Mapping of prosodic structure onto words and phrases in children's and adults' speech production. *Language and Cognitive Processes.*

Goffman, L., & Leonard, J. (2000). Growth of language skills in preschool children with specific language impairment: Implications for assessment and intervention. *American Journal of Speech Language Pathology, 9,* 151–161.

Goffman, L., & Malin, C. (1999). Metrical effects on speech movements in children and adults. *Journal of Speech, Language, and Hearing Research, 42,* 1003–1115.

Goffman, L., & Smith, A. (1999). Development and phonetic differentiation of speech movement patterns. *Journal of Experimental Psychology: Human Perception and Performance, 25,* 649–660.

Green, J.R., Moore, C.A., & Reilly, K.J. (2002). The sequential development of jaw and lip control for speech. *Journal of Speech, Language, and Hearing Research, 45,* 66–79.

Greenfield, P.M. (1991). Language, tools, and brain: The ontogeny and phylogeny of hierarchically organized sequential behavior. *Behavioral and Brain Sciences, 14,* 531–595.

Hall, P.K., Jordan, L.S., & Robin, D.A. (1993). *Developmental apraxia of speech: Theory and clinical practice.* Austin, TX: PRO-ED.

Hill, E.L. (2001). Non-specific nature of specific language impairment: A review of the literature with regard to concomitant motor impairments. *International Journal of Language and Communication Disorders, 36,* 149–171.

Hill, E., Bishop, D., & Nimmo-Smith, I. (1998). Representational gestures in developmental coordination disorders and specific language impairment: Error types and the reliability of ratings. *Human Movement Science, 17,* 655–678.

Hodson, B., & Paden, E. (1991). *Targeting intelligible speech* (2nd ed.). Austin, TX: PRO-ED.

Kamhi, A.G., Catts, H.W., & Davis, M.K. (1984). Management of sentence production demands. *Journal of Speech and Hearing Research, 27,* 329–338.

Kent, R.D. (1992). The biology of phonological development. In C.A. Ferguson, L. Menn, & C. Stoel-Gammon (Eds.), *Phonological development: Models, research, implications* (pp. 65–90). Timonium, MD: York Press.

Leonard, L. (1998). *Children with specific language impairment.* Cambridge, MA: MIT Press.

Leonard, L., Miller, C., & Gerber, E. (1999). Grammatical morphology and the lexicon in children with specific language impairment. *Journal of Speech, Language, and Hearing Research, 42,* 678–689.

Leonard, L., Rowan, L., Morris, B., & Fey, M. (1980). Intra-word phonological variability in young children. *Journal of Child Language, 9,* 55–69.

MacNeilage, P.F., & Davis, B.L. (1990). Acquisition of speech production: Frames then content. In M. Jeannerod (Ed.), *Attention and performance XII: Motor representation and control* (pp. 453–476). Hillsdale, NJ: Lawrence Erlbaum Associates.

MacNeilage, P.F., & Davis, B.L. (2000). On the origin of internal structure of word forms. *Science, 288,* 527–531.

Mills, D.L., Coffey-Corina, S.A., & Neville, H.J. (1993). Language acquisition and cerebral specialization in 20-month-old infants. *Journal of Cognitive Neuroscience, 5,* 317–334.

Molfese, D.L. (1990). Auditory evoked responses recorded from 16-month-old human infants to words they did and did not know. *Brain and Language, 38,* 345–363.

Morris, S.E., & Klein, M.D. (1987). *Pre-feeding skills.* Tucson, AZ: Therapy Skill Builders.

Oller, D.K. (2001). *The emergence of the speech capacity.* Mahwah, NJ: Lawrence Erlbaum Associates.

Paul, R., & Shriberg, L. (1982). Associations between phonology and syntax in speech delayed children. *Journal of Speech and Hearing Research, 25,* 536–547.

Pollock, K., & Hall, P. (1991). An analysis of vowel misarticulations of five children with developmental apraxia of speech. *Clinical Linguistics and Phonetics, 5,* 207–224.

Rice, M., Wexler, K., & Hershberger, S. (1998). Tense over time: The longitudinal course of tense acquisition in children with specific language impairment. *Journal of Speech, Language, and Hearing Research, 41,* 1412–1431.

Schwartz, M., & Regan, V. (1996). Sequencing, timing, and rate relationships between language and motor skill in children with receptive language delay. *Developmental Neuropsychology, 12,* 255–270.

Sharkey, S.G., & Folkins, J.W. (1985). Variability of lip and jaw movements in children and adults: Implications for the development of speech motor control. *Journal of Speech and Hearing Research, 28,* 8–15.

Shriberg, L.D., Aram, D.M., & Kwiatkowski, J. (1997). Developmental apraxia of speech III: A subtype marked by inappropriate stress. *Journal of Speech, Language, and Hearing Research, 40,* 313–337.

Shriberg, L.D., & Campbell, T.F. (Eds.) (2002). *Proceedings of the 2002 childhood apraxia of speech research symposium.* Carlsbad, CA: The Hendrix Foundation.

Smith, A., & Goffman, L. (1998). Stability and patterning of speech movement sequences in children and adults. *Journal of Speech, Language, and Hearing Science, 41,* 18–30.

Smith, A., Goffman, L., Zelaznik, H., Ying, G., & McGillem, C. (1995). Spatiotemporal stability and patterning of speech movement sequences. *Experimental Brain Research, 104,* 493–501.

Smith, A., & Zelaznik, H. (in press). The development of functional synergies for speech motor coordination in childhood and adolescence. *Developmental Psychobiology.*

Smith, B.L. (1994). Effects of experimental manipulations and intrinsic contrasts on relationships between duration and temporal variability in children's and adults' speech. *Journal of Phonetics, 22,* 155–175.

Square, P.A. (1994). Treatment approaches for developmental apraxia of speech. *Journal of Communication Disorders, 4,* 151–151.

Stark, R.E. (1980). Stages of speech development in the first year of life. In G. Yeni-Komshian, J. Kavanagh, & C. Ferguson (Eds.), *Child phonology* (Vol. 1, pp. 73–90). New York: Academic Press.

Stark, R.E., & Tallal, P. (1981). Selection of children with specific language deficits. *Journal of Speech and Hearing Disorders, 46,* 114–122.

Stoel-Gammon, C., & Dunn, C. (1985). *Normal and disordered phonology in children.* Austin, TX: PRO-ED.

Stoel-Gammon, C., Stone-Goldman, J., & Glaspy, A. (2002). Pattern-based approaches to phonological therapy. *Seminars in Speech and Language, 23,* 3–13.

Strand, E.A. (2003). Childhood apraxia of speech: Suggested diagnostic markers for the younger child. In L.D. Shriberg & T.F. Campbell (Eds.), *Proceedings of the 2002 childhood apraxia of speech research symposium* (pp. 75–79). Carlsbad, CA: The Hendrix Foundation.

Thelen, E. (1981). Rhythmical behavior in infancy: An ethological perspective. *Developmental Psychobiology, 17,* 237–257.

Tyler, A. (2002). Language-based intervention for phonological disorders. *Seminars in Speech and Language, 23,* 69–81.

Vargha-Khadem, F. (2003). From genes to brain and behavior: The KE family and the FOXP2 gene. In L.D. Shriberg & T.F. Campbell (Eds.), *Proceedings of the 2002 childhood apraxia of speech research symposium* (pp. 27–36). Carlsbad, CA: The Hendrix Foundation.

Velleman, S. (2003). VMPAC and PEPS-C: Effective new tools for differential diagnosis? In L.D. Shriberg & T.F. Campbell (Eds.), *Proceedings of the 2002 childhood apraxia of speech research symposium* (pp. 81–88). Carlsbad, CA: The Hendrix Foundation.

Velleman, S., & Strand, C. (1994). Developmental verbal dyspraxia. In J. Bernthal & N. Bankson (Eds.), *Child phonology: Characteristics, assessment, and intervention with special populations* (pp. 110–139). New York: Thieme.

Vihman, M.M. (1996). *Phonological development: The origins of language in the child.* Cambridge, MA: Blackwell.

Walsh, B., & Smith, A. (2002). Articulatory movements in adolescents: Evidence for protracted development of speech motor control processes. *Journal of Speech, Language, and Hearing Research, 45,* 1119–1133.

Werner, E.O., & Kresheck, J.D. (1983). *Structured Photographic Expressive Language Test– Preschool (SPELT-P).* DeKalb, IL: Janelle Publications.

Part II

Goal and Target Selection

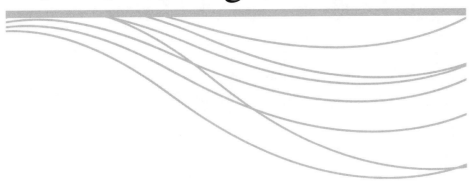

T he selection of goals and targets represents a critical link between assessment/
diagnosis and the intervention process. The goals that a clinician chooses to target
are probably the best reflection of the clinician's theoretical orientation. As a result,
a wide range of approaches are available. Because of its importance, Part II of the book
is devoted to questions about goal and target selection, including

1. What factors influence your selection of treatment goals and targets?

2. How does your selection of goals and targets reflect your theoretical orientation?

3. Do you directly target vowels, perception, syllable structure, prosody, or phoneme
    awareness?

4. How do you integrate language goals with phonological goals?

Part II contains five chapters, reflecting a variety of approaches to goal and target selection.
Chapter 6, by Ann A. Tyler, and Chapter 7, by Janet A. Norris and Paul R. Hoffman,
address all four of these questions. Tyler describes an eclectic approach (developmental
and complexity based) and then illustrates with a case example the steps involved in
selecting goals and targets. Norris and Hoffman frame their approach in a neuro-network
model that views phonology as an integral and inseparable part of the language system.
The remaining chapters focus primarily on the first two questions. In Chapter 8, Barbara
L. Davis highlights the link between assessment outcomes and goal and target selection
and stresses the importance of the clinician's knowledge of developmental milestones in
this process. Next, A. Lynn Williams (Chapter 9) summarizes changes in target selection
practices over the past 25 years that led to the development of her systemic approach
based on a distance metric. In the final chapter in Part 2, Barbara Handford Bernhardt
describes a constraints-based nonlinear approach to goal and target selection that emphasizes the hierarchical nature of phonology. She also reminds us that we need to consider

the whole person when selecting phonological goals and targets, including the child's other cognitive-linguistic abilities, personal-social factors, and oral mechanism structure and function.

Chapter 6

Promoting Generalization

Selecting, Scheduling, and Integrating Goals

ANN A. TYLER

The selection of phonological targets for intervention, although a routine clinical activity, is an aspect of clinical phonology about which considerable efficacy research suggests quite disparate approaches. Approaches to target selection can be broadly classified as *developmental* or *complexity based*. Developmental approaches encompass those that use the normal developmental sequence of phonological acquisition and normative age of acquisition as guidelines for target selection. In contrast, complexity-based approaches focus on the seemingly more complex targets with respect to the child's knowledge, linguistic, or articulatory phonetic factors (Gierut, 2001). Often, targets that would result from these different approaches are diametrically opposed. For example, adherence to the developmental sequence might suggest /f/ as a target for a child missing fricatives, whereas a complexity-based approach would suggest /ð/.

Regardless of the approach, the ultimate goal of a phonological intervention program is generalization, or transfer of learning to other sounds and contexts. Presumably, generalization should allow us to increase intervention efficiency. Within the domain of phonology we can hope to achieve within-class generalization or across-class generalization. On the one hand, within-class generalization involves the transfer of correct production from a target sound to its cognate, to sounds within the same class or sounds affected by the same error pattern, or to the target in an untrained position. Across-class generalization, on the other hand, refers to the correct production of untreated sounds from different manner classes as compared with the target sound. We have considerable evidence that both developmental and complexity-based approaches to target selection lead to generalization (Gierut, 1992; Gierut, Elbert, & Dinnsen, 1987; Gierut, Morrisette, Hughes, & Rowland, 1996; Rvachew & Nowak, 2001; Tyler, Edwards, & Saxman, 1987). It has been shown that developmental target selection approaches facilitate, at a minimum, across-class generalization and complexity-based approaches facilitate across-class as well as within-class generalization. Less well understood is the overall length of intervention time associated with the achievement of these different types of generalization. Furthermore, cross-domain generalization from treatment of other domains of language, that is, effects of language intervention on phonological targets, must also be considered.

Target selection necessarily must begin with a comprehensive analysis of a child's phonological system, involving both independent and relational components (Stoel-Gammon, 1985). Ideally, a computerized analysis program such as PROPH (Computerized

Profiling; Long, 2003) or Computerized Articulation and Phonology Evaluation System (CAPES; Masterson & Bernhardt, 2001) can be used to quickly and accurately provide the following pieces of information: phonetic inventory, syllable structure inventory and match, phonemic inventory, substitution analysis, phonological process analysis, and percent consonants correct (PCC; Shriberg & Kwiatkowski, 1982). This information, along with results of stimulability testing and observation of the child's attention and motivation in that task, is necessary for the selection of intervention targets. When computerized analysis procedures are not available, a "by-hand" analysis of the sample from a standardized articulation test such as the Goldman–Fristoe Test of Articulation–3 (GFTA-3; Goldman & Fristoe, 2000) or the Arizona Articulation Proficiency Scale–3 (AAPS-3; Fudala, 2000) can be completed in a relatively short time and provides valuable information. This analysis should include, at a minimum, the identification of error patterns by position, a phonetic inventory tally, and a word/syllable structure inventory.

A number of phonological process assessment tools are available that identify major error patterns for treatment based either on their severity ranking or percentage of occurrence. For example, both the Khan–Lewis Phonological Analysis (KLPA-2; Khan & Lewis, 2002) and the Hodson Assessment of Phonological Patterns (HAPP-3; Hodson, 2004) provide percentages of occurrences of phonological patterns and recommendations for targeting patterns that apply beyond a specified percentage. The Bankson–Bernthal Test of Phonology (BBTOP; Bankson & Bernthal, 1990) provides severity rankings for processes, and those with rankings of "4" would be potential targets for treatment. It is important to note that all of these standardized tests, a priori, select a finite set of phonological processes to examine and, as such, are constrained in identifying unusual error patterns. In addition, most tests do not provide accurate frequencies for processes that apply primarily in one word position. Identifying the relative frequency of error patterns by position is a benefit of a computerized analysis that is often missed in a standardized phonological process test.

There are three major initial steps to target selection:

1. Choose error patterns that have a major impact on the system with respect to severity and intelligibility.

2. Choose target sounds that can have an impact on those error patterns and/or expand the inventory.

3. Select a goal attack strategy.

The initial focus on error patterns reflects my early training in natural phonological theory and phonological processes; however, my target selection approach is both developmental and complexity based, reflecting my consideration of constraint-based theories and complexity in learning.

The first step involves the selection of error patterns that maximally affect the child's phonological system and distance it from the adult target system. In completing Step 1, a number of additional questions must be answered: How are word/syllable structures affected by error patterns? Which sound classes are proportionally more affected by error patterns? Are there positional constraints? The second step involves selecting one or two key sounds affected by the chosen error patterns to serve as "vehicles" for elimination of the entire error pattern. This is achieved through generalization that should occur from trained exemplars to other sounds in the same class. Although the first two steps involve selecting error patterns for elimination and target sounds as vehicles for this elimination, interplay occurs between selecting targets for expansion of the phonetic inventory versus reduction of error patterns. In completing Step 2, the question of which sounds are absent from the phonetic inventory must be answered with the consideration of stimulability results. It may sometimes be possible to find targets that are absent from the phonetic inventory and that are also good exemplars of the sound classes affected by major error patterns. It may also be the case that target sounds necessary for the elimination of errors resulting from positional constraints are already in the phonetic inventory, so that not all targets would be absent from the inventory.

The final step in the target selection process is the selection of a goal attack strategy or a method for scheduling multiple goals (Fey, 1986). A number of variables must be considered in selecting a goal attack strategy, such as one's theory of language learning, complexity level of goals, interrelatedness of goals, individual characteristics of a child, and intervention setting and agent (Weiss, 2002). Goals can be targeted in one of the following approaches: 1) a vertical strategy in which one goal at a time is focused on until some predetermined level of accuracy is achieved; 2) a horizontal strategy in which several goals are repeatedly targeted within every session; and 3) a cyclical strategy in which several goals are targeted, each for a specified time period independent of accuracy, and the sequence is repeated.

The steps and questions asked in target selection are now addressed in turn through the use of a clinical example. Results from a by-hand analysis of the AAP-3 sample showed that the following major error patterns affected severity/intelligibility: final conso-nant deletion of fricatives and glottal replacement, cluster reduction, velar fronting in the initial and medial positions, and stopping of initial fricatives and affricates. In addition, this child had prevocalic voicing of obstruents, gliding of liquids and /d/, and vocalization of syllabic liquids.

TARGET SELECTION SEQUENCE

Step 1

How Are Word/Syllable Structures Affected by Error Patterns?

To answer this question, both the frequency of different syllable structures (regardless of accuracy) and the match between target and structure productions can be calculated. This child's most frequent syllable structure was CVC (43%) and the match between target syllable shapes and productions was 48%. The primary error patterns affecting syllable structures were final consonant deletion and cluster reduction.

Which Sound Classes Are Proportionally More Affected by Error Patterns?

The sound classes most affected by the major error patterns were fricatives, affricates, and velars. Final consonant deletion applied almost exclusively to fricatives, although two final /g/s were also deleted. Stopping in the initial position affected fricatives and affricates. Velars were affected primarily by velar fronting but also by final consonant deletion and glottal replacement.

Are There Positional Constraints?

In the final position fricatives were deleted (except for two labials that were stopped), and in the initial position fricatives and affricates were replaced by stops. This suggested that fricatives were absent from the phonetic inventory. Similarly, velars were affected either by velar fronting or final consonant deletion/glottal replacement. Furthermore, initial stops were limited to voiced cognates, due to initial voicing. Another noticeable feature of this child's phonology was the frequent occurrence of initial /d/, often because of the interaction of several processes—velar fronting, initial voicing, stopping, and/or cluster reduction.

Step 2

Which Sounds Are Present/Absent in the Phonetic Inventory and What Is Their Stimulability Status?

Our consideration of major error patterns and the sounds affected according to word position has already suggested that our target sounds for intervention may come from the classes of fricatives and velars. In completing Step 2 in the target selection sequence, we must now consider which phones are absent from the phonetic inventory and their stimulability status. There may be a tradeoff between choosing sounds that are absent from the inventory and stimulable and those that are absent and nonstimulable. Presumably, the child has the least amount of knowledge of the nonstimulable absent sounds. Furthermore, evidence exists that nonstimulable sounds are not likely to change without treatment, whereas stimulable sounds will emerge without direct treatment (Miccio, Elbert, & Forrest, 1999; Powell, Elbert, & Dinnsen, 1991). Thus, it would seem that greater change could be induced through the selection of a nonstimulable sound that is absent from the inventory. If a sound is nonstimulable, however, both the child and the clinician often experience frustration and slow progress due to difficulty achieving accurate productions. To aid in the decision of whether to even consider a nonstimulable sound, I observe the child's level of attention, motivation, and persistence during the stimulability task. If these are moderate to high, it may be possible to select a nonstimulable sound. Its potential difficulty may be offset with a stimulable sound absent from the inventory or, in the case of a positional constraint, a target that is already in the inventory but absent in a particular word position.

The child in our example had a phonetic inventory of /h/, /d/, /l/, /w/, /m/, /n/ in the initial position and /p/, /b/, /t/, /n/, /r/ in the final position. Thus, fricatives and affricates were missing from the inventory as were velars and the glide /j/. This child was stimulable in isolation for /g/, /f/, /s/, /ʃ/, /j/ and in syllables for /f/, /s/, /ʃ/, /j/. Now we must decide between treating early developing and stimulable sounds or later developing and nonstimulable sounds. Given that so many sounds are absent from this child's inventory, all targets would be selected from the group missing from the phonetic inventory. Although there is evidence that selecting nonstimulable sounds will lead to greater change in those sounds and in stimulable sounds as well, I would not select only nonstimulable sounds for fear of the child becoming frustrated with his or her beginning experiences in therapy. Instead, I would select a stimulable sound for a new word shape, in this case final position, so final /s/ would be a target. Initial /k/ would also be selected because it is a nonstimulable velar and a voiceless stop, which are not present in the initial position. The final palatal /tʃ/ would also be targeted because it is relatively marked, absent from the inventory, nonstimulable, and represents an absent place of production. If having two nonstimulable targets proves too difficult, we could replace initial /k/ with /g/, which was stimulable. The final target would be a cluster, initial /fl/; this was chosen because /l/ is correctly produced already, and the fricative /f/ is absent from the inventory, but stimulable.

Our goal is to induce as much generalization in the system as possible through within- and across-class generalization. We could predict some of the following generalization patterns: from treatment of final /s/ to other final fricatives, including palatal, and implicationally, stops; from treatment of initial /k/ to its cognate /g/ and possibly these phonemes in the final position; from treatment of /tʃ/ to its cognate /dʒ/ in final and perhaps initial position, and to untrained /j/ identical in place; and from treatment of initial /fl/ to other clusters because it is more marked (Gierut, 1999).

Step 3

I prefer the cycles approach, especially at the initiation of an intervention program, because it mirrors normal phonological acquisition in its brief and gradual presentation of different targets over time and because there are multiple intervention targets. As the child's intelligibility improves through the elimination of error patterns, a horizontal or vertical approach may become more appropriate. This particular cycles approach is modified from Hodson and Paden's (1991) original suggestion in that only four error patterns receive focus as compared with as many as eight to ten. For our case example, the cycle would be 4 weeks, with each target sound receiving focus for 1 week during two sessions in that week.

OTHER TARGETS

Typically I do not target vowels unless children's vowel inventory is severely limited and intelligibility is significantly compromised. In these children, consonant targets would still be the initial focus, with vowels being targeted after approximately two cycles of intervention. Similarly, I do not target prosody, in particular stress patterns and syllable shapes, unless a child is at developmental stages of the continuum where evidence exists that these are constraining productions. For example, if a child is at or around the 50-word point of lexical acquisition and constrained to one stress foot, two-syllable words with strong–weak stress patterns would be targeted (Fikkert, 1994). At the later developing end of the continuum, if a school-age child is unable to produce multisyllabic words that diverge from strong–weak stress patterns, these words would be targeted.

Phonological awareness would be targeted directly only for a child who displayed explicit difficulties in initial sound identification and phoneme segmentation on a standardized instrument and who was in the early elementary grades. Phonological awareness can be targeted indirectly, however, through incorporation of rhyming tasks in sessions that target final phonemes and initial sound alliteration and through identification tasks in sessions that target initial phonemes. It is important to enhance phonological awareness skills, particularly in children whose phonological impairment is more severe, because the likelihood of a phonological awareness problem appears to increase with the overall severity of the phonological impairment (Bird, Bishop, & Freeman, 1995; Larrivee & Catts, 1999).

Perceptual skills would not be directly targeted but would be enhanced indirectly through the use of auditory bombardment and focused recasts of misarticulated sounds in single words. Providing the child with a greater frequency of the target sound in the input, as well as immediate recasts of target errors, may help to increase his or her implicit learning of the phonotactic probabilities in the ambient language (Velleman & Vihman, 2002).

INTEGRATING LANGUAGE AND PHONOLOGY GOALS

Until recently, little has been known about how to integrate language and phonology goals with respect to how much emphasis each domain should receive during intervention (Camarata, 1998). This is an important issue because an average of 60% of children identified with phonological disorders also exhibit language problems, particularly in morphosyntax. Some clinician/researchers advocate a general whole language intervention program under the assumption that organizational changes in higher linguistic levels, induced through focused input and conversational interaction, simultaneously cause changes in lower levels (Hoffman, 1992; Wilcox & Morris, 1995). Yet, we have evidence from a well-controlled group study that a grammatical intervention involving focused stimulation did not lead to significant gains in phonology as measured by PCC for 25 children with moderate-severe morphosyntactic and phonological impairments (Fey, Cleave, Ravida, Long, Dejmal, & Easton, 1994). In contrast, when a child's phonological system prevents accurate production of grammatical morphemes due to error patterns affecting morphophonemic forms, it has been shown that intervention focused on those error patterns leads directly to improvement in the affected grammatical morphemes (Fey & Stalker, 1986; Tyler & Sandoval, 1994).

The goal attack strategies described previously could be used to design an intervention sequence for multiple goals from both phonological and morphosyntactic domains because it appears that both domains may need intervention. For example, phonological and morphosyntactic domains could be treated vertically, with a focus on goals in just one domain until some criterion accuracy is achieved, and then the other domain could become the focus. Goals from the two domains could also be targeted horizontally so that they were both the focus in every session, with targets treated simultaneously within activities. In a cyclical approach, goals from the two domains could be alternated on a weekly basis for a specified cycle.

Tyler, Lewis, Haskill, and Tolbert (2003) used such a variety of strategies in their investigation of phonological and morphosyntactic outcomes in children with co-occurring speech and language impairments. Participants included 47 preschoolers, ages 3;0–5;11, comprising 40 children in an experimental group and 7 in a no-treatment control group. Children were assigned at random to each of four different goal attack strategies: 1 and 2) vertical blocks focused on phonology or morphosyntax goals for 12-week blocks, beginning with different blocks; 3) an alternating strategy in which four phonology and four morphosyntax goals alternated weekly in an 8-week cycle; and 4) a simultaneous strategy with an integrated focus on both phonology and morphosyntactic goals in every session. Data were collected at pretreatment; after the first 12-week intervention block; and post-treatment, after 24 weeks. For the control group, data were collected at the beginning and end of a period equivalent to one intervention block. Change in a finite morpheme composite and target generalization phoneme composite was assessed. The finite morpheme composite reflected the combined percent correct usage of the following finite morphemes: regular past tense –ed; third person singular regular –s; and contractible and uncontractible copula and auxiliary be verbs. The target generalization composite was a percentage reflecting the accuracy of target and generalization sounds selected for each child, from a minimum of three opportunities each in initial and final positions in a citation sample.

Results showed that morphosyntactic change was greatest for children receiving the alternating strategy in comparison with the other strategies after 24 weeks of intervention. No single goal attack strategy was superior in facilitating gains in phonological performance. Ultimately, the selection of a goal attack strategy may be a function of the extent to which a child's morphological problem is due to phonological factors or the extent to which the phonological problem is independent of the morphological problem. When the phonological system affects morphophonemic productions, a vertical goal attack strategy may be preferable because phonology goals can be the sole focus until some predetermined level of accuracy is achieved. When the phonological and morphological problems are relatively independent, however, an alternating cyclical strategy may be the choice. These results provide preliminary evidence that alternating phonology and morphosyntactic goals may be preferable when children have co-occurring deficits in both these domains, although further research regarding cross-domain intervention outcomes is necessary.

REFERENCES

Bankson, N., & Bernthal, J.E. (1990). *Bankson–Bernthal Test of Phonology.* Austin, TX: PRO-ED.

Bird, J., Bishop, D.V.M., & Freeman, N.H. (1995). Phonological awareness and literacy development in children with expressive phonological impairments. *Journal of Speech and Hearing Research, 38,* 446–462.

Camarata, S.M. (1998). Connecting speech and language: Clinical applications. In R. Paul (Ed.), *Exploring the speech-language connection* (pp. 299–318). Baltimore: Paul H. Brookes Publishing Co.

Fey, M.E. (1986). *Language intervention with young children.* San Diego: College-Hill Press.

Fey, M., Cleave, P.L., Ravida, A.I., Long, S.H., Dejmal, A.E., & Easton, D.L. (1994). Effects of grammar facilitation on the phonological performance of children with speech and language impairments. *Journal of Speech and Hearing Research, 37,* 594–607.

Fey, M.E., & Stalker, C.H. (1986). A hypothesis-testing approach to treatment of a child with an idiosyncratic (morpho)phonological system. *Journal of Speech and Hearing Disorders, 51,* 324–336.

Fikkert, P. (1994). *On the acquisition of prosodic structure.* Dordrecht, Netherlands: Holland Institute of Generative Linguistics.

Fudala, J. (2000). *Arizona Articulation Proficiency Scale–Revised.* Los Angeles: Western Psychological Corporation.

Gierut, J.A. (1992). The conditions and course of clinically-induced phonological change. *Journal of Speech and Hearing Research, 35,* 1049–1063.

Gierut, J.A. (1999). Syllable onsets: Clusters and adjuncts in acquisition. *Journal of Speech, Language, and Hearing Research, 42,* 708–729.

Gierut, J.A. (2001). Complexity in phonological treatment: Clinical factors. *Language, Speech, and Hearing Services in Schools, 32,* 229–241.

Gierut, J.A., Elbert, M., & Dinnsen, D.A. (1987). A functional analysis of phonological knowledge and generalization learning in misarticulating children. *Journal of Speech and Hearing Research, 30,* 462–479.

Gierut, J.A., Morrisette, M.L., Hughes, M.T., & Rowland, S. (1996). Phonological treatment efficacy and developmental norms. *Language, Speech, and Hearing Services in Schools, 27,* 215–230.

Goldman, R., & Fristoe, M. (2000). *Goldman–Fristoe Test of Articulation–3.* Circle Pines, MN: American Guidance Service.

Hodson, B.W. (2004). *Hodson Assessment of Phonological Patterns* (3rd ed.). Austin, TX: PRO-ED.

Hodson, B.W., & Paden, E.P. (1991). *Targeting intelligible speech* (2nd ed.). Austin, TX: PRO-ED.

Hoffman, P.R. (1992). Synergistic development of phonetic skill. *Language, Speech, and Hearing Services in Schools, 23,* 254–260.

Khan, L.L., & Lewis, N. (2002). *Khan–Lewis Phonological Assessment–2.* Circle Pines, MN: American Guidance Service.

Larrivee, L.S., & Catts, H.W. (1999). Early reading achievement in children with expressive phonological disorders. *American Journal of Speech-Language Pathology, 8,* 118–128.

Long, S.H. (2003). Computerized Profiling (Version 9.4.1) [Computer software]. Available on-line: http://www.computerizedprofiling.org

Masterson, J., & Bernhardt, B.H. (2001). *Computerized Articulation and Phonology Evaluation System.* Austin, TX: Harcourt Assessment.

Miccio, A.W., Elbert, M., & Forrest, K. (1999). The relationship between stimulability and phonological acquisition in children with normally developing and disordered phonologies. *American Journal of Speech-Language Pathology, 8,* 347–363.

Powell, T.W., Elbert, M., & Dinnsen, D.A. (1991). Stimulability as a factor in the phonological generalization of misarticulating preschool children. *Journal of Speech and Hearing Research, 34,* 1318–1328.

Rvachew, S., & Nowak, M. (2001). The effect of target-selection strategy on phonological learning. *Journal of Speech, Language, and Hearing Research, 44,* 610–623.

Shriberg, L.D., & Kwiatkowski, J. (1982). Phonological disorders III: A procedure for assessing severity of involvement. *Journal of Speech and Hearing Disorders, 17,* 256–270.

Stoel-Gammon, C. (1985). Phonetic inventories, 15–24 months: A longitudinal study. *Journal of Speech and Hearing Research, 28,* 505–512.

Tyler, A.A., Edwards, M.L., & Saxman, J.H. (1987). Clinical application of two phonologically-based treatment procedures. *Journal of Speech and Hearing Disorders, 52,* 393–409.

Tyler, A.A., Lewis, K.E., Haskill, A., & Tolbert, L.C. (2003). Outcomes of different speech and language goal attack strategies. *Journal of Speech, Language, and Hearing Research, 46,* 1077–1094.

Tyler, A.A., & Sandoval, K.T. (1994). Preschoolers with phonological and language disorders: Treating different linguistic domains. *Language, Speech, and Hearing Services in Schools, 25,* 215–234.

Velleman, S.L., & Vihman, M.M. (2002). Whole-word phonology and templates: Trap, bootstrap, or some of each? *Language, Speech, and Hearing Services in Schools, 33,* 9–23.

Weiss, A.L. (2002). Planning language intervention for young children. In D.K. Bernstein & E. Tiegerman-Farber (Eds.), *Language and communication disorders in children* (pp. 256–314). Boston: Allyn & Bacon.

Wilcox, K.A., & Morris, S.E. (1995). Speech intervention in a language-focused curriculum. In M. Rice and K. Wilcox (Eds.), *Building a language-focused curriculum for the preschool classroom: A foundation for lifelong communication* (pp. 73–89). Baltimore: Paul H. Brookes Publishing Co.

Chapter 7

Goals and Targets

Facilitating the
Self-Organizing Nature of a Neuro-Network

Janet A. Norris and Paul R. Hoffman

anguage is defined as comprising semantics, syntax, morphology, phonology, and
pragmatics, but speech-language pathologists often view the phonological aspects
of language as different in nature and thus separate from the other components of
language. In this view of phonology, assessments and treatments are conducted in a manner
separate from other aspects of language. Sounds are assessed in word positions and then
established during treatment in units ranging from sound discrimination; to production in
isolation, nonsense syllables, words, and phrases; and finally to generalized speaking situations.

WHAT FACTORS INFLUENCE YOUR
SELECTION OF TREATMENT GOALS AND TARGETS?

We subscribe to an alternative paradigm that views phonology as an integral and inseparable part of the language system. The constellation model of language processing (Norris,
1998, 2001; Norris & Hoffman, 2002) can be used to profile this view. In this model,
nine levels of processing are arranged in a circle, or constellation, such that all levels are
free to interact and both receive and send input to all other levels within the constellation
(see Figure 7.1). The constellation represents a neuro-network that integrates these processes (Seidenberg, 1994). In this manner, for example, the effects of syntax on coarticula-
tory production during speaking can occur *at the same moment* that sounds are first
organized at the levels of perceptual and categorical processing (Bengio, 1996; Seidenberg & McClelland, 1989). This results in simultaneous left-to-right (input from phonemic
features sending activation to higher language processes in the system) and right-to-left
(input from previous words as well as knowledge about language structures sending
activation to perceptual, categorical, and canonical units) processing during speaking.

When phonological development is viewed from the perspective of a neuro-networking model, specific targets are almost never selected for intervention. Rather, general
goals such as adding six new phonemes to the phonemic inventory, or increasing the
percent consonants correct (PCC) by 40% in spontaneous speech might be chosen. Which
phonemes are added or which consonants are correctly produced are left to emerge

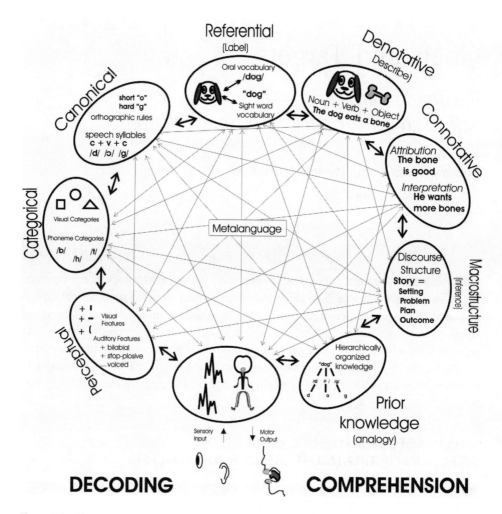

Figure 7.1. The constellation model of language processing, in which nine levels of processing are arranged in a circle, or constellation, such that all levels are free to interact and both receive and send input to all other levels within the constellation. (From Norris, J.A. [2003]. *Phonic faces: Manual and picture cards* (2nd ed.). Baton Rouge, LA: ElementOry; reprinted by permission.)

naturally as an outcome of the self-organizing properties of the child's neuro-network (Lindblom, 1992, 2000). Self-organization occurs as each input received by any of the nine levels of the constellation adds new information that must be assimilated into that level. However, the same input simultaneously reaches each of the other eight levels, all of which in turn send output reflecting any changes to the other nine levels. Thus, a slight change anywhere in the system will cause a change or accommodation throughout the system. In this manner, the system organizes itself so that all units are fine-tuned to each other (Van Geert, 1994). Because the system will naturally reorganize itself to more closely approximate input received from the environment, it is unnecessary for the interventionist to select target phonemes or control the stimuli to focus on specific phonemes when the child's inventory of correct productions is small. Targets only become specific when the child has a nearly adult-like phonological system but exhibits residual errors such as distortion of later developed phonemes.

Goals are selected and outcomes measured using traditional tools such as standardized tests or language sample analyses. A standardized test such as the Goldman–Fristoe Test of Articulation–2 (Goldman & Fristoe, 2000) can be used to elicit and analyze the child's production of consonants to represent phonemes in single words elicited spontaneously and through imitation. This will indicate which phonological and canonical structures have pathways of connectivity already established within the network (i.e., can be imitated) compared with those that are better established (i.e., are spontaneously produced) or those without observable connectivity (i.e., don't appear in any context). This profile will be explored further through phonetic transcriptions of conversational speech or storytelling. The child's phonological performance while engaged in these tasks is likely to be less well organized than single-word productions because the child's system must spread its resources among the other processors. This effect is seen in the well-known finding that articulation of words is better in imitation of single words than in spontaneous production of the words, which is better than production of words during spontaneous speech activities such as storytelling (Dubois & Bernthal, 1978). Sounds produced in single words may not be produced in connected speech, in words with more complex canonical structures, within words that are less familiar to the child, or when the syntactic complexity of utterances increases. Analysis of the child's phonological performance relative to these factors provides insights into the current status of the child's neuro-network.

Complex speech samples can be analyzed for the phonetic inventory of sounds produced and compared with the word-initial, word-final, and cluster inventories produced by typically developing 2- and 3-year-olds (Dyson, 1988). The phonemic inventory of sounds that are nearly always produced appropriately with reference to the adult forms of words would be compared with the phonemic inventories at each age group in Smit and colleagues' (1990) data. PCC serves as an overall metric of phonological development and can be compared with Shriberg, Austin, Lewis, McSweeny, and Wilson's (1997) developmental data. These measurements, coupled with analysis of other levels of language organization, provide a profile of the child's current level of development in both speech and language as well as the dynamics between them.

A child with limited language will have a corresponding limited phonemic inventory. As words and word combinations are acquired, an inventory of consonant and vowel phonemes will necessarily begin to appear in order to enable distinctions between words to be expressed verbally. This is seen as a simultaneous explosion of vocabulary development occurring concomitantly with the appearance of new sound productions (Lindblom, 1992; Reznick & Goldfield, 1990; Studdert-Kennedy, 1991). The contrasts among these early developing phonemes may not necessarily be used conventionally. For example, when a child first adds [t] to the phonetic inventory, it may appear only in word-final position and may not contrast phonemically with [d] in word-initial contexts, resulting in the appearance of prevocalic voicing. As the child learns more words containing a word-initial /t/, the distinction between the two phonemes will be extended to this context as well. Consequently, an increase in the child's correct productions across all phonemes can be expected. That is, phonemes that were already inconsistently produced in some contexts may increasingly appear correctly within conversation. Thus, a 40% increase in correct consonant productions in spontaneous speech might be expected.

A child with greater language development generally will have more phonemes but will also have a far greater number of phonetic contexts in which they must be coordinated.

Words that are semantically more abstract are generally more complex phonologically (Bransford & Franks, 1971), with more consonant clusters and an increasingly greater number of syllables (compare *big, large,* and *giant,* or *cup, glass,* and *crystal*). Morphemes also add phonological complexity to words, ranging from a single additional phoneme (e.g., dog-s) to complex sequences of phonemes to be co-articulated (e.g., indeterminately). As sentences increase in syntactic complexity, the number and complexity of phonological and motor productions increase. The child's phonological and motor speech productions must be coordinated with these multiple language processes to maintain intelligibility, and connected speech may therefore be more unintelligible than short comments or responses within structured activities (Dubois & Bernthal, 1978). This may be especially true of conversations about decontextualized topics, in which past or future events, wants, and ideas are expressed with no support from objects or other visual referents. Words must be used to specify all of the agents, actions, objects, motives, locations, and other information, placing heavy demands on the system to rapidly coordinate all of the processes throughout the constellation (Smith, Norris, & Hoffman, 2001). Intelligibility may be one area affected, and so once again a 40% increase in correct consonant productions in spontaneous speech might be expected as the child masters the phonologically complex words and the consonant cluster sequences that are created by word juxtaposition within increasingly longer sentences.

HOW DOES YOUR SELECTION OF GOALS/ TARGETS REFLECT YOUR THEORETICAL ORIENTATION?

Recall that a neuro-network can be visualized as nine groups of processing units arranged in a circle, or constellation, such that all groups of units are free to interact by both receiving inputs from and sending inputs to all of the other groups within the constellation, as in Figure 7.1. This property is important because it means that any new information or organization entering one group of units has the effect of passing these improvements on to the other eight groups (Elman, Bates, Johnson, Karmiloff-Smith, Parisi, & Plunkett, 1996). For example, when a new vocabulary word is learned (i.e., a referential unit is established) it stands in contrast to other words in meaning (e.g., *cub* versus *bear*). It also must stand in contrast to other words in phonemic structure in the categorical units (e.g., /kʌb/ versus /tʌb/ and /sʌb/). Thus, the meaningful contrasts or features (i.e., perceptual units) between phonemes (i.e., categorical units) within word positions (i.e., canonical units) begin to emerge as a necessary outcome of processing language at the vocabulary or referential level. Once a phonological contrast is established for one word pair, a neurological pattern of connectivity is formed for that phoneme, its features, and its use within a canonical structure (Locke, 1995). This makes it easier (and thus more probable) for other words containing this phoneme to connect to the same neurological units, therefore strengthening the phoneme, its features, and its patterns of occurrence within canonical structures.

This connectivity means that one of the most powerful means for increasing and organizing the phonological inventory is to increase the child's vocabulary and language structures. The more a young child learns about concepts within event structures, the more words enter the lexicon, and the more reorganization occurs throughout the system

(Nelson, 1985, 1996). In this manner, the child's entire system becomes progressively more like the language of the adult speakers, including phonological boundaries between categories of phones and allophones and the canonical structure of words. Similarly, increasingly more complex syntactic forms and constructions motivate the need for refinement in phonological categories to mark plurals, possessives, verb tense, adverbs, and other morphophonemic forms (Hoffman, Norris, & Monjure, 1990, 1996; Tyler, Lewis, Haskill, & Tolbert, 2002). The relationship is reciprocal and interactive. The network builds and refines as more specific phonological forms are needed to reference and distinguish between new elements of meaning in the language. Likewise, the increasing organization of phonology enables the child to hear and begin to determine the meaning of new words and morphosyntactic forms of language (Nelson, 1996). Each new acquisition within the network adds to the information, refines the organization at each of the other points around the constellation, and is in turn refined by these changes within the system.

DO YOU DIRECTLY TARGET VOWELS, PERCEPTION, PROSODY, OR PHONOLOGICAL AWARENESS?

When intervention is viewed from a neuro-networking perspective, vowels, perception, prosody, and phonological awareness are all aspects of language processing. Each affects and is affected by all other points around the constellation. Thus, providing an appropriate context for acquisition and refinement of language processing is critical to facilitating change in any dimension of language.

The context of intervention that is selected will address both the short- and long-term needs of the child. One excellent context is book reading—illustrated storybooks for young children and age-appropriate texts for older children. Books provide a context that can be revisited repeatedly within and across sessions. The illustrations and stories provide an unchanging context that can be talked about from different perspectives and at differing levels of complexity—for example, the focus could change from attention to vowels, sound discrimination, prosody, one or more aspects of phonological awareness, vocabulary, the relationships of meaning expressed through the syntax, or the story plot (Hoffman et al., 1990, 1996). This allows for balance to be maintained across the nine points of the constellation and/or for a systematic focus on one or more points without disconnecting the information from meaningful language.

For example, after interactively reading a page from a storybook to help the child talk about the actions, feelings, and potential future events (i.e., attention to meaning), the focus can shift to attention to form. To assess phonological awareness, the child can be asked to point to individual words in left-to-right sequence as the adult reads the text, establishing the concept of wordness; to listen for and identify the rhyming words in the text; to listen for a target sound within different word positions; and to associate letters with the target sound. The program *Phonic Faces* (Norris, 2001) was developed to help children increase sound awareness and associate sounds with letters. The letters are placed within the mouths of faces to suggest sound production cues (see Figure 7.2). The circle of letter *b* is drawn as the lower lip on the face; children can touch their lower lip while looking at the *b* and see and feel their lip "bounce" as the /b/ sound is produced. The use of these picture cues for sounds and corresponding letters provides children with a visual

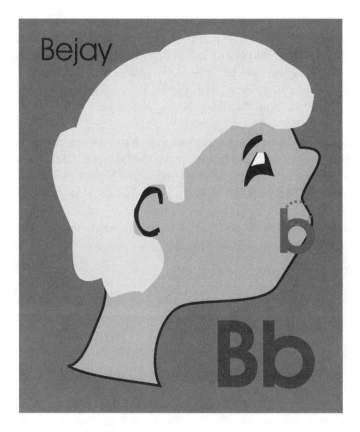

Figure 7.2. Phonic Faces card. The letters are placed within the mouths of faces to suggest sound production cues. The circle of letter "b" is drawn as the lower lip on the face; children can touch their lower lip while looking at the "b" and see and feel their lip "bounce" as the /b/ sound is produced. (From Norris, J.A. [2003]. *Phonic faces: Manual and picture cards.* Baton Rouge, LA: ElementOry; reprinted by permission.)

strategy for increasing awareness of words, sounds, features of sounds, sounds in word position, rhyming words, and sound production—all features related to the processing of phonological aspects of language.

This strategy also can be used to facilitate vowel productions. Stories that embed the vowel sound naturally create a meaningful association of the sound with its production features (see Figure 7.3). A child can be encouraged to produce the /ɪ/ sound along with Iris Iggy in her dislike of carrots (Norris, 2002). Additional sentences can be written to provide further practice with the target vowel within the story, such as "It tastes like ick," "Please lick a little bit," or "Sit still, Iggy." The Phonic Face for Iris Iggy can be held above each relevant word as the child reads or recalls the sentence, thus providing a cue to sound production. The consonant and vowel Phonic Faces can also be used to work on the coarticulation of the entire sound sequence for a difficult word. The child matches his or her own changes in articulatory placement to those shown in the faces. The word then can be attempted immediately within the sentence or phrase context, then within the sequence of sentences that tell the elaborated story. In this manner, sound, sound discrimination, sound feature, word, sentence, and discourse level attention can be focused on as needed, but all remain connected within the constellation because of their meaningful

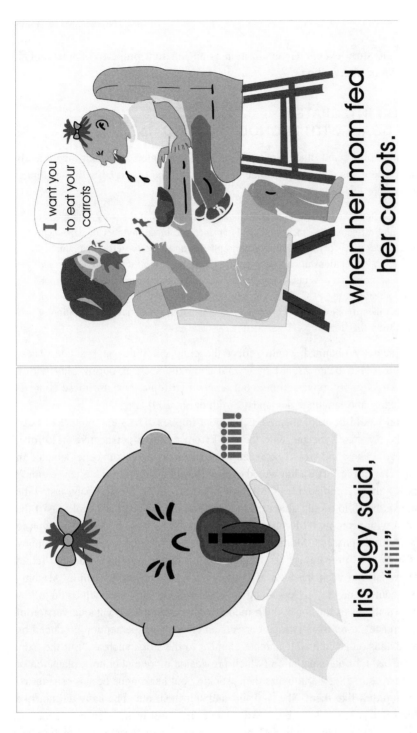

Figure 7.3. The Phonic Faces card for Iris Iggy can be used to create a meaningful association of the sound /I/ with its production features. A child can be encouraged to produce the /I/ sound along with Iris. (From Norris, J.A. [2002]. *Icky Carrots*. Baton Rouge, LA: ElementOry; reprinted by permission.)

relationship to the story events. Generalization is an inherent property of intervention within this model of intervention.

HOW DO YOU INTEGRATE LANGUAGE GOALS WITH PHONOLOGICAL GOALS?

The goals for phonology and other aspects of language are integrated both theoretically and practically. The goals address the refinements that will be observed within a context of language use. For example,

> Given an illustrated storybook, a child will talk about the events of the story with greater complexity and refinement as measured by 1) an increase in the number of dependent clauses used to describe story events, 2) use of morphemes and cohesive terms that establish appropriate temporal relationships between actions, 3) use of attributes, interpretations, and inferences to describe story events, 4) use of specific vocabulary words to refer to information, 5) an increase in the PCC, 6) an increase in the number of consonants produced, and 7) correct identification of the consonant sound heard in the initial word position of noun words from the story.

The measures actually obtained would reflect the child's abilities at baseline. These language changes could be measured in several contexts, such as during play with a specified set of toys or in conversation about a specified topic, because these contexts differ in complexity and language demands (Smith et al., 2001).

Intervention would be implemented as the goal implies. The same picture or page of text would be organized for and with the child from multiple perspectives (Hoffman et al., 1990, 1996). The child would be asked to describe an action or scene depicted in the story, as in "Her eating." The adult would expand the child's utterance ("She is eating") and then model a more complete idea ("Mommy is feeding the baby. The baby tasted the carrots") and ask the child to talk about this new information. The adult would assist the child as needed with prompts ("Mommy . . ."), gestures (pantomime using the spoon to feed the baby), carrier phases ("Mommy is feeding the ___"), phonemic cues ("Mommy is ffff____ the b___"), preparatory sets ("First tell me what mommy is doing" [child responds] "Now tell me what the baby is doing"), or relational terms (child: "Mommy feeding baby"; adult: "and . . ."). Depending on what the child says, the adult could follow the child's turn with an expansion (which models a more complete syntactic version of the child's utterance), a revision (which corrects an error or misperception produced by the child), an extension (which adds another element to the story, such as "But the baby did not like carrots"), or an expatiation (which provides a more elaborate explanation or adds clarification, as in "See her tongue, she is sticking out her tongue because she tasted the carrots. She didn't like them. She said 'iii' and spit them out. The baby did not like carrots"). These intervention techniques will enable the child to develop new concepts and language (semantics, syntax, morphology, and narrative structures) with which to talk about the story (items 1–4 in the goal statement above).

Providing expansions that are specifically targeted at particular syntactic and morphological forms (Fey, Cleave, Long, & Hughes, 1993) or phonological forms (Camarata, 1993) has been shown to be effective in increasing children's production of the targeted forms. In addition, data indicate that targeting development of one of the processors within complex communicative contexts may enhance others. Targeting morphological forms with a combination of modeling, expansions, and eliciting productions through binary choices, cloze procedures, and preparatory sets has been demonstrated to result in phonological improvements (Tyler et al., 2002). Targeting increases in level of semantic complexity appears to result in increased semantic level, increased morphosyntactic complexity, and increased phonological complexity (Bradshaw, Hoffman, & Norris, 1998: Hoffman et al., 1990, 1996). Within these more complex interactions, the sequence of a cloze procedure followed by a child response, followed by an expansion, followed by a request to restate the information resulted in increased semantic and syntactic complexity. The sequence of child phonological error followed by a binary choice presenting a minimal pair contrast resulted in decreased semantic/syntactic complexity with increased phonological complexity (Bellon-Harn, Hoffman, & Harn, 2004). In other words, on a moment-to-moment basis the clinician can manipulate the child's response to increase complexity in either one processor or another, with a related decrease in the complexity of another processor. However, the long-term effect is to strengthen and maintain the temporary increases to promote the development of the overall system.

As these relationships of meaning within the story are being transacted between the clinician and the child, multiple opportunities for phonological refinement are presented. Within the several minutes that a scene is being examined, reexamined, and put into increasingly more complex utterances, the child has multiple opportunities to hear the same words modeled in similar contexts but in utterances ranging from single words to multiple-word sentences. Likewise, the child has multiple opportunities to produce these words in similar contexts and in a range of utterances from simple to complex. This repetitive modeling, redundancy, and immediate recasting or feedback provides the input and the practice needed to refine the phonological system, and many spontaneous instances of new sound production attempts or shifts in productions will occur within a session.

The intensity of the language used to talk about the relatively small amount of information will provide the time and repetition needed to hear new words and begin to categorize their features at multiple constellation points including perception, phoneme categories, and canonical structures. The familiarity, as well as the redundancy between the pictures and the words, helps the child to quickly map the word with its meaning (Dollaghan, 1987; Pangburn, 2002). This, in turn, allows for more processing to be devoted to how the words are produced to express this meaning. In this manner, phonology begins to self-organize without direct attention or focus on articulation training. Thus items 5 and 6 of the goal statement are addressed through the same transactions and are essentially the manner in which we accomplish phonological change in children with delayed development.

A focus on phonology during storybook reading, as with other aspects of language, is addressed from multiple perspectives, including phonemic awareness, print awareness, and sound production. The methods for addressing phonology are described in the previous section. From a neuro-networking perspective, these three aspects of phonology maintain a reciprocal and mutually beneficial relationship (Norris & Hoffman, 2002). In a self-organizing system, any comprehensible input will begin to form patterns or categories that are strengthened by further instances of similar input. The less well-organized the child's phonological system, the more diverse the phonemes explored during book reading.

The associations between sounds and sounds in word positions can be contrasted by both features of the sound and articulatory production using the Phonic Faces as a cue. The multisensory cues enable the child to use the sound, the letter, the visual production cues provided on the Phonic Faces, and the proprioceptive production cues provided as the child imitates the sound to organize the patterns of phonological information (Doyle, Norris, & Hoffman, 2002).

REFERENCES

Bellon-Harn, M.L., Hoffman, P.R., & Harn, W.E. (2004). Use of cloze and contrast word procedures in repeated storybook readings: Targeting multiple domains. *Journal of Communication Disorders, 37,* 53–75.

Bengio, Y. (1996). *Neural networks for speech and sequence recognition.* London: International Thomson Computer Press.

Bradshaw, M.L., Hoffman, P.R., & Norris, J.A. (1998). Efficacy of expansions and cloze procedures in the development of interpretations by preschool children exhibiting delayed language development. *Language, Speech, and Hearing Services in Schools, 29,* 85–95.

Bransford, J.D., & Franks, J. (1971). The abstraction of linguistic ideas. *Cognitive Psychology, 2,* 330–350.

Camarata, S.E. (1993). The application of naturalistic conversation training to speech production in children with specific disabilities. *Journal of Applied Behavioral Analysis, 26,* 173–182.

Dollaghan, C. (1987). Fastmapping in normal and language-impaired children. *Journal of Speech and Hearing Disorders, 52,* 218–222.

Doyle, A., Norris, J.A., & Hoffman, P.R. (2002, November). *Effects of a phonemic alphabet on preschool articulation and print knowledge.* Poster session presented at the American Speech-Language-Hearing Association national convention, Atlanta, GA.

Dubois, E., & Bernthal, J. (1978). A comparison of three methods for obtaining articulatory responses. *Journal of Speech and Hearing Disorders, 43,* 295–305.

Dyson, A.T. (1988). Phonetic inventories of 2- and 3-year old children. *Journal of Speech and Hearing Disorders, 53,* 89–93.

Elman, J.L., Bates, E.A., Johnson, M.H., Karmiloff-Smith, A., Parisi, D., & Plunkett, K. (1996). *Rethinking innateness: A connectionist perspective on development.* Cambridge, MA: MIT Press.

Fey, M.E., Cleave, P.L., Long, S.H., & Hughes, D.L. (1993). Two approaches to the facilitation of grammar in language-impaired children: An experimental evaluation. *Journal of Speech and Hearing Research, 36,* 141–157.

Goldman, R.M., & Fristoe, M. (2000). *Goldman–Fristoe Test of Articulation–Second Edition.* Circle Pines, MN: American Guidance Service.

Hoffman, P.R., Norris, J.A., & Monjure, J. (1990). Comparison of process targeting and whole language treatments for phonologically impaired preschool children. *Language, Speech, and Hearing Services in Schools, 21,* 102–109.

Hoffman, P.R., Norris, J.A., & Monjure, J. (1996). Scaffolded story construction intervention for preschool speech-language delay. *National Student Speech-Language-Hearing Association Journal, 23,* 5–13.

Lindblom, B. (1992). Phonological units as adaptive emergents of lexical development. In C.A. Ferguson, L. Menn, & C. Stoel-Gammon (Eds.), *Phonological development: Models, research, implications.* (pp. 565–604). Timonium, MD: York Press.

Lindblom, B. (2000). Developmental origins of adult phonology: The interplay between phonetic emergents and evolutionary adaptations of sound patterns. *Phonetica, 57,* 297–314.

Locke, J.L. (1995). *The child's path to spoken language.* Cambridge, MA: Harvard University Press.

Nelson, K. (1985). *Making sense: The development of meaning in early childhood.* New York: Academic Press.

Nelson, K. (1996). *Language in cognitive development: The emergence of the mediated mind.* New York: Cambridge University Press.

Norris, J.A. (1998). I could read if I just had a little help: Facilitating reading in whole language contexts. In C. Weaver (Ed.), *Practicing what we know: Informed reading instruction* (pp. 513–553). Urbana, IL: NCTE Press.

Norris, J.A. (2001). *Phonic faces manual and cards.* Baton Rouge, LA: Elementory.

Norris, J.A. (2002). *Icky carrots.* Baton Rouge, LA: Elementory.

Norris, J.A., & Hoffman, P.R. (2001). Language development and late talkers: A connectionist perspective. In R.G. Daniloff (Ed.), *Connectionist approaches to clinical language problems* (pp. 1–109).Fairfax, VA: TechBooks.

Norris, J.A., & Hoffman, P.R. (2002). Phonemic awareness: A complex developmental process. *Topics in Language Disorders, 22,* 1–34.

Pangburn, B.E. (2002). *Experience-based language acquisition: A computational model of human language acquisition.* Unpublished doctoral dissertation, Louisiana State University, Baton Rouge.

Reznick, J.S., & Goldfield, B.A. (1990). *Rapid change in language acquisition during the second year: Naming explosion of knowing explosion.* Unpublished manuscript.

Seidenberg, M.S. (1994). Language and connectionism: The developing interface. *Cognition, 50,* 385–401.

Seidenberg, M.S., & McClelland, J.L. (1989). A distributed, developmental model of word recognition and naming. *Psychological Review, 96,* 523–568.

Shriberg, L.D., Austin, D., Lewis, B.A., McSweeny, J.L., & Wilson, D.L. (1997). The percentage of consonants correct (PCC) metric: Extensions and reliability data. *Journal of Speech, Language and Hearing Research, 40,* 708–722.

Smit, A.B., Hand, L., Frellinger, J.J., Bernthal, J.E., & Bird, A. (1990). The Iowa articulation norms project and its Nebraska replication. *Journal of Speech and Hearing Disorders, 55,* 779–798.

Smith, A. (1997). Dynamic interactions of factors that impact speech motor stability in children and adults. In W. Hulstijn, H.F.M. Peters, & P.M. Van Lieshout (Eds.), *Speech production: Motor control, brain research, and fluency disorders,* Exerpta Medica International Congress Series 1146 (pp. 143–149). Amsterdam: Elsevier.

Smith, E.F., Norris, J.A., & Hoffman, P.R. (2001, November). *Effects of elicitation context on language content and structure.* Technical session presented at the American Speech-Language-Hearing Association national convention, New Orleans, LA.

Studdert-Kennedy, M. (1991). Language development from an evolutionary perspective. In N. Krasnegor, D. Rumbaugh, R. Schiefelbusch, & M. Studdert-Kennedy (Eds.), *Language acquisition: Biological and behavioral determinants* (pp. 5–28). Hillsdale, NJ: Lawrence Erlbaum Associates.

Tyler, A.A., Lewis, K.E., Haskill, A., & Tolbert, L.C. (2002). Efficacy and cross-domain effects of a morphosyntax and a phonology intervention. *Language, Speech, and Hearing Services in Schools, 33,* 52–66.

Van Geert, P. (1994). *Dynamic systems of development: Change between complexity and chaos.* London: Harvester Wheatsheaf.

Chapter 8

Goal and Target Selection for Developmental Speech Disorders

Barbara L. Davis

CHARACTERISTICS OF THE CHILD'S SYSTEM AVAILABLE FROM CLINICAL ASSESSMENT

The gateway for making valid and appropriate clinical choices about goals and targets for intervention is a strong assessment framework. At the most general level, the World Health Organization framework (Wood, 1980), reviewed in Chapter 1 (see Table 1.4), provides a template for consideration of broad issues related to goal selection for the child who demonstrates a developmental speech disorder.

Relative to core aspects of the speech production system, assessment areas most generally include an independent and relational analysis of consonant and vowel production patterns as well as patterns for word and syllable shapes relative to word and syllable position. An independent and relational analysis of prosodic aspects of production patterns forms another fundamental aspect of an assessment framework for developmental speech disorders. Prosody can form either a strength supporting building an intelligible speech production system or it may represent another area that should not be neglected in understanding and forming therapeutic goals to remediate the child's lack of age-appropriate intelligibility (Hargrove & McGarr, 1994). The clinician's theoretical framework may dictate the way(s) in which relational analyses are performed as well as how goals and targets are described for the purposes of intervention. For example, a phonological approach may dictate the use of nonlinear analyses (Bernhardt & Stoel-Gammon, 1994) or phonological process analysis (Hodson & Paden, 1991). A motor-based level of analysis may dictate a traditional substitution, distortion, or omission error analysis framework (Strand, 2002; Van Riper & Irwin, 1959) to understand patterns of relationships between the child's phonetic production abilities and his or her accurate production of language-based targets. Importantly, current theoretically based systems available for relational analysis presume that the level of development of the child's vocal output system is meaning based. If the child is not producing consistent use of vocalizations for communication or is not consistently attaching available vocalization patterns to intelligible meanings, an independent analysis may be more appropriate. (Chapter 1 on the diagnosis of developmental speech disorders contains a more complete description of the clinical assessment framework that forms the gateway for valid selection of clinical goals and targets for these children.)

It is important that the clinician and parents determine whether the behaviors observed in the evaluation process represent a valid sample of the child's typical abilities relative to age-appropriate intelligibility. If problems occur in eliciting valid representations of speech patterns, gathering data in other communication environments must be pursued. Clinicians and primary caregivers should be certain that a valid picture of the child's range of abilities to achieve communication is represented adequately for planning therapy goals and targets. This sample of speech and language behaviors allows for two types of comparisons that are crucial to planning intervention goals and targets. First, normative comparisons with other children at the child's chronological age (assuming that the available test is normed on children who match the child's language and ethnic background). Normative comparison is important to setting expectations for the child relative to the types of behaviors and intelligibility that can be expected as an outcome of therapy. Obviously, normative comparison is not possible for all children who are seen by speech-language pathologists. This is particularly true in the multicultural environment of the United States, in which some clinical settings include children from highly diverse linguistic backgrounds. For these children, Sander's norms (1972), for example, do not represent a valid comparison with their development of consonant accuracy.

If normative comparisons are not possible, comparisons with general expectations for typically developing children provide another avenue for understanding both present level of client function and expectations for clinical outcomes. For example, if a child is producing only open consonant-vowel (CV) syllables with labial and alveolar consonants ("ba" or "do"), he or she is operating at a developmental age range of about 12–15 months old. If the child is 6 years old, comparisons with typical developmental expectations can help in planning initial therapeutic goals and, along with other relevant information, beginning to understand the potential outcomes of therapeutic intervention.

Second, for purposes of planning intervention goals, individual ranges of behaviors, including best possible speech behaviors as well as usual level of verbal intelligibility in spontaneous communication, are important for initial planning. This range of child speech behavioral abilities may be achieved with stimulability testing, by varying the language level of behaviors (e.g., structured sentences instead of spontaneous conversation) or by varying the communication partner (e.g., communicating with the parent rather than with the clinician). These contexts for communication give the clinician basic insights into both the child's initial targets and goals as well as the best ways to facilitate intervention. If the child's performance improves dramatically with visual, auditory, or tactile support, the clinician has important information about teaching strategies. Alternatively, if the child's performance degrades with increase in language complexity or the novelty of utterances required for a topic (e.g., "How do you brush your teeth?" versus a novel response to "What is your favorite school subject and why do you like it?"), the clinician is better prepared to understand the nature of goals and targets appropriate for beginning intervention.

Assessment helps to rule out some areas in which the child may prove able to achieve age-appropriate behaviors. For example, a 5-year-old who produces only glottal consonant closures and back vowels may display appropriate use of stress marking. In this case, stress marking is an area of strength supporting intelligibility relative to lack of mastery of consonants and vowels. In this case, goals and targets selected for intervention can incorporate marking of stress in disyllables as a support for the direct intervention goals involving oral consonant closure and diversification of vowels.

Assessment, at the most general level, provides the raw materials for what should be included in goals and targets for therapeutic intervention. In addition, the assessment process illuminates which behaviors may provide resources for support of intelligibility generally and support for achieving progress with direct intervention goals. Regardless of the system of analysis used, if a relational analysis shows that the child is only capable of producing voiceless velars (e.g., [k] in [duk]) at word-final position when preceded by a back vowel in monosyllables, goals and targets need to be founded on that assessment information. In that case, the clinician might decide to implement a goal of use of voiced [g] in initial position of monosyllables followed by a back vowel (e.g., [go]). Alternatively, the clinician could try to employ the [k] in disyllabic productions (e.g., [kuki]) to achieve increased use of disyllables in the child's repertoire.

Assessment may be based on an initial evaluation or may form an ongoing aspect of intervention as goals and targets are adjusted to respond to the client's pace of progress in therapy. Goals and targets are potentially in need of adjustment, both when the child begins to improve quickly as well as when the child does not improve after a reasonable period of intervention. For example, if the child integrates word initial [g] very quickly into production of monosyllables, then that intervention goal needs to be adjusted to reflect the improvement (e.g., to a goal of integrating velars in initial and final position or into sequences containing diverse vowels). Alternatively, if an initial goal is not successful after a period deemed appropriate for evaluating the child's progress, goals and targets may need to be adjusted downward. If, for example, the goal of expanding to two-syllable utterances using the [k] phoneme as a target is unsuccessful after a period of trial therapy, the clinician may need to try to use [b] plus central vowel (e.g., "bubbles") as a two-syllable target to facilitate two-syllable word productions, assuming [b] is strongly established in the child's production system.

ACCOUNTING FOR LANGUAGE VARIABLES

Interactions of phonetic/phonological patterns and language variables form a crucial consideration for selection of goals and targets for intervention. The most general level of goal in intervention for developmental speech disorders is age-appropriate intelligibility in service of linguistic communication with diverse communication partners. As such, therapeutic goals and targets must always account for language variables at the child's level of developmental function based on the outcome of the assessment process.

If the child is not using his or her voice consistently for communication, the primary initial goal may be "use of the voice for intentional communication" and targets may be related to facilitating communication interactions based on the vocalizations and pragmatic intentions noted to occur in the assessment process. Attachment of available vocalizations to intentional communication will form a first intervention step, a step that implicates language variables implicitly as the ultimate goal for the child but starts intervention at the child's present level of communicative functioning. For example, the child who is producing only vowel-like vocal qualities may be encouraged initially to use those vocalizations consistently for the pragmatic intention of "requesting."

For children who are regularly using their voice for communication and who fall at varied levels of severity relative to expectations for their chronological age, the interface of speech and language variables forms an obviously integral part of planning goals and targets for intervention. In Chapter 1, which is focused on diagnosis of developmental speech disorders, potential language variables related to syntax, morphology, pragmatics/discourse, and semantics were specified as they related to an assessment framework integrating speech and language variables. Figure 8.1 provides a worksheet for integrating these issues in making the link from assessment outcomes to planning for goals and targets in intervention. The worksheet is designed to allow organization of information emerging from the assessment process to determine what types of goals and targets may be logical starting points for intervention. It illustrates a template that records areas of strength and areas of needed improvement. Clearly, noting these areas of potential speech-language interaction and listing areas of strength as well as needed improvements for appropriate developmental intelligibility does not substitute for clinician judgment on the logical selection of initial goals and targets. That judgment may be based largely on the outcome of normative or typical development comparisons as well as on individualized criterion referenced tasks such as stimulability.

BACKGROUND OF TYPICAL DEVELOPMENTAL MILESTONES

The early course of speech acquisition and behaviors observed in children's typical development from earliest vocal attempts through about age 5, when typically developing

	Phonology							Syntax		Semantics			Pragmatics		
	Phonetic inventory—Consonants	Phonetic inventory—Vowels	Phonetic inventory—Syllable/word shapes	Error analysis—Consonants	Error analysis—Vowels	Error analysis—Syllable/word shapes	Prosody	Morphemes	Sentence patterns	Semantic categories	Semantic/syntactic relationships	Vocabulary	Discourse characteristics	Communicative functions	Nonverbal communication
Target															
Strength															
Weakness															

Other dimensions

	Strength	Weakness
Sensorimotor capacities		
Psychosocial		
Processing		

	Strength	Weakness
Academic		
Learning style		

Figure 8.1.   Interface grid for planning goals from assessment results.

children are often 100% intelligible to an unfamiliar listener, have been listed often. They constitute a familiar sequence. However, these behaviors also represent a powerful clinical tool for evaluating the results of clinical assessment to plan goals and targets for children who do not acquire age-appropriate intelligibility and require therapeutic intervention. This body of information enables an ongoing interaction between the assessment and intervention processes. The clinician can compare the child's progress to the expected developmental behaviors for his or her chronological age as a metric of progress in intervention. A child who begins therapy producing labials and alveolars in CV syllables and then begins to achieve use of dorsals and fricatives in CVC forms as well as marking some clusters after 6 months of therapy has made real progress. In this case, the starting behaviors are consistent with the 12- to 15-month age range of typical acquisition patterns. Production patterns that include fricatives and dorsals as well as clusters and final consonants are more consistent with the 18- to 24-month age range of typical development.

Understanding typical developmental milestones also allows consideration of whether goals and targets for intervention are well matched to children who may be exhibiting *delay* or *disorder* in achievement of speech production milestones. The 7-year-old child who is still producing only open CV syllables, typical at 7–18 months, would need a high level of clinical involvement, although he or she is exhibiting delayed rather than disordered patterns. Alternatively, a 4-year-old child who is only producing sequences of glottal closures and singleton vowels might be considered as disordered based on the expectation that glottals and singleton vowels are not expected for speech-like behaviors in the typical developmental sequence. By 7–8 months, typically developing children are producing rhythmic syllables with oral closures that are perceived as labial and alveolar consonants predominantly.

Behaviors expected in the first year of life have been established based on classic research programs (Davis & MacNeilage, 1995; Oller, 1980; Stark, 1980; see Vihman, 1996, for a comprehensive review). Table 8.1 displays the progression of vocal behaviors in the prelinguistic period.

Consideration of typical development milestones allows the clinician to consider very early emerging behaviors for clients who are chronologically young or who demonstrate severe to profound levels of speech delay or disorder. Incorporation of these early milestones in goal planning is based on the premise that acquisition of speech production skill is a continuous process in which the child begins using his or her voice at birth before communication is intentional. Children develop speech production skills based on biological, cognitive, and social foundations resulting in the fully intentional oral communication observed routinely in typically developing children by the middle of the second year of life. Knowledge and use of the prelinguistic vocal milestones in considering developmental speech disorders allow the clinician to start at the level at which the child is presently functioning, especially in the case of young children (i.e., birth to 3 years old) or those who have severe compromise in vocal intelligibility (i.e., a child with cerebral palsy). Generally, the developmental progression begins with undifferentiated vowel-like vocalizations and crying up until about 8 weeks postnatally. Around 8 weeks, infants begin to produce more speech-like vocalizations; vowels often sound like "oooo" and some [g] and [k] closures reliably appear. Pragmatic use of the voice in crying episodes occurs when familiar caregivers are able to distinguish differentiated types of crying (e.g.,

Table 8.1. Characteristics of prelinguistic vocalizations

Reflexive crying and vegetative sounds (0–8 weeks)
Healthy cry
Nasalized vowels
Engagement of pharynx and nasopharynx
Tongue moves mostly back and forth and fills cavity
Physical limitations of vocal tract make it difficult to open and close

Cooing and laughter (8–20 weeks)
Vowel-like "oooo" quality during interactions
"g" and "k" (relationship of tongue to oral cavity)
Crying more variable and goal directed
Three kinds of cry: discomfort, call, request
(Roots of pragmatic intention in the vocal system)
Laughter appears

Vocal play (16–20 weeks)
Respiratory and laryngeal events provide a scaffolding for supralaryngeal maturation
Single syllables without timing regularities
Prolonged vowel and consonant sounds
Articulatory structures begin maturing
Normal vowels: increased separation of oral and nasal cavities so non-nasal vowels can be produced
Raspberries: necessary air pressure in mouth develops because of disengagement of larynx and nasopharynx
Squeal and growl: contrasts in pitch because of descent of larynx into neck makes vocal folds more vulnerable to forces of supralaryngeal muscles
Yelling: better co-ordination of respiratory system and larynx permits loud voice

Canonical babbling (7–8 months)
Rhythmicity: prosodic frame
Spatiotemporal domain meets rigid timing characteristic coordinates with rhythmic motor output in other domains
"bababa" or "daedidaedi" repeated as stereotypes
Reduplicated and variegated from the onset
Reduplicated: same sound qualities
Variegated: change in consonants or vowels or both
Strings of syllables
Rigid timing characteristics for syllables
Real open–close alternations
Mainly self-stimulating rather than social

indicating hunger, pain, or crankiness). Vocal play at 16–20 weeks reveals a production system maturing to begin the process of providing support for largely oral articulatory constrictions as well as respiratory and phonatory control necessary to support development of intelligible speech production. At around 7–8 months, canonical babbling appears reliably. This striking milestone marks the first appearance of speech-like timing rhythmicity that is so apparent in mature speech. True alternation between close and open vocal tract states, which is characteristic of mature speech across languages also emerges in this period. These behaviors (see Oller, 1980, and Stark, 1980, for reviews) form a crucial backdrop for clinical goal setting, because they provide a set of behaviors related to typical chronological age expectations. These expectations are most salient for the client who is not yet using his or her voice to communicate or who is not using the respiratory, phonatory, and supralaryngeal systems in a coordinated fashion to support speech-like behaviors. The 4-year-old noted previously who produces glottal stops for all consonant closures clearly requires clinical goal setting related to the phase of canonical babbling where supralaryngeal close and open alternations form a foundation for later syllable-based speech productions. His use of singleton vowel productions put him in the *vocal play* developmental level (4–6 months in typical development). Clinical goals must thus include moving these vowels into close–open syllabic sequences.

Predictions from early developmental milestones are also available based on a large body of research on characteristics of babbling and early word use. Sample sizes in these studies are smaller than the number of children sampled in large-scale normative studies of speech acquisition. Most classic normative information is based on single-word productions in typically developing English-learning children ages 3–8 years. In contrast, this body of normative data on typical development is mainly based on studies of children from mainstream culture in English language environments. Normative values are only available for consonants by word position, not for vowels, word shapes, or prosody. As such, these norms form a very limited comparison metric for children who are clinically diagnosed with speech delay or disorder in the moderate to severe range, which may include phonotactic complexity compromises related to word and syllable shapes as well as vowel differences or prosodic components. Clinical goal setting based on a discrepancy model must use this general research-based information on typical development when aspects of the child's clinical profile include components in addition to consonant pattern differences or when the child is functioning developmentally younger than 3 years of age.

Table 8.2 contains a summary of available information about this phase of acquisition. This type of information is integral to planning early goals and targets for children who are functioning in this developmental stage relative to speech production skill. Language level may be much higher in some instances in which the child exhibits an intelligibility deficit in the face of more age-appropriate levels of expressive language development.

In this early period of development, consonant place and manner characteristics include stops, nasals, and glides at labial and alveolar places of articulation. Initial and medial consonants are largely voiced and final consonants are voiceless. Vowels are mostly produced in the lower left quadrant of the vowel space. With diversification, high front vowel types occur, often in the second syllable of disyllables. Syllable types include predominant use of CV and CVCV shapes, followed by CVC types, often at very low frequencies (e.g., Davis, MacNeilage, & Matyear, 2002). Words are mostly monosyllables in English, although some studies on languages in which multisyllables predominate show early use of disyllabic or multisyllabic utterances (e.g., see Goldstein, 1995, for a review). Relative to word position, stop consonants are more frequent in initial position and fricative or nasal manner or velar place of articulation in final position, when final consonants occur (Stoel-Gammon, 1985). Within syllables, early vocal forms show lack of movement of the tongue independent of the jaw resulting in labials with central vowels, alveolars with front vowels, and velars with back vowels in English and across languages (Davis & MacNeilage, 2002). In disyllables, reduplication (e.g., "baba") is most frequent, followed by variegation for both consonants and vowels (e.g., "daedi" or "bada"; Mitchell & Kent, 1990; Smith, Brown-Sweeney, & Stoel-Gammon, 1989). When syllables are variegated, consonant manner and vowel height changes may predominate, related to lack of independence of articulators from the jaw cycle in earliest vocal sequences in this period (Davis et al., 2002). If change in consonant place occurs, the labial-alveolar sequence is highest in frequency in English and across languages (i.e., start with initial lip closure, then engage the tongue at the alveolar place; Davis et al., 2002; MacNeilage, Davis, Matyear, & Kinney, 2000). Children may also use idiosyncratic "word recipes" during this period, in

Table 8.2. Phonetic characteristics of babbling and early words

Production variability apparent

Raw materials

Consonants
Manner: stops, nasals, glides /b/, /m/, /d/, /n/, /w/, /j/ + /h/
Place: labial /b/, /m/, /w/ and alveolar /d/, /n/, /j/
Voicing:
  Initial: voiced
  Medial: voiced (between vowels)
  Final: voiceless

Vowels
Lower left quadrant (LLQ)
When vowels change: change in height /ɪ,i/ as in /daedi/
Syllable 1: LLQ; syllable 2: /ɪ,i/ or neutral vowel

General organization

Syllable types
CV, CVCV, CVC, VCV (varies by language)

Word types
Monosyllables, disyllables (varies by language)
Balance of Cs and Vs (indicates use of C and V alternation)
Few clusters

Positional constraints
CV: stop Cs initial
VC: fricative and nasal Cs final
CVC:
  Reduplication most common,
  Use of nasals, fricatives, velars in final position

Within syllables
Labials with central vowels
Alveolars with front vowels
Velars with back vowels
Later stages: look for specific contextual restrictions for C–V associations (may be lexical)

Across syllables
Reduplication most prominent
Variegation
Vowels: height changes
Consonants: manner changes
First C place variegation
Labial-alveolar first
Word recipes
Fits all words into their own pattern
To structure adult forms to agree with word pattern; restructures different adult models in different ways

Prosody

Stress
First syllable stress (language differences here)

Intonation
Falling contour first (language differences here)
Expressive jargon (long strings with language-like prosody)
Use of unanalyzed prosodic single word/sentence contours
Gestalt strategy: "stop it" / "all gone"
(Criteria for interpretation as a gestalt form: child never use components in other contexts)

Changes from babbling to word use

Consonants
Alveolars prominent in babbling; changes to labial prominence in first words

Word/utterance length
Long strings in babbling, first words tend to be mono- or disyllabic
May be multisyllable single words in other languages (e.g., Spanish)

Positional issues
Diversification in final position for consonants and vowels

Key: C, consonant; V, vowel.

which they use a few restricted ways to produce output and word targets fit into their favored production template(s) (Vihman, 1993). Prosodic regularities in this developmental period include first syllable stress and falling intonation contours in English (Pollock, Brammer, & Hageman, 1993; Snow & Stoel-Gammon, 1994). Children learning other languages may show ambient language-related differences in this profile (e.g., Lee, 2003; Teixeira & Davis, 2002). Expressive jargon, intonation contours that are language-like without meaning attached, may also occur contemporaneously in this period. The presence of these jargon sentences when vocal output is otherwise restricted may indicate that the child is capable of producing a series of vocalizations with language-like prosody even if his or her meaning-based output of words is severely restricted. In addition, some prosodic sentences may be observed (e.g., "Stop it" or "All gone") in which the child never uses the individual word components independently of one another.

Although not based on large normative databases, a comprehensive and coherent body of research over the past 15–20 years forms the foundation for these well-attested behaviors. They provide a strong backdrop to facilitate comparing the developmental level of the delayed or disordered speech production patterns of children with behavioral correlates in typical development. Comparative use of this information can support setting goals and targets related to developmental level of function as well as evaluating progress in therapy on an ongoing basis.

One other aspect of early typical development in this period is found in the variability of early productions at the onset of first words. Although variability in tokens of words is usual in this period, it is not the norm for production patterning in children at later developmental periods. As such, it may be an important aspect of planning for early goals and targets, particularly if developmental apraxia of speech is suspected. At present levels of research into this disorder, variability is considered one potential differential diagnostic indicator (Davis, Jakielski, & Marquardt, 1998). Table 8.3 displays a matrix for considering variability in the child for whom this issue is salient in considering goals and targets for therapy. In planning goals and targets for a child who is variable in realizations of word targets, two types of considerations are relevant related to the interface of speech production and language variables. In one type of goal, the clinician might wish to keep the language level constant (e.g., simple sentence types with a mean length of utterance of two to four words) and center on segmental, syllable or word, or prosodic accuracy. In a higher level

Table 8.3. Variability in spontaneous speech

Language level constant	Segmental accuracy
(Relational analysis type/token)	Syllable/word complexity[a]
	Prosodic
Language level change	Segmental
	Syllable/word complexity[a]
	Positional complexity
	Prosodic

Areas of change in language complexity
1. Syntactic
2. Semantic
3. Pragmatic
4. Topic
   a. Familiar
   b. Novel

[a]Number of syllables in a word, number of words in an utterance.

goal, the clinician might wish to vary aspects of language level and center therapeutic goals around consistency in speech production as language level is varied. Both options require careful planning for intervention for the goal of maintaining consistency of productions.

GENERAL FACTORS FOR GOAL AND TARGET SELECTION

In addition to factors related specifically to speech production variables and the interface of speech and language variables in goal and target selection for remediation, some general factors must be integrated into the decision matrix (see Table 8.4). These general factors are a part of the assessment process, as are the other more central factors relative to sound system goals. General factors may be based on direct observations of the child via standardized testing or informal assessments, parent or teacher reports via interview or case history, as well as available medical and educational records. All of these pieces of information form a background for decision making that integrates the primary speech and language variables chosen for remediation into the complex of individual internal variables (e.g., hearing, motor, or peripheral structure status) and individual external variables (e.g., family cultural background and nuclear family structure and expectations) that are important to success in intervention at the general level.

In some instances, these factors constitute important etiological factors that may guide the types of goals selected as well as prognosis for intervention. Hearing loss,

Table 8.4.   Factors related to goal setting for developmental speech disorders

Motor abilities
General motor skills
Oral-facial motor skills

Structural differences
Minor
  Lips
  Tongue
  Teeth
  Hard palate
Major
  Lips
  Tongue
  Teeth
  Hard palate
  Soft palate
  Nasopharynx

Perceptual abilities
Hearing loss
Speech sound perception

Neuromotor differences
Dysarthria
Apraxia

Cognitive–linguistic abilities
Intelligence
Language level
Academic performance

Psychosocial abilities
Age
Gender
Family background
Sibling influences

dysarthria, or major peripheral structural differences such as cleft palate are examples of etiological factors that may strongly affect the types of goals and targets selected for intervention. Minor structural variations form an example of a factor that may or may not have an impact on planning for therapeutic intervention, depending on their effects on the clinical speech patterns observed. For example, a child may have a shortened lingual frenulum that may not affect speech production.

Background factors influencing the course of therapy and the types of goals selected include intelligence and academic performance issues. Psychosocial factors may influence prognosis and, in the case of family factors, may strongly influence the types of goals and targets selected relative to the families' conceptualizations about disability and how differences from typical behavior should be handled. These issues are particularly relevant to planning for children and families from diverse cultural and linguistic backgrounds.

In every instance, these general factors should be included in planning for goals and targets. Singly or in combination, they may have profound implications, in the case of major etiological factors, or be ruled out as aspects of therapeutic intervention. Indeed, some general factors can be considered as resources the child brings to the therapeutic intervention process. For example, a child with very high intelligence may be very motivated to change minor or mild speech pattern differences to achieve social acceptance. In contrast, the child whose family does not believe that intelligibility is an important issue in their acceptance of the child within their culture may change the nature of goals chosen for intervention dramatically toward functional rather than developmental goals for that child.

SUMMARY

A thorough and valid clinical assessment is the most important gateway to appropriate selection of clinical goals and targets for developmental speech disorders. Characteristics of the child's clinical profile compiled from the assessment process form the foundation for the clinician in determining initial goals. Ongoing changes in goals and intervention targets are dependent on interaction between assessment results and progress in intervention. The child's clinical profile, in the areas of core sound system characteristics, in associated aspects of each child's overall language development, and in general descriptive variables, is important to selection of clinical goals and targets. Family and cultural values and expectations may also potentially affect the types of goals selected.

The clinician's knowledge of typical developmental milestones forms a backdrop for understanding where the child's present level of function lies relative to expectations for his or her chronological age. Understanding the discrepancy between developmental and chronological age emerges from the clinician's knowledge of typical development as well as understanding of the impact of etiological factors on speech patterns. This discrepancy will motivate the choice of goals selected, regardless of the theoretical stance of the clinician in implementation of intervention.

REFERENCES

Bernhardt, B., & Stoel-Gammon, C. (1994). Non-linear phonology: Introduction and clinical application. *Journal of Speech, Language, and Hearing Research, 37,* 123–143.

Davis, B.L., Jakielski, K.J., & Marquardt, T.P. (1998). Developmental apraxia of speech: Determiners of differential diagnosis. *Clinical Linguistics and Phonetics, 12*(1), 25–45.

Davis, B.L., & MacNeilage, P.F. (1995). The articulatory basis of babbling. *Journal of Speech and Hearing Research, 38,* 1199–1211.

Davis, B.L., & MacNeilage, P.F. (2002). The internal structure of the syllable: An ontogenetic perspective on origins. In T. Givon & B. Malle (Eds.), *The rise of language out of pre-language* (pp. 135–148). Amsterdam: Benjamin.

Davis, B.L., MacNeilage, P.F., & Matyear, C.L. (2002). Acquisition of serial complexity in speech production: A comparison of phonetic and phonological approaches to first word production. *Phonetica, 59,* 75–107.

Goldstein, B. (1995). Spanish phonological development. In H. Kayser (Ed.), *Bilingual speech-language pathology: An Hispanic focus* (pp. 17–38). San Diego: Singular Publishing.

Hargrove, P.M., & McGarr, N.S. (1994). *Prosody management of communication disorders.* San Diego: Singular Publishing.

Hodson, B.W., & Paden, E. (1991). *A phonological approach to remediation: Targeting intelligible speech* (2nd ed.). Austin, TX: PRO-ED.

Lee, S. (2003). *The phonetic basis of early speech acquisition in Korean.* Unpublished doctoral dissertation, The University of Texas at Austin.

MacNeilage, P.F., Davis, B.L., Matyear, C.M., & Kinney, A. (2000). Origin of speech output complexity in infants and in languages. *Psychological Science, 10,* 459–460.

Mitchell, P., & Kent, R. (1990). Phonetic variation in multisyllabic babbling. *Journal of Child Language, 17,* 247–265.

Oller, D.K. (1980). The emergence of the sounds of speech in infancy. In G. Yeni-Komshian, J. Kavanagh, & C. Ferguson (Eds.), *Child phonology, Vol. 1: Production* (pp. 93–112). New York: Elsevier.

Pollock, K., Brammer, D.M., & Hageman, C.F. (1993). An acoustic analysis of young children's productions of word stress. *Journal of Phonetics, 21,* 183–203.

Sander, E. (1972). When are speech sounds learned? *Journal of Speech and Hearing Disorders, 37,* 55–63.

Smith, B., Brown-Sweeney, S., & Stoel-Gammon, C. (1989). A quantitative analysis of reduplicated and variegated babbling. *A First Language, 17,* 147–153.

Snow, D., & Stoel-Gammon, C. (1994). Phrase final lengthening and intonation in early child speech. *Journal of Speech and Hearing Research, 37,* 831–840.

Stark, R. (1980). Stages of speech development in the first year of life. In G. Yeni-Komshian, J. Kavanagh, & C. Ferguson (Eds.), *Child phonology, Vol. 1: Production* (pp. 113–142). New York: Elsevier.

Stoel-Gammon, C. (1985). Phonetic inventories, 15–24 months: A longitudinal study. *Journal of Speech and Hearing Research, 28,* 505–512.

Strand, E. (2002). Childhood apraxia of speech: Suggested diagnostic markers for the younger child. In L.D. Shriberg & T.F. Campbell (Eds.), *Proceedings of the 2002 childhood apraxia of speech symposium.* Carlsbad, CA: Hendrix Foundation.

Teixeira, E.R., & Davis, B.L. (2002). Early sound patterns in the speech of two Brazilian Portuguese speakers. *Language and Speech, 45*(2), 179–204.

Van Riper, C., & Irwin, J. (1959). *Voice and articulation.* Englewood Cliffs, NJ: Prentice Hall.

Vihman, M.M. (1993). Variable paths to early word production. *Journal of Phonetics, 21,* 61–82.

Vihman, M.M. (1996). *Phonological development: The origins of language in the child.* Cambridge, MA: Blackwell.

Wood, P. (1980). Appreciating the consequences of disease: The classification of impairments, disabilities, and handicaps. *The World Health Organization Chronicles, 34,* 376–380.

Chapter 9

From Developmental Norms to Distance Metrics

Past, Present, and Future Directions for Target Selection Practices

A. Lynn Williams

Target selection factors have changed significantly over the 25 years of my career as a speech-language pathologist (SLP). Although these changes mirror the shift in the way that I select target sounds for intervention, I believe the transformation reflects a broader change in the way I view speech disorders in children now as compared with when I first started practicing. I began my career as an SLP in 1980, which was at the beginning of the phonological process revolution that was largely created by the publication of Ingram's (1976) book, *Phonological Disability in Children.* With the introduction of phonological processes, SLPs began to view the rule-governed, patterned aspects of children's speech errors that implied a cognitive aspect to the learning of a sound system. Prior to this view, I had been trained to simply list children's sound errors by word position according to substitutions, omissions, distortions, and additions (SODA), which could take as much as a page of a report for children who had multiple sound errors! With the change in assessment, there was also a change in selection of treatment targets. With the sound-by-sound approach, I chose targets based primarily on developmental norms with secondary consideration given to stimulability and consistency of errors. Specifically, I selected early developing sounds that were stimulable and were inconsistently in error. The premise of this approach to target selection was that ease of learning was based on phonetic, or articulatory, factors. That is, children learned early, stimulable, inconsistent sounds more easily than they did more complex targets that were later, nonstimulable, and consistently erroneous sounds.

With the shift to a pattern analysis that described sound errors in terms of phonological processes, I shifted my selection of treatment targets to factors related to intelligibility, such as frequency of occurrence of phonological processes. Developmental norms could still be used, but with regard to age of *suppression* of processes rather than age of *acquisition* of sounds.

A series of studies was conducted in the 1980s and 1990s that questioned the traditional approach to target selection that largely underpinned both the sound-by-sound and phonological process frameworks. Based on these studies, the construct of phonological complexity was proposed that represents a fundamental shift in traditional methods of target selection and, on the surface, seems counterintuitive to principles of learning. Results from a number of studies indicated that greater systemwide change occurred when targets were selected that were more phonologically complex than when phonologically simpler targets were selected. Collectively, the studies reported that greater systemwide change occurred when targets were later developing, nonstimulable, consistent errors that represented least phonological knowledge. This approach to teaching the most difficult aspects first has been discussed by Gierut (2001) with regard to teaching mathematics (Yao, 1989, as cited in Gierut, 2001). Specifically, teaching the most complicated math concepts of division first facilitated learning of the easier concepts of addition, subtraction, and multiplication. However, teaching addition first did not facilitate learning of the other mathematical concepts.

CURRENT APPROACHES TO TARGET SELECTION

Recent research has addressed challenges to the nontraditional approach of phonological complexity. For an interesting debate between traditional approaches to target selection and the construct of phonological complexity, the reader is referred to a recent exchange of Letters to the Editor by Gierut and Morrisette (2003) and Rvachew and Nowak (2003). It seems that the claims of both perspectives are valid when the type of change or phonological learning is considered. With regard to *sound learning,* children learn the simpler targets easier and faster, similar to the math analogy. In terms of *system shifting,* children have more difficulty learning the more complex targets, similar to learning the more complex mathematical concepts; yet, they evidence greater systemwide change. Gierut (2001) made a similar distinction in discussing "local generalization" versus "global generalization." Local generalization has an impact on a more narrow aspect of the phonological system in that change is limited to the target sound in untreated words or different contexts. Global generalization, however, reflects a broader aspect of change that is systemwide in which both treated and untreated aspects of the sound system are changed as a result of intervention.

The selection factors and rationales that underlie the traditional and nontraditional approaches to target selection were summarized by Williams (2003b) and are presented in Table 9.1. In my own clinical work and research, it seemed that target selection factors that were based on broad, dichotomous categorizations (i.e., early versus later developing sounds; stimulable versus nonstimulable; consistent versus inconsistent; most knowledge versus least knowledge) did not capture the unique and individual phonological organizations that each child presented or the specific learning needs of an individual child. As a consequence, I have moved away from the characteristics of individual *sounds* to the characteristics of an individual child's *sound system* in selecting treatment targets. This shift is an outgrowth of the assessment and intervention models that I have worked on, namely, Systemic Phonological Analysis of Child Speech (SPACS; Williams, 2001, 2003a) and the multiple oppositions treatment approach (cf. Williams, 2000a, 2000b).

SPACS is a child-based assessment model that maps a child's sound system onto an adult system in terms of phoneme collapses. For example, a child might substitute [t]

Table 9.1. Selection factors and rationales in traditional and nontraditional approaches to target selection

Selection factor	Traditional approach	Nontraditional approach
Stimulability	Select sounds that are stimulable. *Rationale:* Sounds that are stimulable are easier to learn (Hodson & Paden, 1991; Winitz, 1975).	Select sounds that are not stimulable. *Rationale:* Stimulable sounds will emerge without direct intervention (Miccio et al., 1999).
Developmental norms	Select early developing sounds. *Rationale:* Early developing sounds are acquired first (Khan & Lewis, 1990; Shriberg & Kwiatkowski, 1982).	Select later developing sounds. *Rationale:* Training later developing sounds will result in greater system-wide change (Gierut et al., 1996).
Consistency	Select sounds that are inconsistently produced in error. *Rationale:* Variability may be an important indicator of flexibility, change, and potential growth (Forrest et al., 1994; Tyler & Saxman, 1991).	Select sounds that are consistent in their error productions. *Rationale:* Consistent errors represent stable underlying representations, which will result in across-the-board change (Forrest et al., 2000).
Knowledge	Select sounds for which the child has most knowledge. *Rationale:* Sounds for which the child has some knowledge will be easier to learn.	Select sounds for which child has least knowledge. *Rationale:* Training least knowledge results in greater systemwide change (Gierut et al., 1987).

From Williams, A.L. (2003). Target selection and treatment outcomes. *Perspectives on Language Learning and Education, 10*(1), 12–16; reprinted by permission. *Perspectives* is the newsletter of Division 1, Language Learning and Education of the American Speech-Language-Hearing Association (ASHA). The table is reprinted with permission from the publisher, ASHA.

for /k/, /ʧ/, /f/, /s/, /ʃ/, /st/, /tr/, /kl/, and /kr/ word-initially. Thus, the child collapses several adult phonemes to one sound in her sound system. This one-to-many phoneme collapse can be diagrammed as follows:

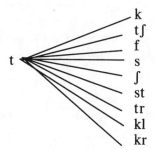

The systemic approach is based on the *function* of the sound in the child's rule set and its potential for having the greatest impact on phonological restructuring. The function of a sound is a concept that assumes that the importance of target sounds is broader than the characteristics of the sound itself. As discussed previously, sounds can be characterized as early or later developing, stimulable or nonstimulable, and most or least knowledge. However, the function of a sound is dependent on the role it plays in a particular child's unique phonological system, and it will therefore vary from child to child. Consequently, the *function* of a particular sound is independent of the *characteristics* of that sound.

The systemic approach to target selection is based on a distance metric that incorporates two parameters: maximal classification and maximal distinction. Maximal classification involves selection of sound members from different manner classes, different places of production, and different voicing. Maximal distinction is the selection of target sounds that are maximally distinct from the child's error in terms of place, voice, manner, and linguistic unit (singleton versus cluster). Selection of targets that are more distinct from the child's error (maximal distinction) makes them more salient and therefore presumably more learnable. Furthermore, selection of targets that are representative of the sound classes collapsed across a phoneme collapse (maximal classification) provides focused training across a rule set. I make an analogy to assembling a puzzle with regard to these two components of the distance metric. If we think of the child's sound learning task in terms of a jigsaw puzzle, the input we give them in the form of the treatment targets serves as the puzzle pieces. I believe that the distance metric provides the critical corner pieces of the puzzle through the use of salient, focused input that is intended to facilitate the child's phonological learning and reorganization. The distance metric selects sounds that represent the extremes of the child's rule set. This primes the child for maximal learning and phonological reorganization in a way that allows him or her to fill in the less salient puzzle pieces or targets. I think it is a more difficult learning task for the child to be given an inside puzzle piece—a target that has no specific connection to the sound system but was selected based on non–child-specific characteristics such as developmental norms, stimulability, consistency, or phonological knowledge.

In the 1:9 phoneme collapse, for example, the target sounds selected using a systemic approach might include [t] ~ [k], [tʃ], [f], and [st]. The sounds are maximally classified and maximally distinct from [t] in terms of *place* (alveolar versus velar, palatal, labioden-tal), *manner* (stop versus affricate, fricative), and *linguistic unit* (singleton versus cluster). These targets were selected based on their function within the phoneme collapse regardless of their individual characteristics of early or later developing phonemes, stimulability or nonstimulability, or most or least phonological knowledge. The systemic approach to target selection is used with the multiple oppositions treatment approach (Williams, 2000a, 2000b, 2003a) in which several sounds are targeted simultaneously in larger contrastive treatment sets. Using this example, the contrastive sound pairs for multiple oppositions would include the following treatment exemplars for the target sounds:

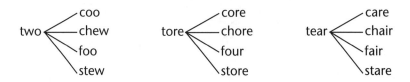

I believe that the systemic approach to target selection using the distance metric reflects my current work to find the "order within the disorder" of children's speech disorders. We are truly working in an amazing time in which we attempt to identify the unique "languages" of children who have disordered speech. Each child is unique and individual, and each has his or her own sound system that is logical, rule-governed, and predictable. Through my clinical work, I am realizing the validity of parents' descriptions of their children's disordered speech as being "their own language." To me, it is very exciting to discover the rules of a child's language and use the puzzle analogy with the distance metric to help them learn the sound system of the ambient language. Therefore, the function of target sounds within a given child's system will be unique from any other child and independent of the characteristics of sounds within adult-based categorizations of sounds.

ADDITIONAL TREATMENT TARGETS

Although I target consonants primarily for intervention, I target vowels directly under two circumstances. Some children produce vowel errors in addition to their consonant error productions. In those situations, I contrast the child's vowel substitute with the target vowel. For example, one child produced the lax vowel [ɘ] for the tense vowel [e]. These vowels were contrasted in sound pairs, as shown here:

    wet   ~ wait
    bread ~ braid
    sell   ~ sail

A second situation in which vowels are specifically targeted involves the presence of a phonological rule that the production of the consonant is conditioned by the vowel environment. An example is a child who exhibited an allophonic rule of complementary distribution in which his production of alveolar and velar stops was conditioned by the following vowel. Specifically, if the following vowel was a back vowel, the child produced the velar stop. Conversely, if the following vowel was a front vowel, he produced the alveolar stop. In treatment, alveolar and velar stops were crossed with front and back vowels in order to eliminate the asymmetry in the child's distribution of alveolar and velar stops.

Perception is another aspect of intervention that is addressed frequently with children who have speech disorders. Although perception is an important prerequisite to production, it is very difficult to assess a child's perceptual skills, especially in younger, preschool-age children. I do not address perception directly in intervention because the research studies have been equivocal in their findings related to the benefits of perception training. Given the nature of the contrastive sound pairs, perception is addressed indirectly in treatment. Furthermore, I begin intervention at an imitative word level so the child has numerous opportunities to hear the distinction of sound pairs in the clinician's models as well as to reproduce that distinction in their own productions.

Phonological awareness is frequently addressed within my intervention sessions with children who have speech disorders. Indirectly, the rhyming contrasts of the sound pairs increase the children's phonological sensitivity and awareness of rhyme. However, I also target specific phonological awareness goals in intervention if the child exhibited deficits in these skills based on standardized or nonstandardized testing. I frequently include rhyme identification and rhyme generation as early phonological awareness goals. Recently, I have addressed a broad spectrum of phonological awareness skills through brief classroom activities with preschool children. These activities are fun, play-based activities that are based on children's literature, music, and games and include opportunities to address sound identification and matching, sound substitution, rhyming, and sound and syllable segmentation. The activities are conducted three times per week for approximately 20 minutes for each classroom lesson. The children are actively engaged and enjoy the activities. Our results have shown that the children who received these classroom activities demonstrated increased phonological sensitivity compared with children who did not receive the classroom activities (Williams & Coutinho, 2003).

AFTER TARGET SELECTION:
LEXICAL FACTORS IN SELECTION OF TREATMENT STIMULI

According to studies conducted since the late 1990s (cf. Gierut & Morrisette, 1998; Gierut, Morrisette, & Champion, 1999; Gierut & Storkel, 2002; Morrisette, 1999; Morrisette & Gierut, 2002; Storkel & Rogers, 2000), evidence indicates that after the target sounds have been selected for treatment, word frequency and neighborhood density are important factors in choosing the target words that will be used in treatment. Frequency refers to the number of occurrences of a given word in a language. Morrisette (1999) defined a high-frequency word as one that occurred in the language 100 times or more. High-frequency words are recognized faster than low-frequency words and they are more resistant to slips of the tongue. Neighborhood density refers to the number of phonetically similar counterparts that exist for a word based on one sound substitution, deletion, or addition. For example, the word *feet* is in the neighborhood with *fleet, meet, fee,* and *eat.* Morrisette (1999) defined a high-density word as having 10 or more phonetically similar counterparts. Similar to high-frequency words, words from low-density neighborhoods are recognized faster than those from high-density neighborhoods and they are resistant to slips of the tongue.

Based on a series of studies (Gierut & Morrisette, 1998; Gierut & Storkel, 2002; Morrisette, 1999; Morrisette & Gierut, 2002; Storkel & Rogers, 2000), Gierut and her colleagues recommended that target sounds should be trained in words that are either high frequency or low density. Treatment words that have either of these characteristics are more facilitative of generalization than words that are low-frequency or high-density words. Examples of good treatment words would be *drive, house,* and *mouth,* which are low-density (i.e., fewer than 10 phonetically similar counterparts) and high-frequency words (i.e., more than 100 occurrences). Examples of poor treatment words would be *duck, boot,* and *catch,* which are high-density (i.e., more than 10 phonetically similar counterparts) and low-frequency words (i.e., fewer than 100 occurrences).

Studies that have examined lexical characteristics related to generalization are intriguing extensions of word recognition studies in adults for whom the two lexical parameters of frequency and density were found to have psychological reality. However, additional studies are needed to determine the clinical relevance of lexical factors given the constraints of determining the frequency and density of potential treatment words, as well as selecting words that are meaningful and can be represented for the target sounds selected for intervention.

SUMMARY AND FUTURE RESEARCH

Target selection factors provide an important opportunity for SLPs to engineer the input we present to children to be more teachable and therefore more learnable. Examining each child as a unique speaker of an exotic language makes our work more challenging and infinitely more interesting because we need to select targets that are functional within that child's sound system, which will help the child put together the new puzzle of speech in less time and with less effort. The focus on treatment is not exclusively on consonants but can extend to additional targets such as vowels and phonological awareness skills.

SLPs consider a variety of variables in selecting treatment targets, of which only a few have been discussed in this chapter. Powell (1991) listed more than 20 factors that are relevant in making clinical decisions related to treatment targets. Many of these factors, including frequency of the sound in the language, visual cues of target sounds, and functionality of targets in a child's daily interactions, have not been investigated in terms of treatment outcomes.

Our clinical decision making may also extend to the selection of words that will be used in working with children on the target sounds. Although the lexical factors of word frequency and neighborhood density hold some appeal, it is not clear whether the clinical payoff will be realized in the amount of time and effort required to select treatment exemplars that incorporate low-density or high-frequency words.

REFERENCES

Forrest, K., Elbert, M., & Dinnsen, D.A. (2000). The effect of substitution patterns on phonological treatment outcomes. *Clinical Linguistics & Phonetics, 14,* 519–531.

Forrest, K., Weismer, G., Dinnsen, D.A., & Elbert, M. (1994). Spectral analysis of target appropriate /t/ and /k/ produced by phonologically disordered and normally articulating children. *Clinical Linguistics & Phonetics, 8,* 267–282.

Gierut, J.A. (2001). Complexity in phonological treatment. *Language, Speech, and Hearing Services in Schools, 32,* 229–241.

Gierut, J.A., Elbert, M., & Dinnsen, D.A. (1987). A functional analysis of phonological knowledge and generalization learning in misarticulating children. *Journal of Speech and Hearing Research, 30,* 462–479.

Gierut, J.A., & Morrisette, M.L. (1998). Lexical properties in implementation of sound change. In A. Greenhill, M. Hughes, H. Littlefield, & H. Walsh (Eds.), *Proceedings of the 22nd annual Boston University conference on language development* (pp. 257–268). Somerville, MA: Cascadilla Press.

Gierut, J.A., & Morrisette, M.L. (2003). Unified treatment recommendations: A response to Rvachew and Nowak (2001). *Journal of Speech, Language, and Hearing Research, 46*(2), 382–385.

Gierut, J.A., Morrisette, M.L., & Champion, A.H. (1999). Lexical constraints in phonological acquisition. *Journal of Child Language, 26,* 261–294.

Gierut, J.A., Morrisette, M.L., Hughes, M.T., & Rowland, S. (1996). Phonological treatment efficacy and developmental norms. *Language, Speech, and Hearing Services in Schools, 27,* 215–230.

Gierut, J.A., & Storkel, H.L. (2002). Markedness and the grammar in lexical diffusion of fricatives. *Clinical Linguistics & Phonetics, 16*(2), 115–134.

Hodson, B.W., & Paden, E.P. (1991). *Targeting intelligible speech: A phonological approach to remediation* (2nd ed.). Austin, TX: PRO-ED.

Ingram, D. (1976). *Phonological disability in children.* London: Edward Arnold.

Khan, L.M., & Lewis, N.P. (1990). Phonological process therapy in school settings: The bare essentials to meeting the ultimate challenge. *National Student Speech, Language, and Hearing Association Journal, 17,* 50–58.

Miccio, A.W., Elbert, M., & Forrest, K. (1999). The relationship between stimulability and phonological acquisition in children with normally developing and disordered phonologies. *American Journal of Speech-Language Pathology, 8,* 347–363.

Morrisette, M.L. (1999). Lexical characteristics of sound change. *Clinical Linguistics & Phonetics, 13*(3), 219–238.

Morrisette, M.L., & Gierut, J.A. (2002). Lexical organization and phonological change in treatment. *Journal of Speech, Language, and Hearing Research, 45,* 143–159.

Powell, T.W. (1991). Planning for phonological generalization: An approach to treatment target selection. *American Journal of Speech-Language Pathology, 1,* 21–27.

Rvachew, S., & Nowak, M. (2003). Clinical outcomes as a function of target selection strategy: A response to Morrisette and Gierut. *Journal of Speech, Language, and Hearing Research, 46*(2), 386–389.

Shriberg, L.D., & Kwiatkowski, J. (1982). Phonological disorders II: A conceptual framework for management. *Journal of Speech and Hearing Disorders, 47,* 242–256.

Storkel, H.L., & Rogers, M.A. (2000). The effect of probabilistic phonotactics on lexical acquisition. *Clinical Linguistics & Phonetics, 14*(6), 407–425.

Tyler, A.A., & Saxman, J.H. (1991). Initial voicing contrast acquisition in normal and phonologically disordered children. *Applied Psycholinguistics, 12,* 453–479.

Williams, A.L. (2000a). Multiple oppositions: Case studies of variables in phonological intervention. *American Journal of Speech-Language Pathology, 9,* 289–299.

Williams, A.L. (2000b). Multiple oppositions: Theoretical foundations for an alternative contrastive intervention approach. *American Journal of Speech-Language Pathology, 9,* 282–288.

Williams, A.L. (2001). Phonological assessment of child speech. In D.M. Ruscello (Ed.), *Tests and measurements in speech-language pathology* (pp. 31–76). Woburn, MA: Butterworth-Heinemann.

Williams, A.L. (2003a). *Speech disorders resource guide for preschool children.* Clifton Park, NY: Thomson Delmar Learning.

Williams, A.L. (2003b). Target selection and treatment outcomes. *Perspectives on Language Learning and Education, 10*(1), 12–16.

Williams, A.L., & Coutinho, M. (2003, November). Contexts for facilitating emergent literacy skills. Miniseminar presented at the annual convention of the American Speech-Language-Hearing Association, Chicago, IL.

Winitz, H. (1975). *From syllable to conversation.* Baltimore: University Park Press.

Yao, K. (1989). *Acquisition of mathematical skills in a learning hierarchy by high and low ability students when instruction is omitted on coordinate and subordinate skills.* Unpublished doctoral dissertation, Indiana University, Bloomington.

Chapter 10

Selection of Phonological Goals and Targets

Not Just an Exercise in Phonological Analysis

Barbara Handford Bernhardt

Phonological intervention, as with other goal-oriented activities, operates within a sphere of optimistic uncertainty. Goals and targets are set based on what is learned about a child during the assessment process and according to the frameworks used by the speech-language pathologist (SLP). It is impossible, however, to foretell whether and when those goals and targets will be mastered. What can be done to optimize opportunities for efficient progress at the point of goal and target selection? This chapter describes an approach to goal and target selection derived from 1) constraints-based nonlinear phonological analysis and 2) the integration of other factors concerning the child (e.g., cognition, motor skills, perception, environment). The phonological analysis can identify needs and strengths of the child's phonological system, but selection of goals and targets depends on consideration of other factors concerning that person.

The first part of this chapter outlines a framework for proposing goals and targets derived from the application of constraints-based nonlinear phonological theories, following Bernhardt and Stemberger (2000). Since the 1920s, linguistic theories have provided many frameworks for phonological analyses. Recent constraints-based nonlinear phonological theories have provided a much more comprehensive view of the function and structure of phonological systems. Evidence from clinical studies supports the application of these theories in phonological intervention (Bernhardt, 1990, 1992; Bernhardt & Major, in press; Bernhardt & Stemberger, 2000; Edwards, 1995; Major & Bernhardt, 1998; Von Bremen, 1990). Computer applications (e.g., Masterson & Bernhardt, 2001) have sped up the process of analysis for clinical application.

Speech-language pathology has a variety of standard and nonstandard procedures for deriving information about a child's abilities and contexts outside the domain of phonology. In conjunction with information gained from family members and other professionals, this information provides a context for selection of specific goals and targets. The second part of this chapter describes how various factors about the child affect the selection of goals and targets. The orientation that drives this part of the process derives from client- and family-centered approaches to speech-language pathology and reflects concepts influenced by the World Health Organization (WHO) International Classification of Functioning, Disability and Health (ICF; World Health Organization, 2001). The WHO classification divides functioning into three levels: the level of a person's bodily structure and function (e.g., the phonological system), a person's activities (e.g., communication with others, related activities such as literacy), and a person's participation in society (e.g., attending preschool). Goals of phonological intervention may include not only speech production (and perception) but also the client's general communication, literacy skills, and integration into the community.

CONSTRAINTS-BASED NONLINEAR PHONOLOGICAL THEORY AND GOAL AND TARGET SELECTION

Three major concepts underlie the Bernhardt and Stemberger (2000) applications of constraints-based nonlinear phonological theory: phonological constraints, hierarchical structure, and the independent or autonomous aspect of phonological units. What is meant by these three concepts and what are their implications for goal and target selection?

Constraints

Human communication reflects a tension between the desire for comprehensibility and the effort required to overcome limitations of the cognitive, perceptual, and motor systems. Depending on the degree of phonological impairment, the limitations (or negative constraints) may have an excessive impact on comprehensibility (the positive constraints or objectives). In the jargon of one major constraints-based theory known as *optimality theory,* limitations of the system are designated as *not* or *markedness* constraints. Comprehensibility comes through mastery of phonological form that is faithful to the form of the ambient language. These positive constraints are designated as *survival* (of underlying form) or *faithfulness* constraints (see Barlow & Gierut, 1999; Bernhardt & Stemberger, 1998). The overall goals of phonological intervention in terms of constraints-based theory are twofold: 1) to promote the positive objectives and constraints (what is currently *not* in the system) and 2) to reduce the impact of the limitations on production (demotion of the negative constraints), as in the examples that follow.

Constraints analysis I:
(where >> equals more important than, greater than, higher ranked than)

High-ranked positive constraints:	Survived(Consonant)	Must produce some consonant (no deletion allowed)
>>		
High-ranked negative constraint:	Not(Fricative)	No fricatives allowed
>>		
Medium-ranked positive objective:	Survived(Fricative)	Wants fricatives, can't produce them
>>		
Lowest ranked negative constraint:	Not(Stop)	Default stop substitution allowed

(Even though the negative constraint against stops is still part of the phonology, because this constraint is lowest ranked, stops are permitted; the negative constraint has no power in the set of identified constraints.)

Goal and targets I: Change the relative ranking of Not(Fricative) and Survived(Fricative) so that fricatives can be produced.

This analysis is relatively straightforward and, as with a process analysis, identifies and targets stopping of fricatives. However, a more complex constraint analysis can be invoked that integrates additional aspects of the child's feature and segmental systems. Both fricatives and stops are obstruents ([–sonorant]). If a child uses stops for fricatives, the child does not have to learn that fricatives are obstruents (the [–sonorant] feature is present in the stop substitution) but rather that they are [+continuant]. If this same child produces [+continuant] glides, fricatives could potentially be shaped from glides by a narrowing of the air stream in the oral cavity. Bringing the fricatives into the [+continuant] category means paying attention to positive constraints in addition to negative constraints. A positive constraint (faithfulness to glides) is used as a scaffold to approach the new targets (fricatives). An expanded constraints analysis follows below.

Constraints analysis II:

High-ranked positive constraints:	Survived(Consonant)	Must produce consonant (no deletion allowed)
	Survived(Glides)	Must produce [+continuant]
>>		
High-ranked negative constraint:	Not(Fricative)	Prevents fricatives
>>		
Medium-ranked positive objective:	Survived(Fricative)	Wants fricatives, can't produce them
>>		
Lowest ranked negative constraints:	Not(Stop)	Default stop substitution allowed
	Not(Glide)	Glides allowed

Goals and targets II:

1. Change the relative ranking of Not(Fricative) and Survived(Fricative)

2. Promote Survived(Fricative) to the level of Survived(Glide) through relating the two constraints in treatment as [+continuant] segments (speech sounds)

In the usual case, the mere facilitation of new targets helps overcome negative constraints. Sometimes, however, the negative constraints stem from other factors (e.g., misperception of a particular contrast, a structural deficit in the oral mechanism, memory limitations for long words). In such cases, the conditions leading to the negative constraints may themselves need to be targeted. Further discussion of other factors and their implications for goal selection is given in the second half of this chapter.

Phonological Defaults and Nondefaults

Another aspect of phonological constraints that affects goal and target selection concerns the notion of default and nondefault phonological forms. Phonological forms vary in the amount of resources required for speech production (the number and complexity of negative constraints that need to be overcome). Some phonological forms require a considerable investment of articulatory and cognitive resources (have strong negative constraints), for example, voiced fricatives, complex consonant sequences, or the English /r/. These highly constrained forms are often called nondefault (marked) forms. Because they require more resources and are later developing, they are commonly among the set of possible intervention targets. Other phonological forms are relatively easy to produce because they require fewer articulatory or cognitive resources, for example, stops, labials, alveolars, open monosyllables, and singleton consonants versus clusters. These less-marked default forms tend to appear in place of (substitute for) other more complex forms and to develop earlier, and they are less frequent intervention targets (see Chapter 9, and Bernhardt & Stemberger, 2000). Constraints-based theory implies that nondefault forms should be targeted in intervention because they are the forms that require the most learning (e.g., fricatives, liquids, complex consonant sequences, words with initial weak syllables). Default forms are often present in the child's productions before intervention, or, if some are absent, they may develop spontaneously once the more challenging nondefault targets are acquired (see Chapter 9, and Gierut, 1998). Of course, the child may have a default form that does not match that of the ambient language (e.g., a child who uses velars instead of alveolars). In such cases, the target may need to be an adult default (alveolars). Similarly, a child may have virtually no phonological forms (only a few central vowels, no consonants). In such cases, the first step may be to help the child produce phonological forms that require few resources (the defaults).

Phonological Hierarchy

While acknowledging that speech sounds occur in sequence, nonlinear phonological theory emphasizes the hierarchical nature of phonological form. The major division in the hierarchy is between higher level *phrase and word structures* and lower level *segments* and *features* (lowest level) (see Figure 10.1), with many levels contained within each of those broad sectors. Phonological patterns reflecting the hierarchical organization show both top-down and bottom-up effects. A top-down pattern is deletion of all material below the level of the unit deleted, for example, if a syllable is deleted because of constraints on stress patterns, all segments and features from that syllable are also deleted (e.g., *balloon* as [lun], *bed* as [bɛd], *butter* as [bʌdə]). The child cannot produce an initial weak syllable, and consequently the [b] and [ə] of that syllable disappear, even though the child can produce [b] or [ə] in other contexts. A bottom-up pattern is deletion of material above the level of the problematic unit (e.g., *giraffe* as [wæf], *jay* as [eɪ], but *balloon* as [bəwun]). The child can produce initial weak syllables and consonants but does not produce them if they contain segments that are not in his or her system, in this case, /ʤ/.

What are the implications of constraint theory and nonlinear phonology for goal and target selection? Figure 10.2 relates negative constraints to positive goal types. Negative constraints can prohibit single elements (an individual feature, a stress pattern, a word structure) or combinations of elements. Goals and targets need to reflect the two types of negative constraints. If a constraint prohibits all final consonants or all velars, the goal is to introduce that target into the system in any and/or all available contexts. If a constraint targets combinations of elements, the goal is to target that specific combination. Constraints on combinations of elements can occur simultaneously (features in combination, segments in various word positions) or in sequence (no labials after velars). For example, two

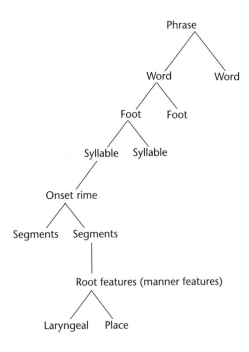

Figure 10.1. Basic phonological hierarchy.

Constraint type	High-ranked negative (markedness) constraints on individual structures or features ↓	High-ranked negative (markedness) constraints on combinations of existing elements (simultaneous or sequential combinations) ↓
Goal type	Faithfulness to new individual structures or features (e.g., Word shape such as CV)	Faithfulness to multiple existing elements at the same time (e.g., Combination of [+continuant] and [Coronal] for /s/, /z/)

Figure 10.2. Constraints and goal types. Negative or markedness constraints prohibit the production of elements. Positive (faithfulness) goals are set to overcome the negative markedness constraints. Constraints affect individual elements, such as single features or word structures. They can also affect simultaneous and/or sequential combinations of elements, such as feature-word position co-occurrence (e.g., fricatives word initially), or sequences (e.g., [Labial]–[Coronal] sequences as in the word *boat*). Goals need to be considered for both single elements and the combination of elements. Different types of constraints lead to different types of goals, as indicated by the downward-pointing arrows. (*Source:* Bernhardt & Stemberger, 2000).

features may be present independently in a child's inventory but not in combination, that is, labiodental fricatives and alveolar stops may occur, but alveolar fricatives may be missing from the inventory. The goal is to combine the features of place (alveolar) and manner (fricative). Constraints can also prohibit interactions of structure and features. A child may be able to produce velar stops word-finally but not word-initially, even though that child produces other word-initial stops. It is the simultaneous combination of word-initial position and velars that is prohibited.

Figure 10.3 shows a summary diagram of areas to evaluate for goal and target selection, including both individual elements (outlined in column 1) and combinations of elements (outlined in column 2). The rows show the major hierarchical divisions for potential goals: structural units such as word and phrase levels, and features (and related segments). Four quadrants show four types of goals, addressing the hierarchical division between structure and features, and constraints on individual elements versus combinations of elements.

Potential new targets at the phrase and word structure levels (quadrant A, Figure 10.3) include: 1) new phrasal stress and intonation (prosodic) patterns, 2) new word lengths, 3) new word stress patterns, and 4) new word shapes in terms of consonant (C) and vowel (V) sequences, for example, CVC (as in *hat*) or CCV (as in *blue*). Word shapes are the most common targets within that group, although word stress patterns may be targeted directly for older children, and both word and phrasal stress (prosody) may be targeted directly where needs indicate, for example, if there is restricted use of unstressed grammatical morphemes that appears to have a phonological basis (deletion of weak syllables in sequences, or monotonic production, with inaccurate phrasal stress timing). Some word structure positions may be limited in terms of features and segments and, thus, positional or sequence goals for features and segments may need to be targeted, as exemplified in quadrant C of Figure 10.3.

Potential feature targets may include manner, place, and laryngeal features (voicing, glottal features), both as new individual features for the system (quadrant B, Figure 10.3) and in new feature combinations (quadrant D, Figure 10.3). For example, if a child has no /l/, the feature [+lateral] would be a new individual feature target. If a child shows partial development of a category (e.g., only one fricative [f]), additional members may need to be added to that category by combining features already in the system. For example, if a child produces [f], and also has voiceless alveolar stops, the existing feature [Coronal] (from /t/) can be combined with the existing fricative ([+continuant]) to produce /s/. Features from different areas of the consonant and vowel feature systems are considered

Goal type	New individual structures or features	New combinations or sequences of existing elements
Structural goals	A. *New structures in:* Phrasal stress, intonation Word length in syllables Word Stress Word shape: No final C *Goal: CVC*	C. *New combination, word position or sequence for existing elements* *e.g., Child has singleton /l/, but clusters only with glides.* *Goal: /l/ in clusters*
Segmental (or feature) goals	B. *New individual features* *e.g. No palatoalveolars* *Goal: [-anterior] for palatoalveolars /ʃ,/tʃ/ /dʒ/ /ʒ/*	D. *New combinations of features* *e.g., Child has fricative /f/ and coronal stop /t/:* *Goal: [+continuant] (from /f/) with [Coronal] from /t/ > /s/, /z/*

Figure 10.3. Areas of the phonological hierarchy to consider for goal selection. As observed for Figure 10.2, goals need to be considered for both single elements and the combination of elements, reflecting constraints on single and multiple elements. They also need to address the two major divisions of the phonological hierarchy: structure (quadrants A and C), and features, with their related segments (quadrants B and D). The table differentiates goal type by single element (quadrants A and B) or combination of elements (quadrants C and D), and by the phonological hierarchy division (the rows). (*Source:* Bernhardt & Stemberger, 2000).

potential targets, with nondefault features considered higher priority, as discussed in the previous section on constraints. Both consonants and vowels may be targeted, although consonants are more frequent segmental targets (vowels showing fewer problems overall).

The relative importance of the identified needs within the four quadrants depends on that individual's system and other contextual factors (discussed in the next section). If many top-down patterns are found, more attention may need to be given earlier in the program to higher level phrase and word structures in order to reduce the impact of those general constraints. If many bottom-up patterns, or, comparatively speaking, more segmental than structural deficiencies are found, more attention may need to be given to segments and features.

Evidence has been garnered over the past 16 years to support goal selection based on the phonological hierarchy and the quadrant approach (e.g., Bernhardt, 1990, 1992; Edwards, 1995; Major & Bernhardt, 1998; Von Bremen, 1990). Children typically progress in at least one of the targeted hierarchical levels within the first block of treatment (Bernhardt, 1990, 1992; Edwards, 1995; Von Bremen, 1990). Progress at one level of the hierarchy facilitates change at the other levels (success breeds success), even for more complex targets. It is impossible to say at the outset what will be the most successful early target for a given child. By covering the entire phonological system in the goal proposal, each child has the best chance for success.

Independence (Autonomy) of Phonological Units

The third major concept underlying goal and target selection is the autonomy of phonological units. Although linked together in the phonological hierarchy, each unit has its own set of possible phonological operations or patterns. An example of feature autonomy is the migration of a single feature from one syllable position to another. To illustrate, if a child has two strong constraints, a negative one prohibiting final consonants and a positive one promoting survival of the feature [Labial], words such as *sleeve* and *time* are problematic. How can [Labial] survive if the final /v/ or /m/ are impossible? [Labial] can migrate elsewhere in the word, leaving a blank final position: thus, the pronunciations might be [fli] for *sleeve* and [paɪ] for *time*.

What does this notion of phonological independence imply for goal and target selection? First, goals can be set for various levels of the system, as noted previously. In addition, autonomy suggests the potential for scaffolding support from level to level. While targeting a new form at one level, it may be advantageous to use existing form at other levels. When targeting C2 of CVC, for example, existing segments from C1 can be used to create C2. This scaffolding approach has been demonstrated to be effective (Bernhardt, 1990, 1992; Bernhardt & Gilbert, 1992, Major & Bernhardt, 1998; Von Bremen, 1990). This is not to say that goals cannot be doubled up (new structures, new features), but such an approach assumes that all other factors are positive, as discussed below.

SELECTING GOALS AND TARGETS: CONSIDERING THE WHOLE PERSON

A phonological analysis provides a picture of a child's phonological production from the feature to the phrase, but it does not define the goals and targets for treatment. Certain structures, segments, and features may be seen as developmental concerns; other forms may be identified that are strengths of the system. However, the identification of concerns is not the identification of goals and targets. That determination requires integration of other information about the child into the selection process.

Among the possible targets, the main argument in the literature at the current time is whether targets should be chosen on a developmental basis or on the basis of markedness. Evidence from some researchers (Barlow & Gierut, 1999; Gierut, 1998) suggests that more marked (severely constrained) forms may be the optimal targets because their mastery will facilitate the mastery of less marked targets. Other researchers have found evidence to support the selection of goals based on a developmental sequence (e.g., Rvachew & Nowak, 2001) or on the child's own system (see Chapter 9). The latter view is more consistent with the process of goal and target selection presented in this chapter. In addition, information gleaned during assessment about the child's cognitive, motor, perceptual, and language abilities, and personal and social contexts, is taken into account in the goal selection process described here. A systematic approach to decision making still eludes us in this regard; clinical process remains an art (but see McLeod & Bleile, 2004, for a more systematic approach to the WHO, 2001, model of functioning and its implications for assessment and goal setting).

In this section, the importance of contextual factors in goal and target selection is highlighted through case illustrations. These particular examples highlight the importance of considering a child's other cognitive and linguistic abilities, personal-social factors, and oral mechanism function and structure. Other major factors that need to be taken into account (but are not exemplified here) are literacy needs, perception, voice, and fluency.

Cognitive-Linguistic Factors

How do cognitive and linguistic abilities interact with goal and target selection? On the one hand, if a child has minimal use of language and/or a cognitive impairment, it may be important in early word development to promote the defaults of the phonological system rather than the nondefaults. By keeping demands low for phonology, the child may have more resources to use for semantic and syntactic learning. Certainly, children at the one- or two-word stage of development tend to have few nondefault features and structures (Bernhardt & Stemberger, 1998). Developmental choice of goals and targets appears appropriate in this case. In older children with language impairment and limitations in working memory or attention, it may also be necessary to choose goals, targets, and strategies that do not overtax the lexical or syntactic systems when addressing phonology (Baker & Bernhardt, 2004).

What can we expect, however, from someone with high ability in cognition and language? Can we choose goals solely based on the phonology, targeting challenging nondefaults, for example, clusters with /s/, when no fricatives or final consonants are produced? This did appear to be effective and efficient for Dylan, a 4-year-old with a moderately severe phonological impairment (described in detail in Bernhardt & Stemberger, 1998, 2000). Dylan showed needs at many levels of the hierarchy, from word structure (multisyllabic words, CVC, CVCV) to segments and features (fricatives, liquids), to sequences (Coronal–Labial). In the first period, goals included the developmentally early word shapes CVC and CVCV, targeted with existing stops, nasals, and glides, and the later-developing manner categories of fricatives and liquids. To teach fricatives, two later-developing targets were selected: /v/ and /s/. The /v/ (with three nondefault features) was targeted in the existing syllable shapes CV and CV/m/; /s/ (with one nondefault feature) was targeted in the syllable shape CCV. Although CCV was in the system in stop–glide sequences, /s/-stop sequences differ in sonority sequence, and thus, the CCV was only a weak scaffold for the /s/-stop cluster. Progress was rapid for all targets, with fricatives showing fast generalization to other members of the fricative category and across word positions. Coronal–labial sequences appeared spontaneously.

Why did this child progress so quickly? His cognitive and language skills were strong, meaning that phonological learning could proceed unimpeded by constraints in other language systems. He had no perceptual or oral-motor considerations. In addition, some of his phonological awareness skills were well developed (segmentation, sound–symbol correspondence). Dylan's rapid progress may have reflected the goal and target selection based on the constraints-based nonlinear phonological theories. His results appear to support the selection of targets at different levels of the phonological system and at different levels of development for the first intervention period (early developing CVC, CVCV versus later developing fricatives and liquids). It also appeared efficacious to use existing forms at one level of the system, to support learning at other levels, and to target more than one element per category. In addition, Dylan's strong cognitive and language skills may have also helped him move quickly through a set of phonological targets. Furthermore, he had other predisposing factors for change. His parents reported that he liked to be a leader at preschool and was finding his leadership slipping because his peers did not understand him very well. Thus, he was motivated to change. He also enjoyed speech therapy and eagerly participated in practice activities, both in the clinic and at home. The importance of such personal-social factors for outcomes and for goal and target selection is discussed in the next section.

Personal-Social Factors

Unlike Dylan, two other children with similar profiles in terms of cognitive, linguistic, perceptual, and oral-motor abilities and good home support did not show this kind of rapid change (Brandy, age 3; Bill, age 5). At assessment, factors other than phonology appeared positive for both of these children; thus, challenging nondefaults were targeted (i.e., word-initial clusters rather than singletons). After the first 8 weeks of treatment, neither child showed any changes in spontaneous speech, even though they could articulate their various cluster targets within words during treatment sessions.

Considering the children's general abilities, and in comparison with other children in the nonlinear intervention studies, this was considered insufficient progress. Thus, for the second block of treatment, less challenging targets were selected. For Bill, voiceless initial stops were second-block targets (he used [h] for all word-initial consonants except liquids and voiced stops, plus he showed deletions in other word positions). For Brandy, word-initial stops were targeted in stop–nasal sequences (CVCV, then CVC), in order to eliminate regressive nasal assimilation (e.g., *ten* as [nɛn]). Treatment frequency was also increased (six to seven sessions per month instead of four). Both children showed immediate success after changes were made in targets and session frequency. In fact, Bill showed mastery of the phonological system within 3 months. Brandy did not show immediate mastery of the subsequent goal (velars); thus, the increase in treatment frequency was not solely responsible for change, at least in her case.

In hindsight, personal-social factors appeared relevant for goal and target selection. At assessment, both Brandy and Bill appeared to have very positive personal-social attributes. However, after a few treatment sessions, it appeared that neither was highly motivated to change. Although Bill was highly unintelligible, he was a leader in his kindergarten peer group and claimed that his friends already understood him. He enjoyed practicing the activities in clinic and at home but showed no changes in conversational speech until the developmentally earlier, voiceless initial stops were targeted, and treatment frequency was increased. Brandy, unlike Bill, was not confident about her speech; she was quiet at preschool, and although she would attempt the challenging targets in treatment and could produce them in words, she was somewhat reluctant to do so, appeared embarrassed about her speech, and was reluctant to practice at home. Once the easier targets were presented in therapy, both children mastered them immediately, used them in conversation, and went on to attempt other, more challenging targets with their confidence bolstered.

Negative personal-social factors (such as lack of motivation and confidence) can be barriers to change. It is difficult to assess such nebulous constructs in one or two assessment sessions. If change does not occur within a reasonable time period and all other factors appear positive, the goals of intervention may need to include enhancement of motivation and confidence. One way to do that is to choose phonological targets that are more easily attainable.

Other Factors, with a Note on Articulatory Competency

Many other personal and contextual factors are relevant for goal and target selection. Space prohibits a detailed discussion of all of them. Note, however, that if a child misperceives a particular contrast, it may be important to target the perceptual contrast directly, before or during production training (Rvachew, 1994). If a child shows limitations in phonological awareness, it is important to target those areas directly when the desired improvement in awareness does not occur as a result of phonological intervention (Bernhardt & Major, in press; Major & Bernhardt, 1998). Children with deficits in language comprehension and production generally need direct attention to those areas. Some children do gain rapidly in morphosyntax as a result of phonological intervention (Bernhardt & Bopp, 1996), although Tyler, Lewis, Haskill, and Tolbert (2002) have noted that approaches that alternate morphosyntactic and phonological goals may be more effective across a wider range of children.

Finally, in terms of other factors, the issue of articulatory competency (structure and function) is discussed with respect to goal and target selection. In the following examples, targets were selected based solely on phonological theory. However, articulatory considerations may have been relevant in the positive outcomes.

Two 6-year-olds (Charles and Gordon) had interdental fricative substitutions for all coronal fricatives and affricates (see Bernhardt, 1992, and Bernhardt & Stemberger, 1998, 2000, for details about Charles, and Bernhardt & Stemberger, 1998, 2000, for details about Gordon). The interdental tongue position was their default place of articulation for coronal sibilants. In terms of articulatory abilities, both boys had difficulty producing a tongue groove, a necessary feature of alveolar and palatoalveolar sibilants. Tongue grooving for sibilants was thus a general goal ([+grooved] or, alternatively, [+strident]). None of the segments was stimulable at assessment. The targets selected to achieve the goal were the nondefault [–anterior] grooved palatoalveolars /ʃ/ and /dʒ/, in accordance with implications of constraints-based nonlinear theory. The [–anterior] place of the palatoalveolars was considered a more distinct and distant phonological contrast with interdentals than the [+anterior] place for /s/ and /z/ (which is actually shared by the interdentals). The boys acquired the palatoalveolars, and, through generalization, gained the ability to produce /s/ and /z/ without dentalization. The results suggest support for an approach that targets nondefault features in this context.

Looking further, there may be more than a phonological interpretation. The oral mechanism assessment indicated that both boys had tongue coordination difficulties and a tongue thrust during swallowing. The tongue groove for the palatoalveolar sibilants is broader than that for the alveolars and is at the region of the tongue blade rather than the tongue tip (use of which is crucial for the alveolar sibilants); thus, the palatoalveolars may be easier to produce than /s/ and /z/, which require control of the tongue tip.

The probable congruence between articulatory ease and phonological contrast was fortuitous in the above cases for the palatoalveolars. In other cases, phonological needs and articulatory ease may conflict. For example, the phonology might identify certain targets, but the child might lack the oral structures or the motor implementation abilities to produce these targets due to orofacial anomalies or lags in articulatory development. Thus, conflict could occur between phonological needs and potential for change, without additional strategies to address the oral structure and function relative to the specific targets (e.g., surgery, dental appliances, visual feedback in speech habilitation, allowance of time for physical growth and motor development). Articulation and phonology are not mutually exclusive categories; speech is a motor activity, but it requires representation and processing. Phonological and articulatory competencies and needs must necessarily be considered together in assessment and treatment.

SUMMARY

If all factors converge positively, the goals and targets of phonological intervention can be achieved in a timely fashion. Constraints-based nonlinear phonological analyses identify the child's various needs and strengths at various levels of the phonological hierarchy. In the optimal case, nondefault, marked (often later developing) forms at the various levels are preferred goals and targets, and scaffolds can be found within the child's system to assist learning of the new forms. Progress may be limited, though, unless attention is paid to other critical factors about the child during goal selection: cognitive-linguistic, personal-social, perceptual, and articulatory. These other factors may suggest less marked, developmentally incremental goals and targets, or the need to include goals for vowels, prosody, perception, or phonological awareness. The future is always uncertain; there are constraints on our ability to predict what will happen. Nevertheless, a comprehensive approach to goal and target selection has the potential to change a child's constraint rankings in a positive direction.

REFERENCES

Baker, E., & Bernhardt, B. (2004). From hindsight to foresight: Working around barriers to success in phonological intervention. *Child Language Teaching and Therapy, 20,* 287–318.

Barlow, J., & Gierut, J. (1999). Optimality theory in phonological acquisition. *Journal of Speech, Language, & Hearing Research, 42,* 1482–1498.

Bernhardt, B. (1990). *Application of nonlinear phonological theory to intervention with six phonologically disordered children.* Unpublished doctoral dissertation, University of British Columbia, Vancouver.

Bernhardt, B. (1992). The application of nonlinear phonological theory to intervention with one phonologically disordered child. *Clinical Linguistics & Phonetics, 6,* 283–316.

Bernhardt, B., & Bopp, K. (1996, November). Cost-effective treatment: Language production improvement through phonological intervention. Poster presented at the ASHA Convention, Seattle, WA, *ASHA Abstracts,* 76.

Bernhardt, B., & Gilbert, J.H. (1992). Applying linguistic theory to speech-language pathology: The case for nonlinear phonology. *Clinical Linguistics & Phonetics, 6,* 123–145.

Bernhardt, B., & Major, E. (in press). Speech, language and literacy skills three years later: Long-term outcomes of early phonological and metaphonological intervention. *International Journal of Language and Communication Disorders.*

Bernhardt, B.H., & Stemberger, J.P. (1998). *Handbook of phonological development from the perspective of constraint-based nonlinear phonology.* San Diego: Academic Press.

Bernhardt, B.H., & Stemberger, J.P. (2000). *Workbook in nonlinear phonology for clinical application.* Austin, TX: PRO-ED.

Edwards, S.M. (1995). *Optimal outcomes of nonlinear phonological intervention.* Unpublished master's thesis, University of British Columbia, Vancouver.

Gierut, J.A. (1998). Treatment efficacy: Functional phonological disorders in children. *Journal of Speech, Language, and Hearing Research, 41,* S85–S100.

Major, E.M., & Bernhardt, B. (1998). Metaphonological skills of children with phonological disorders before and after phonological and metaphonological intervention. *International Journal of Language and Communication Disorders, 33,* 413–444.

Masterson, J., & Bernhardt, B. (2001). *Computerised articulation and phonology evaluation system.* San Antonio, TX: Harcourt Assessment.

McLeod, S., & Bleile, K. (2004). Integrating goal setting with children with speech impairment. *Child Language Teaching and Therapy, 20,* 199–219.

Rvachew, S. (1994). Speech perception training can facilitate sound production learning. *Journal of Speech and Hearing Research, 37,* 347–357.

Rvachew, S., & Nowak, M. (2001). The effect of target selection strategy on phonological learning. *Journal of Speech, Language, and Hearing Research, 44,* 610–623.

Tyler, A., Lewis, K., Haskill, A., & Tolbert, L. (2002). Efficacy and across-domain effects of phonological and morphosyntactic interventions. *Language, Speech, and Hearing Services in Schools, 33,* 52–66.

Von Bremen, V. (1990). *A nonlinear phonological approach to intervention with severely phonologically disordered twins.* Unpublished master's thesis, University of British Columbia, Vancouver.

World Health Organization. (2001). *ICF: International classification of functioning, disability and health.* Geneva: Author.

Part III

Intervention

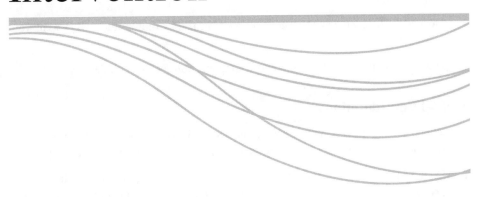

For Part III, on intervention, we were interested to discover how contributors structured intervention programs, the techniques and materials they used, and how they might modify their interventions for developmental level, severity of the disorder (e.g., developmental apraxia of speech), and language or dialect spoken. The specific questions posed to contributors are shown here.

Structure of Intervention Programs

1. When should a child receive individual therapy as opposed to group therapy?

2. How do you determine when a child needs direct phonological intervention and when they need more general language stimulation?

3. To what extent do you include parents in therapy?

4. Are there certain types of therapy that can be conducted through a collaborative classroom model?

5. How often do you need to see a child to make progress?

6. How do you monitor progress?

7. What do you do when your intervention plan is not working?

8. When do you dismiss a child from services?

Intervention Techniques and Materials

1. There are many published/packaged programs available today for phonological intervention. Which, if any, of these do you use, and how do you adapt or modify them?

2. What specific intervention techniques do you find most useful?

3. What types of materials (e.g., word lists, picture sets, toys, computer programs) do you recommend?

4. Do you include perceptual (auditory) training and/or oral-motor exercises in your intervention? If so, when?

5. How do you integrate language and communication into speech therapy?

Special Considerations

1. Which special procedures and/or techniques would you recommend for articulation/ phonological intervention with children of different ages or developmental levels?

2. Do you recommend specific approaches for different subgroups of children? For example, if you differentiate between articulation disorders, phonological disorders, and/or developmental apraxia of speech, how does your intervention approach differ?

3. How would intervention differ for a child who speaks a different language or a nonstandard English dialect at home?

Part III consists of seven chapters on intervention. Chapter 11 (by Ann A. Tyler) and Chapter 12 (by Paul R. Hoffman and Janet A. Norris) address the first two sets of questions. Although their approaches are vastly different, both provide excellent discussions of service delivery choices and other structural and/or programmatic considerations. Tyler describes a hybrid approach to intervention for children with co-occurring speech and language impairments. Hoffman and Norris focus on play, daily routines, and storybook reading activities designed to facilitate the child's refinement and reorganization of his or her neuro-network. In Chapter 13, Shelley Velleman considers the third set of questions, describing special considerations in the treatment of specific groups, including children with childhood apraxia of speech and children who speak other languages or nonmain-stream English dialects.

The remaining four chapters in Part III present specific approaches to phonological intervention and in doing so address many of the questions in the first and second categories (program structure and materials/techniques). Adele W. Miccio (Chapter 14) presents a program designed to enhance stimulability, Susan Rvachew (Chapter 15) outlines a three-phase program utilizing computer-based activities, A. Lynn Williams (Chapter 16) describes her systemic (multiple oppositions) approach, and Judith A. Gierut (Chapter 17) provides an overview of her complexity-based approach.

Chapter 11

Planning and Monitoring Intervention Programs

ANN A. TYLER

W hen faced with planning and monitoring intervention programs, speech-language professionals must consider numerous variables in decision making. The structure of intervention programs is influenced by variables such as the focus of therapy, service delivery model, inclusion of parents, frequency of sessions, and criteria for monitoring progress and dismissal—elements about which we have limited efficacy data. In contrast, considerable efficacy data suggest that a variety of different intervention approaches can be used to successfully improve a child's sound system. Furthermore, myriad techniques and materials are available. These elements are discussed in the sections that follow.

FOCUS OF THERAPY: PHONOLOGY OR LANGUAGE?

The focus of therapy, whether it is directly on phonology or more generally on language, is one of the first clinical decisions that must be made. Tyler (2002) discussed language-based intervention for phonological disorders and considered which children are appropriate candidates for a language-based approach. Children diagnosed with phonological disorders often display difficulties in other domains of language and are at risk for academic problems. Estimates of the co-occurrence of phonological and language deficits average approximately 60% in clinical samples of children with speech and/or language impairments (Shriberg & Austin, 1998). In addition, one of the largest subgroups of children identified with language impairment has both phonological and morphosyntactic deficits (Rapin & Allen, 1983, 1988). Clearly, language-based approaches seem to be most appropriate for this subgroup of children with both speech and language (morphosyntactic) impairments.

Research in the area of cross-domain effects of language interventions on phonology, however, is inconclusive and suggests that not all children will make gains in phonology as a result of language intervention. Fey, Cleave, Ravida, Long, Dejmal, and Easton (1994), for example, found that 25 children who received a 5-month focused-stimulation language intervention did not improve their phonology, as measured by percent consonants correct (PCC; Shriberg & Kwiatkowski, 1982b), despite large gains made in grammar. In contrast, Tyler, Lewis, Haskill, and Tolbert (2002) investigated the cross-domain effects of both a morphosyntax and a phonology intervention and found that the morphosyntax intervention led to gains in phonology that were similar to those achieved by the phonology intervention. The morphosyntax intervention addressed primarily finite morphemes that mark tense and agreement because these have been shown to be especially problematic for children with speech-language impairments (Bedore & Leonard, 1998; Rice, Wexler, & Cleave, 1995; Rice, Wexler, & Hershberger, 1998). Other language interventions that focus on narrative skills and indirectly on phonology in natural conversational interactions have also been shown to be effective in facilitating phonological gains (Hoffman, Norris, & Monjure, 1990; Wilcox & Morris, 1995). The conflicting findings, especially from the two studies with larger sample sizes and control groups (Fey et al., 1994; Tyler et al., 2002), may be due to differences in intervention targets and techniques and to different outcome measures of phonological performance.

The equivocal findings regarding the effects of language interventions on change in phonological performance also suggest that individual children may respond differently to an intervention depending on the interaction of the goals with their phonological-morphosyntactic systems as well as with each child's unique characteristics. The question then becomes, "For which specific children with both speech and language impairments will a language-based intervention be effective in changing phonology?" Tyler (2002) suggested that children whose systems show greater inconsistency in the use of *all* phonemes, as well as greater severity, as measured by pretreatment PCC, may be most likely to demonstrate gains from a morphosyntactic intervention such as one that focuses on finite morphemes (Haskill, Tyler, & Tolbert, 2001). This remains to be tested empirically; however, it is possible that language-based intervention is effective for children with highly inconsistent phonological errors because it provides exposure to all phonemes across positions in the context of conversational speech and thus offers more varied stimuli than a phonological approach that focuses only on specific phonemes.

In addition to considering severity (as measured by PCC) and inconsistency of errors, it is vitally important to consider the phonological error patterns and their interaction with morphology in determining which children would benefit from a language-based approach. When children have phonological error patterns such as final consonant deletion and/or cluster reduction, these errors may prevent accurate production of grammatical morphemes. Research has shown that elimination of such error patterns should lead to improvement in grammatical morphemes involving the critical morphophonemic alternations (Fey & Stalker, 1986; Tyler & Sandoval, 1994). Thus, if a child's morphological problem appears to be due to phonological factors, phonological and not language-based intervention would be the choice.

In addition to certain children with both phonology and language impairments, other children with concomitant impairments may be appropriate candidates for language-based intervention. Children with phonological impairments and fluency concerns and children with phonological impairments and cognitive limitations both may benefit from a language-based approach because of its lack of direct attention to the production of speech sounds (Conture, Louko, & Edwards, 1993).

Thus, to summarize the decision-making process with regard to whether a child needs direct phonological intervention or a language-based approach, the following questions must be considered:

1. Does the child have both phonological and expressive (or, less often, receptive) language difficulties?

2. If the child has both phonological and expressive (or receptive) language difficulties, is there interaction between the child's phonological error patterns and the morphological system?

3. If both phonology and expressive language are impaired, how severe is the child's phonological disorder and how inconsistent are errors for all phonemes?

4. Does the child have a phonological disorder and other concomitant deficits such as fluency concerns or cognitive limitations?

SERVICE DELIVERY MODEL

When structuring intervention programs, decisions must be made about service delivery models with respect to whether the intervention is provided through the traditional pull-out model, in the classroom, or through collaborative consultation. The intervention can also be provided individually or in a group. In addition, the role of parents in the intervention program must be evaluated.

The decision regarding service delivery model is inherently related to the focus and directness of the intervention procedures. If, on the one hand, a drill-play activity focused on target phonemes is selected, for example, the collaborative consultation model would be a less likely choice due to the time-intensive training of the teacher that would be necessary. On the other hand, if a naturalistic intervention focused on multiple phonemes is selected, the collaborative consultation model is a good candidate because the intervention can be accomplished in naturalistic communicative contexts by using frequent models and recasts and no direct elicitations or reinforcement. The speech-language pathologist (SLP) and teacher can assess the language arts curriculum and select activities in which target sounds can be modeled and recast. In addition, the SLP could provide materials and activities designed around target sounds. The collaborative consultative model lends itself particularly well to language-based intervention approaches that involve auditory awareness activities, focused stimulation, and conversational interactions.

The choice of service delivery model may also depend on where in the training sequence an individual child is working. If a child is working on carryover in conversational speech, a classroom setting may provide communication opportunities within the ideal intervention location. In contrast, a child who is just beginning therapy and has numerous sounds that are nonstimulable may benefit most from the pull-out model. Ideally, an SLP will have a continuum of service delivery models to choose from precisely because different individual clients will lend themselves better to one model or another.

Another important aspect of service delivery is whether intervention should be conducted in an individual or group setting. Data from the National Outcomes Measurement System (NOMS) implemented by the American Speech-Language-Hearing Association (ASHA, 2002) suggest that when preschoolers received individual therapy they showed greater articulation progress as compared with those who received group therapy. This was the case when progress was scored on functional communication measures (FCMs) for articulation only. When children with articulation problems were also scored on other FCMs, there was no longer an effect of service delivery model on articulation progress. It is likely that the greater progress achieved in the individual model is related to the SLP's ability to focus on the unique aspects of an individual child's phonological system, rather than having to sacrifice the choice of goals for those of other children in a group. Furthermore, some evidence indicates that group treatment needs to be conducted for a longer time to achieve results similar to those of individual treatment.

The role that parents should play in the intervention process is another aspect of service delivery. Parents can be intervention agents, assisted through a collaborative model, or they may be instructed to provide a structured home program that augments the SLP's direct intervention.

Research indicates that parents as intervention agents facilitate significant improvement in their children's speech production skills as compared with skills attained when their children received no intervention, as well as with those of a no-treatment control group (Broen & Westman, 1990). In this parent training program, called Project Parent, parents were taught both what to teach and how to teach in weekly parent classes that involved group discussion as well as individual parent–child time with a clinician. Evidence also indicates that enlisting parents' support with a structured home program facilitates additional change in speech production skills. NOMS data indicate that the percentage of children making functional changes is at least doubled when they participate in a structured home program. An even greater percentage of children showed multiple levels of progress on articulation FCMs when they completed a structured home program as compared with when they did not have a program or did not complete the program provided for them (ASHA, 2002).

For most families, we ask that they participate in a home program that consists of primarily naturalistic activities. At a minimum, we recommend that parents provide auditory stimulation for target sounds through modeling. We recommend that parents read books that we have selected for target sounds because they provide alliteration or rhyming patterns involving those target sounds. We also recommend that parents provide recasts of the child's incorrect productions of target sounds during normal conversation, in the form of a single-word response. If parents desire to do more and seem able to do so, we suggest simple, naturalistic activities in which parents can model target sounds but children are not expected to repeat or practice correct productions. Parents and child could play with play-dough, for example, pretending to be a che*f* and to flu*ff*, stu*ff*, and pu*ff* the dough when the target sound is a final /f/. We typically do not recommend that parents drill the child or teach target sound productions until a child has achieved correct productions at the single-word level in treatment. At that point, parents may be provided with stimulus picture cards to review with the child once per day before the next scheduled session.

The frequency, or the intensity, of service delivery must also be considered. Limited data are available with regard to the optimal number of sessions per week needed to make a reasonable amount of progress. Not surprisingly, NOMS data suggest that more treatment time, especially in individual sessions, is associated with a greater proportion of children showing functional gains. Ideally, I try to schedule intervention sessions twice a week for 45 minutes to 1 hour. For the first 6–8 months of an intervention program, it seems that optimal progress is made if sessions occur at least twice weekly. After some marked changes are made in a child's phonological system, it may be possible to decrease the frequency of sessions to once a week, particularly if there is an accompanying home program. If caseload size dictates that children must be grouped, I prefer to see children for one group session but keep one individual session. NOMS data further suggest that more individual treatment time, in combination with successful completion of a structured home program, contributes to a greater percentage of children making progress in articulation outcome measures (ASHA, 2002).

INTERVENTION TECHNIQUES AND MATERIALS

Although numerous published phonological intervention programs are currently available, I use few of them and even then I adapt and modify them from their intended usage. Stimulus picture cards, for example, sometimes in the form of minimal pairs, are often necessary and the following are programs from which I may select some: *Contrast Pairs for Phonological Training* (Palin, 1992); *Contrasts: The Use of Minimal Pairs in Articulation Training* (Elbert, Rockman, & Saltzman, 1980); *SPARC for Phonology* (Thomsen & Donnelly, 2000); and *Metaphon Resource Pack* (Dean, Howell, Hill, & Waters, 1990).

One difficulty with published contrast materials is that the sounds selected for contrasting an error and target may not be those on which a particular child needs to work. The published contrast pair may be, for example, initial /t/ versus /s/, but the child substitutes /j/ for /s/ and thus needs pairs that contrast these initial sounds. In addition, most published picture materials do not represent contrasts involving multiple oppositions or maximal oppositions, with sounds differing by major class (Barlow & Gierut, 2002; Gierut, 1989, 1990; Williams, 2000). Thus, it is often necessary to generate one's own word list and then search for the appropriate stimulus pictures, and most published materials are less than optimal.

There are, however, several resource manuals for incorporating literature and naturalistic activities in phonological intervention that I find useful. *Phonogroup* (Kelman & Edwards, 1994), for example, provides naturalistic activities designed for the remediation of common phonological processes, along with probe lists and stimulus materials. The activities and procedures are succinctly described and easy to implement. *Once Upon a Sound* (Smith-Kiewel & Claeys, 1998) is another resource that incorporates children's literature and songs and provides home practice suggestions for common target sounds. *Phonobuilding* (Vicino & Wenger, 1993) is a manual of stories with pictographs designed to target a variety of phonological patterns in a cycles approach.

I find a variety of techniques most useful in phonological remediation and classify them broadly as those oriented toward perception or production. From research on normal phonological acquisition, we have come to recognize that children acquire phonological oppositions gradually, primarily through an auditory-perceptual based process, supported by the early use of vocal motor schemes and subsequent refinement of articulatory gestures. Children with phonological disorders may encounter difficulties at peripheral auditory or articulatory levels, as well as at a higher organizational level. It is important, therefore, to provide these children with auditory-perceptual information regarding the target contrasts, articulatory practice, and information regarding the organization and function of sounds in the ambient language. Linguistic approaches to phonological intervention that have flourished in the past emphasize the function of the phonological system to support communication and, thus, the pragmatic limitations of unintelligible speech. They also tend to focus on the contrastive nature of phonemes and the use of contrast training to facilitate reorganization of the system.

As part of a large project investigating different goal attack strategies for sequencing both phonological and morphosyntactic goals in children with co-occurring speech and language impairments (Tyler, Lewis, Haskill, & Tolbert, 2003), my colleagues and I developed phonological intervention procedures that represent a combination of auditory-perceptual, production oriented, and organizational features that we had used successfully over the years. The intervention is "hybrid" because it involves a combination of activities that are child-centered, or more naturalistic, and clinician-directed, or more direct. The four components to the intervention are listed here:

1. Auditory awareness activities designed to heighten children's awareness of target sounds and direct their attention to the auditory-acoustic attributes of the sounds

2. Conceptual activities designed to develop children's awareness of the differences and similarities between target sounds and their contrasts

3. Production practice activities, both drill-play (i.e., drills in the context of games) and naturalistic, that are designed to help establish production of a new sound, to facilitate practice of that sound in communicative contexts, and to increase awareness of the success/failure in communicating an intended message

4. Phonological awareness activities designed to stimulate preliteracy skills by increasing children's awareness of the speech sound system.

Each of these components is described in more detail and examples are provided in the sections that follow.

Perceptual and Conceptual Focused Activities

Auditory awareness activities require that a child listen to auditory material that has a high frequency of models of the target sound. For example, a target sound may be highlighted by simply reading a list of words containing that sound in the relevant position while the child is engaged in a quiet activity such as coloring (Hodson & Paden, 1991). Auditory awareness activities in our intervention involve reading a book containing a high frequency of exemplars of the target sound, as well as target sound identification and discrimination. My colleagues and I developed a list of children's literature for a variety of target sounds and begin sessions by reading the book for the target sound to be focused on in the session. Next, to introduce children to the target sound and illustrate the sound, pictureable items are used to represent each sound. The book *Four Famished Foxes and Fosdyke* (Edwards, 1995), for example, is used to provide auditory bombardment for the target initial /f/, and the sound is represented as the "fan" sound. The SLP produces the target while pointing to a picture of a fan and asks the children to name the sound and name the letter that represents the sound. In addition, the major perceptual feature differentiating the sound from its error replacement is described. For example, the fan sound is long and air keeps coming out. In a sound discrimination task, children are instructed to listen to a list of sounds produced in isolation and to identify when they hear the target sound by dropping a block in a can that is labeled with the picture representing the sound. The child should achieve approximately 80% correct identification of the six target sounds randomized among 15 sounds in the list that differ by major class features from the target.

Conceptual activities are designed to develop children's awareness of the differences and similarities between target sounds and their contrasts. Activities used in Metaphon (Howell & Dean, 1994), for example, focus on helping children establish vocabulary to talk about sounds and to explore the differences between their productions and the target sounds. Activities of this type begin by translating phonological terms into child-centered vocabulary; for example, long and short are used to contrast fricatives and stops, respectively. Next, these concepts are extended to discussion about nonspeech elements and finally to discussion about the relevant target and error contrast. Children might first glue long and short hair on paper dolls. Next the SLP and child might take turns being speaker and listener and experiment with making long and short sounds as directed by cue cards that are drawn from a pile of pictures representing long and short objects. Finally, children may be required to listen to sounds in the two contrasting categories in isolation or in words, to reflect on what is heard, and to classify the SLP's productions as long or short.

Production Focused Activities

In our intervention program, production practice activities take two forms: drill play and naturalistic. Responses are thus elicited from the children in clinician-directed activities or recast and re-embedded in naturalistic activities that involve environmental manipulation of materials and input. Initially, a target sound may need to be established in the child's system through more traditional phonetic placement, shaping, and auditory–visual–tactile cueing techniques. Depending on the child's level of accuracy with the sound, activities graduate in difficulty from production of the sound in isolation to syllables, words, sentences, and conversational speech. Some children may need to begin training with nonsense syllables, which can be represented by made-up characters. For many children, careful selection of stimulus words will facilitate correct production of the target sound at the word level, and activities can begin with word imitation. Care should be taken to choose stimulus words that contain the target sound in the position being trained but that also contain sounds that the child produces correctly in other word positions. Facilitory vowel contexts and simple syllable structure should also be considered in constructing stimulus words. When the child correctly produces the target sound, then his or her entire word production matches the adult target and communication has been successful.

The elicitation of imitated and, subsequently, of spontaneous productions of target sounds can take place in a variety of drill-play activities (i.e., drills in the context of games) that lend themselves to a model/imitation format. Some examples of such activities are feeding picture cards to a clown or puppet; playing hide and seek with picture cards or objects in the room; or shopping for items in a store, which are named as they are bought, bagged, and unpacked. Shriberg and Kwiatkowski (1982a) found that drill-play activities were preferred by SLPs and were more effective in comparison with less structured play-based activities. Our goal would be to elicit 24–32 productions, using 8–10 stimulus words, in approximately a half hour of therapy.

During drill-play activities designed to elicit imitative and spontaneous productions of target sounds in words, the SLP should provide auditory, tactile, or visual cues that are necessary to help the child achieve a correct production. To elicit /s/ clusters, for example, the SLP may provide the tactile cue of running her finger down the child's arm during the production of /s/ and tapping on the wrist at the segmentation for the remainder of the word. If the child is working on eliminating the error pattern of initial voicing, the SLP should manipulate her auditory model by prolonging the aspiration phase of voiceless stop targets. The child should be reinforced not only for correct target sound productions but also for responses that are close, because they involve suppression of the target error pattern, although the sound may not be the targeted one. When the child is working on final /f/ to eliminate the error pattern of stopping and produces a bilabial fricative, for example, the SLP can respond positively by saying, "I heard a long air sound at the end." Such close-to-target productions should be followed by a correct model of the target.

If a child's targets involve syllable or word structure—such as onsets, rhymes or codas—or stress and the number of syllables in a word, chaining techniques described by Bernhardt (1994) are particularly useful. For example, if a child does not produce a consonant in the final position but does so in the initial position, it can be introduced to the opposite part of the syllable through sequences of alternating syllables. In singing "Little Bunny Foofoo" the sequence of *foofoo* can be repeated until the /u/ is prolonged and followed by a final /f/ for *oof*. In general, activities that highlight the rhyme through rhyming, or the initial consonant through alliteration, are useful when focusing on syllable structure and the addition of codas or onsets, respectively.

We have also incorporated a naturalistic activity within each session and find it particularly useful for children who will not readily imitate words in a drill-play format. Naturalistic intervention for speech sound disorders is accomplished within natural conversational interactions by using excessive models and recasts, few direct elicitations, and no direct reinforcement, while at the same time providing opportunities for verbal interaction. Some of the models provided should take the form of "recasts" of the child's prior production at just the single-word level, when the opportunity arises. In addition to modeling, the following methods can be used to encourage productions: 1) giving children an opportunity to make a choice, when both choices involve target words; or 2) producing lexical errors for target words, thus providing children an opportunity to correct your "error"; and 3) constructing activities so that children must name the target to achieve the stated goal of the activity. Activities are usually designed around a theme and a group of stimulus words containing the target sound; art, snack, or dramatic play activities can all be designed to provide increased numbers of models of targets and opportunities for the child's productions. Naturalistic activities are particularly well-suited for groups because responses are not explicitly required, but children can be given the opportunity to produce targets and their productions can be recast and re-embedded in the conversational context.

Minimal Pairs

Minimal pair contrasting is a technique often associated with phonological intervention approaches because it highlights the semantic confusion caused when the child produces a sound error that results in a pair of homonyms (e.g., both *fin* and *tin* produced as [tɪn]). Traditionally, this minimal pair technique involves contrasting a pair of words that have phonemes differing by one feature, such that one word contains the child's error sound and the other contains the target. The goal of this technique is to help the child recognize that the target sound is required to signal a difference in meaning between the two words that he or she produces similarly. In many minimal pair approaches, the child is instructed to make both perceptual and productive contrasts involving the target and error sounds.

We have found minimal pairs are a useful technique only at a specific point in the treatment hierarchy. That point is when the child can achieve some accurate productions of the target sound in words with a model but is not yet able to produce the sound spontaneously in single words. We have found that a child is not ready for minimal pair activities until he or she has achieved approximately 40% accuracy for target sound productions in words after a model. If a child is unable to produce the target sound in words and the SLP presents the child with a semantic confusion resulting from the error, the child is likely to experience frustration and failure because he or she is unable to correct the production to disambiguate the message.

We have also found that it is important to plan minimal pair activities so that the child must produce the word in the pair containing the target sound but not necessarily the word containing the error; the child can already produce the error. It is more important that the child attempt to produce the minimal pair word with the target and be faced with the confusion resulting from a homonymous production if he or she makes an error. Thus, an example of a minimal pair activity would be "Go Fish" in which a child is dealt picture cards representing *only* words containing the target sound and the SLP has cards representing both minimal pair words. The child is instructed to ask for cards to match those in his hand and form pairs. If the child produces the target sound in the word, he receives the card that matches; however, if he produces the error sound, he will receive the card representing the minimal contrast and will not be able to form a pair until he corrects the production. Once the child understands that his incorrect production causes communicative confusion and is able to correct the production, minimal pair activities quickly facilitate increased accuracy of target sound productions. This, in turn, often leads to correct spontaneous word productions. When the child can accurately produce the target sound in words and is beginning to generalize productions to more complex contexts, minimal pair activities are no longer useful.

Oral-Motor Exercises

I strongly advise against the use of oral-motor exercises for children with phonological-articulatory disorders for two primary reasons. First, no research base supports the premise that part–whole training will transfer to the production of speech or that speech develops from earlier oral nonspeech movements, both key rationales for the use of these exercises. Second, no efficacy data exist to show that oral-motor exercises result in improvement in speech production skills.

Many practicing SLPs use oral-motor exercises for all of their clients with phonological-articulatory difficulties on the assumption that practicing nonspeech oral movements will increase coordination and strengthen the musculature for speech production because speech movements originate in nonspeech movements. Considerable evidence shows, however, that even in as early a function as babbling, the coordinative organization of lip and jaw movement is distinct from that in nonspeech behaviors such as chewing

(Green, Moore, Higashikawa, & Steeve, 2000; Green, Moore, Ruark, Rodda, Morvee, & Van Witzenburg, 1997; Moore & Ruark, 1996; Ruark & Moore, 1997). Although the structures used in speech and nonspeech movements are similar, they differ in how they are used.

I believe that oral-motor exercises also are promoted by SLPs because there is some inherent appeal for parents and other consumers in practicing movements of the articulators because "they must not be working properly" if speech is unintelligible. Simple observation and practice of oral-motor exercises demonstrate that many have no relevance to speech. In my graduate phonological assessment and remediation class, for example, each student selected a card from the Oral-Motor Fun Deck (Super Duper Publications, 1997), demonstrated the exercise, and asked the class to decide which phoneme the exercise was designed to stimulate. We could find little resemblance to speech sound productions in exercises such as putting the tongue tip on the farthest back top tooth and then moving the tongue from tooth to tooth around the mouth; placing the tongue on the roof of the mouth while raising and lowering the jaw; and pulling lips apart from a tightly sealed position, making a smacking noise. Such exercises do not break the speech task down into smaller independent units that can later be integrated into a whole, but rather disintegrate the final target. Thus, if our goal is to improve speech production and intelligibility, we should target the correct production of speech sounds in words and conversation—we should work on speech.

Of even greater concern with respect to the use of oral-motor exercises in phonological-articulatory treatment is the lack of data showing that they are effective in improving speech production skills. Numerous anecdotal accounts exist of the effectiveness of oral-motor exercises, suggesting that their use leads to greater improvement in speech sound productions than would be obtained from an articulation-phonological approach alone. No well-controlled efficacy studies have been conducted, however, in which oral-motor exercises as a form of isolated treatment have been shown to be effective in changing phonological-articulatory behaviors. Colone and Forrest (2000) applied oral-motor treatment and phonological treatment to each of a pair of monozygotic twin boys, age 8;11. The twin receiving the oral-motor treatment showed no improvements, whereas the twin receiving phonological treatment showed positive gains. When phonological treatment was provided for the twin who initially had oral-motor treatment, gains were similar to those observed for the other twin.

In almost all anecdotal accounts, as well as a few experimental studies, oral-motor exercises are used in combination with some other type of phonological or articulation treatment. Thus, it is impossible to know what accounted for the reported gains in performance: the treatment techniques in isolation or the combination of techniques. Polmanteer and Fields (2002), for example, compared the performance of two groups, containing four children each, on the *Structured Photographic Articulation Test–Dudsberry II* (SPAT-D II; Dawson & Tattersall, 2001) after the children received either phonological-articulation therapy or phonological-articulation therapy with oral-motor therapy. Each group received 20 minutes of therapy, twice weekly, for 6 weeks; the group receiving oral-motor treatment had 10 minutes devoted to those exercises. Results suggested that children who had received the oral-motor combination treatment had fewer errors; however, these results should be interpreted with caution due to the extremely small sample size and use of parametric statistics. A further difficulty in interpreting these results stems from the combined presentation of oral-motor exercises with typical articulation therapy, underscoring the importance of separating oral-motor therapy for experimental scrutiny.

MONITORING PROGRESS, MODIFYING PLANS, AND DISMISSAL CRITERIA

My approach to monitoring treatment progress is entirely data based (Olswang & Bain, 1994). Both quantitative data (measurable behaviors) and qualitative data (subjective interpretations) are useful in evaluating change and making clinical decisions regarding whether the client is responding or how long to focus on a therapy target. Quantitative data may take the form of percent accuracy from treatment or generalization probes, or a more global measure such as PCC or an intelligibility calculation. Qualitative data may be in the form of clinical observations, parent/teacher report, client/family satisfaction surveys, or a severity rating.

First, to determine whether a child is responding to the intervention program, probes for the target sound in the trained position can be administered on a weekly or biweekly basis at the beginning of the session. The cue can be manipulated from a direct model for every stimulus to intermittent models or to indirect models. For example, if the target is initial /f/ as an exemplar to eliminate the error pattern of stopping of fricatives, the clinician may present eight to ten words used in treatment with differing levels of cues. Results from this type of probe allow the clinician to determine whether he or she is using the appropriate cue level and whether the child is making progress in response to the intervention. Simultaneously, the clinician may observe the child's level of attention, motivation, and satisfaction in the task and ask the parents if the child is participating willingly in therapy (Olswang & Bain, 1994). If the child shows a progression from requiring direct levels of cueing to less direct cues and his or her accuracy shows a steady increase, we can assume that the response to treatment is positive. If, however, there is minimal change in accuracy, direct cues continue to be required; if the child also does not appear motivated or attentive, the intervention plan is not working and a modification is necessary. In this case, the clinician could present the target in syllables or at a simpler contextual level or change the target based on the child's other errors.

Equally important is the assessment of whether significant change is occurring through generalization or the transfer of learning. Different types of generalization have been documented and might be expected. Stimulus generalization refers to the use of treatment targets in other contexts and environments from which they were trained. Response generalization refers to the use of targets in words and positions that were not trained. Response class generalization refers to the use of untrained exemplars of a sound class or error pattern from which a target was trained. Furthermore, systemwide change might be predicted based on linguistic relationships among targets and sounds from other sound classes. Finally, between-domain generalization, such as change in an untreated linguistic domain other than phonology, might also be possible.

To assess response and response class generalization, it is critically important at the beginning of the intervention program to plan to administer a probe of the target sound in untrained words, as well as related but untrained sounds affected by the same error pattern. Typically, we use five untrained words, both single and multisyllabic, for the target and all related sounds in the trained position. So, for example, with initial /f/ as a target to eliminate stopping of fricatives, we would present five untrained words containing initial /f/ and five for each of the other initial fricatives affected by stopping (Tyler, Edwards, & Saxman, 1987). These words remain as our probe items and may not be used as stimuli during treatment. Typically, once the child has displayed 75%–90% accuracy in the production of the target in untrained words, we might expect some response class generalization. To evaluate whether this is occurring, the generalization probe for untrained sounds in the same class should be administered every 4–6 weeks. If results from the generalization probe show that no other sounds in the class from which the target is a member are changing, then additional targets representing that class should be selected. In our example, if no other fricatives are beginning to appear, then additional fricatives should become treatment targets.

We may also evaluate the significance of change occurring through stimulus generalization to conversational speech, that is, through parent report of the use of trained words, with the target produced correctly in conversation outside of the therapy setting. Similarly, generalization of untrained words and sounds in conversation can be assessed in the therapy setting through the use of seminaturalistic conversation probes. For example, materials for a dramatic play activity could be provided such that the representative words contain the target initial /f/ and other untrained initial fricatives. The clinician could then tabulate the correct production of targets in conversational speech. The parents' observation of the use of untrained sounds in conversation would also be an indication that response class generalization, and thus important change, is occurring.

If a point is reached in the intervention program at which change has occurred for the target sound in untrained words and for some related, untrained sounds, but no generalization has been made to conversational speech, correct productions in more complex speech contexts such as sentences may need to be targeted. In addition, less structured tasks may need to be implemented so that productions occur in more naturalistic contexts. For an older child, a self-monitoring program may need to be implemented.

At what point should intervention on a particular target be discontinued, and when should a child be dismissed from an intervention program? These two questions are among the most difficult to answer because so many individual differences are due to temperament and environmental factors. Olswang and Bain (1994) recommend that when a child correctly produces more than 40% of untrained probe items for a target and productions are observed in conversational speech, treatment on the target can be discontinued. The target should be monitored, however, to ensure its continued use and progress both in the clinical setting and at home. Others recommend that a target sound should reach 75% accuracy in treatment before it is discontinued. Certainly, the often-noted high accuracy of 90% correct production in single words is likely not necessary for a target to be eliminated from treatment, at least at the single-word level. Once a target is produced correctly in untrained words at least half of the time, it should be advanced to some more difficult level or monitored in more naturalistic contexts.

The decision about when to dismiss a child from treatment should be made with consideration of numerous factors, not limited to the child's

1. Initial starting severity level

2. Years in treatment

3. Overall motivation, tolerance, and satisfaction with the treatment program

4. Comparison of articulation performance with age-matched peers through norm-referenced measures

5. Number and type of errors remaining in conversational speech, as well as stimulability status of these error sounds

Quantitative data can take the form of standard scores from phonological-articulation tests. If these scores place the child within 1 *SD* of the mean performance for his or her age group, this is good justification for dismissal. Significant clinical change may also be marked by a dismissal standard score that exceeds the 95% confidence interval for the initial pretreatment standard score. Quantitative data in the form of the number of errors remaining in the child's conversational speech and comparison of those sounds in error with developmental norms for sound acquisition (Smit, Hand, Freilinger, Bernthal, & Bird, 1990) may also be useful in justifying a decision for dismissal. Qualitative data often used in deciding whether to dismiss a client, even temporarily, include the child's and parents' overall satisfaction with the treatment program as assessed by a questionnaire or the child's current level of motivation and tolerance for the program as indicated from behavioral observation during therapy and at home. It is not unusual, for example, to find a child who has made considerable progress in treatment as demonstrated by standard scores that represent improvement beyond the 95% confidence interval but that do not yet fall within the normal range. This child, however, has become disenchanted with therapy, is not highly motivated, and has few errors remaining that fall outside developmental norms. For such a child, a dismissal decision would be warranted. As this example illustrates, decisions regarding dismissal must always be made by weighing the quantitative and qualitative data for the individual case.

REFERENCES

American Speech-Language-Hearing Association. (2002). National Outcome Measurement System (NOMS). Retrieved September, 2002, from the ASHA Web site: http://professional.asha.org/resources/NOMS/treatment_outcomes.cfm

Barlow, J.A., & Gierut, J.A. (2002). Minimal pair approaches to phonological remediation. *Seminars in Speech and Language, 23,* 57–68.

Bedore, L.M., & Leonard, L.B. (1998). Specific language impairment and grammatical morphology: A discriminant function analysis. *Journal of Speech, Language, and Hearing Research, 41,* 1185–1192.

Bernhardt, B. (1994). Phonological intervention techniques for syllable and word structure development. *Clinics in Communication Disorders, 4,* 54–65.

Broen, P.A., & Westman, M.J. (1990). Project parent: A preschool language program implemented through parents. *Journal of Speech and Hearing Disorders, 55,* 495–502.

Colone, E., & Forrest, K. (2000, November). *Comparison of treatment efficacy for persistent speech sound disorders.* Poster presented at the American Speech-Language-Hearing Association meeting, Washington, DC.

Conture, E., Louko, L., & Edwards, M.L. (1993). Simultaneously treating stuttering and disordered phonology in children: Experimental therapy, preliminary findings. *American Journal of Speech-Language Pathology, 2,* 72–81.

Dawson, J.I., & Tattersall, P.J. (2001). *Structured Photographic Articulation Test–Dudsberry II.* DeKalb, IL: Janelle Publications.

Dean, E.C., Howell, J., Hill, A., & Waters, D. (1990). *Metaphon Resource Pack.* London: NFER-Nelson.

Edwards, P.D. (1995). *Four famished foxes and Fosdyke.* New York: HarperCollins.

Elbert, M., Rockman, B., & Saltzman, D. (1980). *Contrasts: The use of minimal pairs in articulation training.* Austin, TX: Exceptional Resources.

Fey, M., Cleave, P.L., Ravida, A.I., Long, S.H., Dejmal, A.E., & Easton, D.L. (1994). Effects of grammar facilitation on the phonological performance of children with speech and language impairments. *Journal of Speech and Hearing Research, 37,* 594–607.

Fey, M.E., & Stalker, C.H. (1986). A hypothesis-testing approach to treatment of a child with an idiosyncratic (morpho)phonological system. *Journal of Speech and Hearing Disorders, 51,* 324–336.

Gierut, J.A. (1989). Maximal opposition approach to phonological treatment. *Journal of Speech and Hearing Disorders, 54,* 9–19.

Gierut, J.A. (1990). Differential learning of phonological oppositions. *Journal of Speech and Hearing Research, 33,* 540–549.

Green, J.R., Moore, C.A., Higashikawa, M., & Steeve, R.W. (2000). The physiologic development of speech motor control: Lip and jaw coordination. *Journal of Speech, Language, and Hearing Research, 43,* 239–255.

Green, J.R., Moore, C.A., Ruark, J.L., Rodda, P.R., Morvee, W.T., & Van Witzenburg, M.J. (1997). Development of chewing in children from 12 to 48 months: Longitudinal study of EMG patterns. *Journal of Neurophysiology, 77,* 2704–2727.

Haskill, A., Tyler, A., & Tolbert, L. (2001). *Months of morphemes.* Eau Claire, WI: Thinking Publications.

Hodson, B., & Paden, E. (1991). *Targeting intelligible speech: A phonological approach to remediation* (2nd ed.). Austin, TX: PRO-ED.

Hoffman, P.R., Norris, J.A., & Monjure, J. (1990). Comparison of process targeting and whole language treatment for phonologically delayed preschool children. *Language, Speech, and Hearing Services in Schools, 21,* 102–109.

Howell, J., & Dean, E. (1994). *Treating phonological disorders in children: Metaphon—Theory to practice.* London: Whurr Publishers.

Kelman, M., & Edwards, M.L. (1994). *Phonogroup.* Eau Claire, WI: Thinking Publications.

Moore, C.A., & Ruark, J.L. (1996). Does speech emerge from earlier appearing motor behaviors? *Journal of Speech and Hearing Research, 39,* 1034–1047.

Olswang, L.B., & Bain, B. (1994). Data collection: Monitoring children's treatment progress. *American Journal of Speech-Language Pathology, 3,* 55–65.

Palin, M. (1992). *Contrast pairs for phonological training.* Chicago: Riverside Publishing.

Polmanteer, K.N., & Fields, D.C. (2002, November). *Effectiveness of oral motor techniques in articulation and phonology treatment.* Presented at the annual convention of the American Speech-Language-Hearing Association, Chicago.

Rapin, I., & Allen, D.A. (1983). Developmental language disorders: Nosalgic considerations. In U. Kirk (Ed.), *Neuropsychology of language, reading, and spelling* (pp. 155–184). New York: Elsevier.

Rapin, I., & Allen, D.A. (1988). Syndromes in developmental dysphasia and adult aphasia. In F. Plum (Ed.), *Language, communication, and the brain* (pp. 57–75). New York: Raven Press.

Rice, M., Wexler, K., & Cleave, P. (1995). Specific language impairment as a period of extended optional infinitive. *Journal of Speech and Hearing Research, 38,* 850–863.

Rice, M., Wexler, K., & Hershberger, S. (1998). Tense over time: The longitudinal course of tense acquisition in children with specific language impairment. *Journal of Speech, Language, Hearing Research, 41,* 1412–1430.

Ruark, J.L., & Moore, C.A. (1997). Coordination of lip muscle activity by 2-year-old children during speech and nonspeech tasks. *Journal of Speech and Hearing Research, 40,* 1373–1385.

Shriberg, L.D., & Austin, D. (1998). Comorbidity of speech-language disorder: Implications for a phenotype marker for speech delay. In R. Paul (Ed.), *The speech–language connection* (pp. 73–117). Baltimore: Paul H. Brookes Publishing Co.

Shriberg, L.D., & Kwiatkowski, J. (1982a). Phonological disorders II: A conceptual framework for management. *Journal of Speech and Hearing Disorders, 47,* 242–256.

Shriberg, L.D., & Kwiatkowski, J. (1982b). Phonological disorders III: A procedure for assessing severity of involvement. *Journal of Speech and Hearing Disorders, 47,* 256–270.

Smit, A.B., Hand, L., Freilinger, J.J., Bernthal, J.E., & Bird, A. (1990). The Iowa articulation norms project and its Nebraska replication. *Journal of Speech and Hearing Disorders, 55,* 779–798.

Smith-Kiewel, L., & Claeys, T.M. (1998). *Once upon a sound.* Eau Claire, WI: Thinking Publications.

Thomsen, S., & Donnelly, K. (2000). *SPARC for Phonology.* East Moline, IL: LinguiSystems.

Tyler, A.A. (2002). Language-based intervention for phonological disorders. *Seminars in Speech and Language, 23,* 69–81.

Tyler, A.A., Edwards, M.L., & Saxman, J.H. (1987). Clinical application of two phonologically-based treatment procedures. *Journal of Speech and Hearing Disorders, 52,* 393–409.

Tyler, A.A., Lewis, K.E., Haskill, A., & Tolbert, L.C. (2002). Efficacy and cross-domain effects of a morphosyntax and a phonology intervention. *Language, Speech, and Hearing Services in Schools, 33,* 52–66.

Tyler, A.A., Lewis, K.E., Haskill, A., & Tolbert, C. (2003). Outcomes of different speech and language goal attack strategies. *Journal of Speech, Language, and Hearing Research, 46,* 1077–1094.

Tyler, A.A., & Sandoval, K.T. (1994). Preschoolers with phonological and language disorders: Treating different linguistic domains. *Language, Speech, and Hearing Services in Schools, 25,* 215–234.

Vicino, J., & Wenger, L. (1993). *Phonobuilding.* Eau Claire, WI: Thinking Publications.

Wilcox, K.A., & Morris, S.E. (1995). Speech outcomes of the language-focused curriculum. In M.L. Rice & K.A. Wilcox (Eds.), *Building a language-focused curriculum for the preschool classroom, Vol. 1: A foundation for lifelong communication* (pp. 171–180). Baltimore: Paul H. Brookes Publishing Co.

Williams, A.L. (2000). Multiple oppositions: Theoretical foundations for an alternative contrastive intervention framework. *American Journal of Speech-Language Pathology, 9,* 282–288.

Chapter 12

Intervention

Manipulating Complex Input to
Promote Self-Organization of a Neuro-Network

PAUL R. HOFFMAN AND JANET A. NORRIS

W hether a child receives individual or group therapy depends mainly on the resources available and the type of clinical setting, such as private practice, a university clinic, or a school with a large caseload. Any child can benefit from individual therapy, including intervention within group activities as an individual speech-language pathologist (SLP) prompts the child to participate and respond with greater complexity. Most children can, however, improve their language skills when participating in group settings of three to six children when provided input at a level appropriate to their learning needs and frequent turns to respond and receive feedback. The therapist must therefore be skilled at providing the same information at multiple levels of complexity as the group explores a topic and at providing feedback appropriate to the responses elicited from each child.

Children who require individual therapy are those who

- Cannot stay socially engaged within a group (including those who are developmentally very young)

- Would be considered to fall within the category of *relatively severe* on the pervasive developmental disorder (PDD) spectrum

- Cannot process auditory information unless it is accompanied by overlapping visual information and thus appear to have attention-deficit/hyperactivity disorder (ADHD) to a severe degree and behave in a socially inappropriate way in most situations

- Have significant sensory impairments that prohibit them from learning when the input is presented at even a small physical or temporal distance

- Have a learning rate and needs that are so different from other group members that little benefit is being gained from group participation. Fortunately, this is a relatively small population of children

HOW DO YOU DETERMINE WHEN A CHILD NEEDS DIRECT PHONOLOGICAL INTERVENTION AND WHEN GENERAL LANGUAGE STIMULATION IS NEEDED?

As described in Chapter 7, when intervention is approached from a neuro-networking perspective, phonology is recognized as one component of language (along with semantics, syntax, morphology, and pragmatics). Phonology is an integral and inseparable part of the language constellation. Language must have a form for words to inhabit so that they can have existence, serve as a tool for thought through reference to concepts, and function as a code that can be externalized and thus shared with others through listening and speaking (Nelson, 1985, 1996). Phonological form without meaning and function is a useless shell. Phonology is only useful when it is integrated with language throughout the network. Phonology refines when there is new information that must be organized within the system and when there is a social need for a revision of previously organized categories. Thus, the goal of intervention is to help children simultaneously refine the many aspects of language around the constellation in order to communicate their message to others with specificity, clarity, intent, and accuracy. With each turn in a therapy session, the interventionist must make a decision regarding what may be interfering with the successful communication of a message and focus attention on that element when providing feedback to the child.

For children with limited or very delayed language, insufficient phonological data exist within the system to have the need (neurological or social) for many categories of phonemes or phoneme productions within canonical structures. A child who falls within this group does not yet have sufficient vocabulary or morphosyntactic forms to necessitate a large number of phonological categories to differentiate between words. The child is not experiencing what Piaget (1952, 1954) calls "disequilibrium." The existing phonological categories and corresponding productions are sufficient to distinguish between, reference, and code the existing language without ambiguity for the child. However, as more language is learned and more words begin to overlap within the existing phonological categories, a need arises for reorganization and refinement. This occurs as a result of the self-organizing properties of a neuro-network and as an outcome of social consequences when the child's message is not understood and frustration or disequilibrium ensues (Lindblom, 1992, 2000). At that moment the system is primed to make an accommodation to existing categories, and so recasts, expansions, and modeling of language without specific emphasis on production cues are valuable input to the child and will generate phonological changes. Each element of the constellation receives the input and each makes accommodations to restructure the information to more closely match the feedback (Saffran, Newport, Aslin, Tunick, & Barrueco, 1997). This doesn't mean that recasts with specific emphasis on production cues should never occur, but they should not occur disproportionately in relationship to the other needs around the constellation.

Some children with motor disorders such as developmental apraxia may need more frequent production cues (including some time devoted to oral-motor exercises) than do children with a phonological delay without the motor component. The principles and intervention strategies do not differ greatly for these children with apraxic characteristics, however. By definition, the characteristic associated most frequently with developmental apraxia of speech is at least a 1-year discrepancy between receptive and expressive language (Blakeley, 2001). This suggests that a phonological delay is a contributing factor to the articulation difficulties. Furthermore, a 1-year language delay for a young child is a highly significant delay that is shown to be consistent with long-term language delays and disorders; delays in written language acquisition including reading, writing, and spelling; and social-pragmatic disorders of language (Conti-Ramsden & Botting, 1999;

Stothard, Snowling, Bishop, Chipchase, & Kaplan, 1998). It is important that therapy address all of the child's concerns and not just the motor component. The motor component of developmental apraxia must integrate with the other components of the constellation for the motor changes to be used by the child when communicating.

Motor skills developed in isolation have few points of connection to the complex processes that must simultaneously occur when communicative speech is produced. A child must formulate the proposition of the message; determine the intent of the message (i.e., to inform, request, demand) and anticipated social consequence; select appropriate vocabulary words to code the message and achieve the goals; organize the relationships of meaning between words using syntactic and morphological strategies; organize the sentences relative to shared prior knowledge with the listener, previous sentences, and successive sentences using appropriate discourse structures; select and sequence the correct phonological and prosodic patterns to express the meaning and intent of the utterance; and execute the corresponding motor patterns that are connected within the neuro-network. The child will use those motor patterns that receive input from units around the constellation. When intervention addresses the motor speech differences independent of a communicative context, the child will default to the motor patterns that are connected within the network rather than using those practiced in therapy. A lack of generalization, often extending for months or even years, results (see Bernthal & Bankson, 2004, for a review). Compounding the problem, the language difficulties experienced by these children are not addressed, and thus the entire network fails to refine and add complexity. This is observed as the persistent and often increasing expressive language delay that characterizes developmental apraxia. By school age this delay further manifests itself in poor readiness for the development of written language so that the child is often relabeled as having a learning disability (Blakeley, 2001; Hickman, 1997).

Even when there is a strong neuromotor component to a child's speech intelligibility problems, intervention must address the phonological and other language needs of the child and must integrate sensorimotor changes with the other elements of the language constellation. The prognosis for these children indicates that early intervention must be both remedial for current delays and deficits and preventive to limit future learning problems at school age. Once again, storybook reading surfaces as a context for intervention that can serve to address these multiple goals.

TO WHAT EXTENT DO YOU INCLUDE PARENTS IN THERAPY?

With fairly extensive training, parents can be taught to conduct articulation training (Bowen & Cupples, 1999; Shelton, Johnson, Willis, & Arndt, 1975). However, these types of activities are not natural parent–child interactions, nor do they easily fit into the busy schedules of most families. Conversely, activities such as storybook reading are part of the daily routines of many families. Encouraging parents to engage in repeated readings of the same books for many successive days, taking time to talk about the pictures and explain story events, will provide experiences the child can use to organize phonological information as well as the multiple other levels of the language constellation. In addition, teaching parents to either repeat the child's utterance before adding a response or recast the child's utterance with an expansion is an easy technique parents can learn to use throughout the day in naturally occurring interactions. The parent generally will require a few sessions of training (10 minutes at the end of the child's therapy session for several sessions) for this communicative pattern to feel less foreign and become more automatic.

van Kleek (1996) has shown that books read by parents to young children generally fall into either the category of a storybook or an alphabet book. When a storybook is read, parent–child interactions focus primarily on meaning, with very little attention to the form of print such as individual letters, letter sounds, or punctuation or to the identification of individual words within the text. In contrast, when an alphabet book is read, parent–child interactions focus primarily on the form of print, identifying letters of the alphabet by name and naming pictures that are associated with that letter of the alphabet. Thus, most spontaneous parent–child storybook readings are focused either on meaning or print, with neither type of book eliciting a focus specifically on sound.

With training that specifically encourages a focus on print, parents can and do spend more time during storybook reading attending to print. Ezell and Justice (2000) showed that following a 5-week clinic-based book-reading program in which parents were trained to use particular behaviors with reading and were provided books for home use, parents did increase their print focus during reading. Most of the children also showed increases in emergent literacy skills following the 5-week period. In a follow-up study with a control group, parents taught to use print-focused behaviors did attend more to print during book reading and their children demonstrated greater gains in emergent literacy knowledge compared with a control group that did not receive the parent training (Justice & Ezell, 2000). A further study (Justice & Ezell, 2002) showed that when print-focus behaviors were taught to teachers in the Head Start program, the groups receiving the print-focused book reading made significantly greater emergent literacy gains compared with control group children who received a focus on pictures.

Without this specialized training, however, control groups did not attend to print or emergent literacy skills and children did not increase in this knowledge just from being read to. This limits the positive potential of such shared book readings and does not focus attention on sounds or other aspects of phonological information. The prolonged periods of parent training required to instill these changes in parent behavior limit the feasibility of providing such training to many parents. To remedy these problems, *Phonic Faces Alphabet Storybooks* were developed (Norris, 2001). Each alphabet storybook focuses on the production of a specific sound as a natural part of a story. *Icky Carrots* (Norris, 2002) (see Figure 7.3) tells the story of Iris Iggy who does not like the carrots her mother is feeding her. On each page of the story, children are encouraged to produce the /ɪ/ phoneme that the baby makes as she rejects how they sound, taste, feel, smell, and so forth. Each page has words containing the /ɪ/ in the beginning, and/or middle word position. The stories follow traditional story grammar; some such as *Icky Carrots* are written as simple reactive sequences, whereas others have complete story structure (setting, character, problem, plan, attempt, and outcome). Our preliminary studies with parents and Head Start teachers show that adults focus on helping children produce these sounds and identify the sounds in word positions following a 5-minute introduction to the purpose and form of the alphabet storybooks (Carter-Brazier, Norris, & Hoffman, 2003; Norris & Hoffman, 2003). This focus on sounds does not generalize to other storybooks with similar plots read immediately following the training, indicating that the structure of the alphabet storybooks naturally directs attention and talk to sounds.

CAN CERTAIN TYPES OF THERAPY BE CONDUCTED THROUGH A COLLABORATIVE CLASSROOM MODEL?

At the preschool level the majority of intervention goals can be conducted through a collaborative classroom model. Preschool activities, such as symbolic play, block play, art, snack, storybook reading, music, and outdoor play provide activities in which the child is engaged in hands-on learning with visual and other multisensory input that can support auditory input (Norris & Hoffman, 1990). The same intervention activities described in Chapter 5 can be used (i.e., modeling, expansion, extension, expatiation, prompts, gestures, cloze, phonemic cues, preparatory sets, and relational terms, in addition to coaching during which the adult provides words the child can use to communicate with peers). As language is used by the child and recast by the adult to describe ongoing actions and events, the self-organizing properties of a neuro-network operate in the same manner as described for storybook reading.

The continuous opportunities for peer interaction in the preschool classroom provide the forum for social consequences to prompt refinements of phonology and speech production. If a child's communicative attempt is not understood by a peer, the adult can explain, "He didn't understand you—try saying the word like this (provide a model with emphasis on a salient phoneme within the word)." Similarly, recasting the utterance with a request for the child to try communicating the message again implies that a change is needed, generating the disequilibrium needed to motivate a change.

Most kindergarten classrooms are more structured and have fewer opportunities for peer interactions, although the intervention strategies can be applied during learning centers or other less structured activities. Kindergarten, however, is the time when auditory discrimination (i.e., listening for the sounds of the letters of the alphabet), canonical structures (i.e., learning sounds in word positions), coarticulation (i.e., sound blending), rhyme, and other aspects of phonological awareness and sound production are an everyday focus of the curriculum (Ehri, Nunes, Willows, Schuster, & Shannahan, 2001; Norris & Hoffman, 2002). This is an ideal context for collaboration because most teachers do not have coursework in phonetics, phonology, or language development. The relationships between sound production, sound discrimination and awareness, and printed letters is unfamiliar to most kindergarten teachers. Collaboration offers SLPs the opportunity to model how to maximize learning during regular classroom activities that focus on sound awareness and letter learning. Special emphasis can be placed on developmental sounds such as /s/, /l/, /r/, and /θ/ that comprise the majority of residual articulation errors for children in this age group. A focus on these sounds and their production can be incorporated into the classroom lesson plans each week throughout the year rather than just a single letter-of-the-week exposure. This can occur in the form of listening for the words in the current reading book containing these sounds in various word positions, finding the letters corresponding to these sounds, and using the letters to prompt correct production of these sounds as these words are read within the story. *Phonic Faces* (Norris, 2001) cards, on which the letter is drawn as the tongue, lip, or other articulator within the face of a character, can prompt these correct productions when paired with the letter in the book.

In first and second grade, the curriculum continues to focus on sound discrimination, coarticulation/sound blending, and other phonological and speech production skills in the form of phonics instruction. The focus on sound-in-syllable position intensifies as children learn the rules or patterns of phonic principles during reading and spelling instruction.

This provides ideal contexts for collaboration, as the SLP can work within the classroom with children showing phonological disorders using the curriculum they need to master for language arts. The program *Phonic Faces* has separate faces for 42 phonemes, including consonant and vowel digraphs as well as long and short vowels. Short vowels are pictured as babies, whereas long vowels are pictured as adults. Stories are used to help children understand, see, and manipulate vowel shifts in spelling. For example, the adult Mister E does not like babies in his words. When he appears at the end of a word or syllable, he starts to complain. The child is thus allowed to "silence" him by turning him over (thus the "silent e" rule), but in exchange, the adult vowel must agree to stand in for the baby (thus the vowel shifts to the long vowel sound; Norris, 2001).

To blend sequences of sounds to form words, children who have difficulty remembering the sounds, phonic rules, or sequence of sounds only need to place their mouths in the same positions as those shown on the succession of *Phonic Faces*. If they can't hear the resulting word, the child is provided a binary choice either auditorily ("Is your mouth saying 'cat' or 'can'?") or through a picture choice. Thus, the SLP working with children in such activities can work on a range of phonological skills that will help the child achieve curriculum benchmarks in language arts while simultaneously achieving goals in speech. The same tools and strategies can be used for older children who are exhibiting reading delays related to learning disabilities, including dyslexia, or other disabilities affecting written language acquisition.

HOW OFTEN DO YOU NEED TO SEE A CHILD TO MAKE PROGRESS?

We know of no conclusive research to support or refute choices in service delivery. Many factors influence progress, and our field is just beginning to engage in evidence-based practice. However, given that all children cannot receive hourly sessions three times weekly over extended periods of time, when resources are limited our preference is for block scheduling, or limited periods of longer (60–120 minutes), intensive intervention delivered in cycles (e.g., 6-week cycles of intervention once or twice weekly alternating with 6 weeks of no intervention; Van Hattum, 1969). Children with severe delays might participate in several continuous cycles before entering a no-intervention phase; children with less severe delays would be monitored for maintenance and generalization following the no-intervention cycle at which point a decision would be made to either enter another intervention cycle or continue in the monitoring phase.

In addition to our clinical success with this model, the reason for this preference is theoretical. For a neuro-network to build and organize, the system requires sustained exposure to comprehensible input (Seidenberg & McClelland, 1989). For example, few people can write a paper or study for an exam in 20-minute blocks of scattered time. It takes sustained periods of focused attention to a topic or problem for new information to become assimilated, and for new patterns and reorganizations to form. For children learning the complexities of a phonological system, including all of the many language processes it is derived from and must integrate with, sustained attention is required. In typical development, children from a professional family are exposed to more than 1,500 spoken words per hour. Extrapolating this verbal interaction to a year, a child in a professional family would hear 11 million words (Hart & Risley, 1995). Typically developing children exposed to less language input in turn learn less language. Hart and Risley's (1995) data show that children from low-income families hear only 3 million words per year and thus could start kindergarten having heard 32 million fewer words than their wealthier classmates. Children with speech and language learning disabilities have similarly impoverished experiences even with rich language exposure because they do not benefit from everyday language input to the extent that typically developing children do.

Talk during intervention differs from everyday talk in important ways. Everyday talk is characterized by a distance between words and their corresponding visual events. Parents make comments or ask questions that precede the visual action by several seconds or even minutes or longer. For example, parents might say, "Are you ready to eat lunch?" before the lunch preparations have even begun. "Get your coat," is followed by changing locations and the passage of time before the coat is found. When the coat is located, the message is rarely recast nor is the child required to put the message into words. In typical development, the child may hold the message in memory and spontaneously comment, "I found my coat," but children who have delays are less likely to maintain this topic. This causes the adult to become more directive and the child more passive. In contrast, intervention places the child in the speaker role in which the child is asked to talk about an action or change of state occurring at the current moment or in a future that occurs immediately. Thus the auditory words and the visual event provide overlapping input to the neuro-network. This enables the meaning and form of words to be processed in integration within the network (Norris & Hoffman, 2001; Pangburn, 2002; Roy, 2000). Intervention strategies prompt the child to use words that fit the visual context and also maintain the topic for a sustained time period. Recasting and requiring the child to revise the same message, often several times during the interaction, provide the redundancy needed by the system to sufficiently process the information to result in a change or refinement.

Once the system has more information, and greater organization and refinement, it begins to function more normally. The system may have needed different timing or more visual or multimodality support to build, organize, and refine its structures, but once the neuro-network is expanded it begins to function more "normally." This will be observed in changes throughout the system, as the child produces more pragmatically appropriate, semantically specific, syntactically complex, and phonologically intelligible talk.

HOW DO YOU MONITOR PROGRESS?

As with any intervention, progress is monitored through changes in the products of speech and language. Long-term progress can be determined through changes in standardized measures such as articulation and/or language tests, as well as through speech and language samples. Short-term progress can be monitored using probes, which are short samples of the output from the system. Probes may be taken at the end of a session or on a weekly schedule. For example, a probe for a preschool child might be telling a story from a picture or picture sequence. Depending on the needs and abilities of the child, this may be a picture previously explored in intervention or a novel picture accompanied by an adult-modeled story, or, at a higher level, a novel picture with no support provided for the story. The ideas that comprise the main points of the story as well as several details can be typed on a scoring form. As the child tells the story, the adult checks off the ideas from the story told by the child and indicates each sentence that is longer than the child's current mean length of utterance (MLU). These behaviors can usually be recorded as the child is telling the story. The child is then prompted to create and/or imitate several sentences about the picture from which several phonemes will be judged for omission, sound substitution, or distortion. Thus, in a few minutes a fairly representative sample of the child's articulation and language can be obtained that can be compared with a baseline as well as with the previous probe to ascertain whether progress is observed.

For older children, the principle is the same. The child can be asked to read a passage at the current instructional level. Miscues are marked on-line and comprehension questions are answered following the reading. Because the graded readability of a passage is determined by measures of syntactic and semantic complexity (Fry, 1968), changes in probes for number of miscues, words read per minute, and comprehension questions answered correctly represent measurable changes in language processing. Asking the child to "sound out" words missed in the probe can provide a measure of change in phonological information related to reading. Asking the child to reread an easy passage but attending to correct speech production for sounds can provide a quick measure of the speech production within a complex structured context.

WHAT DO YOU DO WHEN YOUR INTERVENTION PLAN IS NOT WORKING?

When intervention is not working it means that input is not comprehensible to the system and cannot be assimilated into the neuro-network in order to achieve the needed reorganizations and refinements. Usually this means the input is too difficult on one or more dimensions, or as Vygotsky (1978) proffered, not within the child's zone of proximal development (ZPD). New information must be familiar enough to be assimilated into existing structures but have sufficient novel or contrasting elements to create the discontinuity needed to effect change. For some children the zone or range of input between the known and the incomprehensible is very limited. For example, some children can learn when a picture is located immediately in front of them (i.e., the child is seated at a table with the clinician immediately next him or her, pointing to salient information) but not when the same picture is at a distance (i.e., the child is seated in a chair with the adult holding the picture in front of him or her, as in group storybook reading; Norris, 2000). The picture viewed by itself can be too difficult for the child to comprehend when there is not sufficient information in the illustration for the words and the visual images to overlap within the neuro-network (e.g., the story is about a girl who lost her dog, but the picture only shows her talking to her friend). In this case the picture and text maintain a distanced relationship and the words alone may be insufficient for the child to derive meaning. Likewise, the picture may be comprehensible but the adult may be using an MLU or vocabulary choices that are too complex for the child to internalize. Conversely, the child may not be able to see changes in states or action from pictures and may need input in which props show the actions represented in the picture.

Intervention is a process of monitoring whether changes are occurring and which aspects of language within the constellation are or are not reorganizing and refining.

Decisions are then made to intensify the level of focus on one or more elements such as increasing the frequency of sound production cues, changing the level of input by modifying materials, providing stronger support or more multimodality support for one or more elements (e.g., incorporating a tool such as *Phonic Faces* or oral-motor exercises), or reducing the level of language input. The continuum must be recognized between what the child is currently doing and what changes intervention needs to effect. Finding the tools and strategies that will enable the child to move forward on the continuum is the art of effective intervention.

WHEN DO YOU DISMISS A CHILD FROM SERVICES?

When a neuro-network has sufficient organization and complexity it begins to function more typically. The network for a child with phonological disorders needs different input to learn and organize, but what is learned and organized can be used for future learning. The network that is created has a structure similar to that of a typically developing network (or is structured to compensate for differences) and thus functions more normally. A more complex network is capable of learning from input that is more displaced along all dimensions, such as requiring less overlap between visual and auditory features from input, or attending to information presented at greater distances in time and space. The system begins to learn independently. Monitoring progress following periods of no intervention during block scheduling is one way to determine whether sufficient independent learning is occurring for maintenance, generalization, and new acquisitions to be manifested.

A neurologically different system remains different throughout the lifespan, however. Whereas some children compensate for these differences and may never require further intervention, others will manifest difficulties when new phonological skills must be learned, such as reading and spelling. At these times, intervention should be reinstated by an SLP (Norris, 1998a). These children instead are typically seen by a reading or special education specialist who most often is not trained to recognize or provide intervention for the language problems underlying the reading disability.

Recognizing the complexity and long-term effects of a phonological delay will enable the SLP to understand the course of development that may be observed. Early intervention, therefore, should be enacted that will intervene for current presenting problems but also focus on preventing or limiting problems the child is at risk for displaying at school age. School-age intervention should address phonological issues using written language to enable the child to function within the classroom environment. This may include compensatory strategies for children with severe or persistent problems, such as assistive technology for writing and spelling.

MANY PUBLISHED/PACKAGED PROGRAMS ARE AVAILABLE FOR PHONOLOGICAL INTERVENTION. WHICH, IF ANY, DO YOU USE, AND HOW DO YOU ADAPT OR MODIFY THEM?

Published or packaged programs can be useful, depending on the nature of the problem and the manner in which the programs are used. For example, a less experienced clinician may need a systematic program to follow in order to acquire the skills and knowledge needed to eventually conduct more dynamic intervention. This may be true particularly in cases in which speech aides or other paraprofessionals are providing intervention. Packaged programs can also be used for engaging the child in independent learning. Programs or materials may be placed in a learning center or language laboratory and the child trained to use the program, with monitoring conducted by the SLP. Empowering a child to be in charge of his or her own learning can serve as a motivator for change and limit the learned helplessness children may show when independent learning is difficult. Programs also may be effective for addressing problems such as distortions of /s/ or /r/ phonemes in which an incorrect production may be habituated and repetitive practice may be needed to change or refine the existing patterns within the neuro-network.

WHAT SPECIFIC INTERVENTION TECHNIQUES DO YOU FIND MOST USEFUL?

The goal of intervention is to facilitate the expansion, reorganization, and refinement of the neuro-network to result in maximum phonological and articulation development. When the network is fully integrated, the spontaneous speech of the child will reflect these changes because the phonological and motor patterns are integrally connected to the semantic, syntactic, morphological, discourse, and pragmatic aspects of language. To accomplish this, the techniques used in intervention must address these multiple aspects of speech and language. Contexts such as play, daily routines, and storybook reading are ideal for this purpose.

Figure 12.1 provides a model for intervention conducted within these complex contexts. In this model, adapted from the situational-discourse-semantic model (Norris, 2000; Norris & Hoffman, 1996, 2001, 2002), four dynamics are profiled, each along a continuum. The goal is to work as close to the center—or the most integrated level of the model—as the child can coordinate. In the upper left corner, a continuum is displayed for the nature of intervention task, or the level of *social and cognitive displacement* (i.e., the situational context). On the outside pole of this continuum is picture naming or word drills, which are devoid of communicative meaning (pictures and words are spoken to practice production of a target phoneme rather than to express a message) or social intent (the words are spoken to comply with an adult request, with no expected social outcome). The purpose, meaning, and consequences are the adult's. On the innermost pole of the continuum is spontaneous talk, in which the child must communicate information that is relevant, truthful, and appropriate to the needs of the listener. The child must ensure that meaning, purpose, and consequence are shared with the listener. Using this model, intervention might begin with a structured action-based activity, such as making a peanut butter sandwich. In this case the actions and outcomes to be talked about are the child's own, so there is minimal cognitive distance between the child's sensory experience and the ongoing social talk. Such a context provides the forum for talk that is meaningful and social, activating input throughout the constellation but sufficiently structured to control the amount and type of input to be processed. This same event might be enacted later in a more difficult context such as play or storybook reading, in which the child's talk must focus on the actions of the dolls or storybook characters. In time, the difficulty of the context can be increased

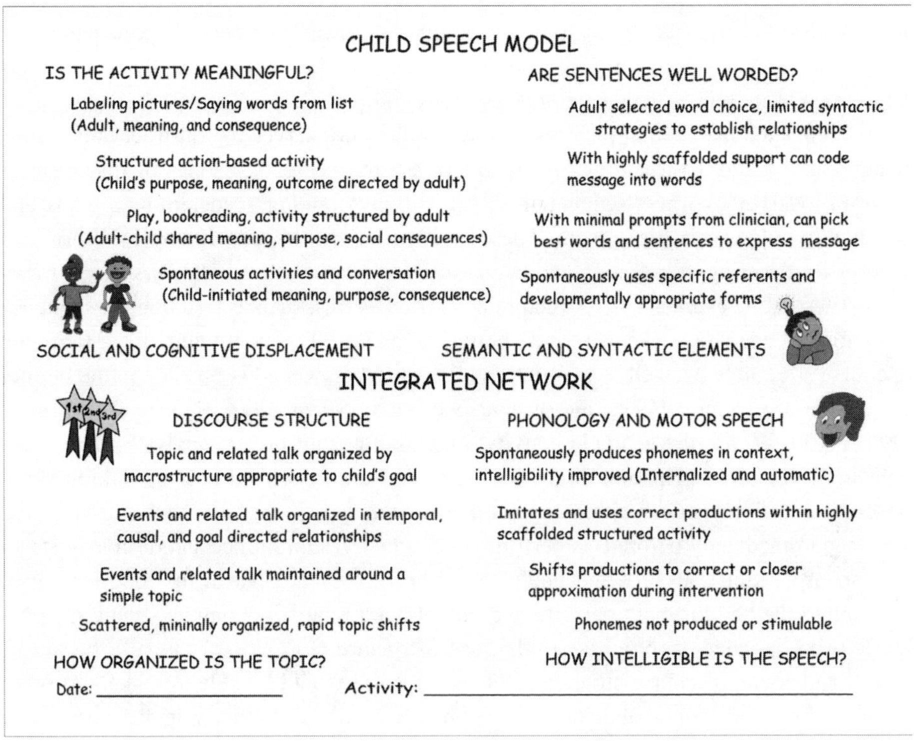

CHILD SPEECH MODEL

IS THE ACTIVITY MEANINGFUL?

Labeling pictures/Saying words from list
(Adult, meaning, and consequence)

Structured action-based activity
(Child's purpose, meaning, outcome directed by adult)

Play, bookreading, activity structured by adult
(Adult-child shared meaning, purpose, social consequences)

Spontaneous activities and conversation
(Child-initiated meaning, purpose, consequence)

SOCIAL AND COGNITIVE DISPLACEMENT

ARE SENTENCES WELL WORDED?

Adult selected word choice, limited syntactic
strategies to establish relationships

With highly scaffolded support can code
message into words

With minimal prompts from clinician, can pick
best words and sentences to express message

Spontaneously uses specific referents and
developmentally appropriate forms

SEMANTIC AND SYNTACTIC ELEMENTS

INTEGRATED NETWORK

DISCOURSE STRUCTURE

Topic and related talk organized by
macrostructure appropriate to child's goal

Events and related talk organized in temporal,
causal, and goal directed relationships

Events and related talk maintained around a
simple topic

Scattered, mininally organized, rapid topic shifts

HOW ORGANIZED IS THE TOPIC?

Date: _____

PHONOLOGY AND MOTOR SPEECH

Spontaneously produces phonemes in context,
intelligibility improved (Internalized and automatic)

Imitates and uses correct productions within highly
scaffolded structured activity

Shifts productions to correct or closer
approximation during intervention

Phonemes not produced or stimulable

HOW INTELLIGIBLE IS THE SPEECH?

Activity: _____

Figure 12.1. In the intervention model, adapted from the situational-discourse-semantic model, four dynamics are profiled, each along a continuum. The goal is to work as close to the center of the model as the child can coordinate, or the most integrated level of the model. Adapted from J. Norris, E.C. Healey, et al. (1998).

to conversation about the event with no support from the actual objects, play objects, or pictures.

During the activity the adult and child must engage in talk using appropriate *semantic and syntactic elements,* or the top right continuum of the model (Norris, 1998b, 2000; Norris & Hoffman, 2001). On the outside pole of this continuum is picture naming or similar adult-selected responses, produced in isolation with no syntactic context to relate the word to actions or states. In many approaches to articulation, this is the primary context of stimulus presentation (i.e., single words containing the phoneme in a given word position). On the innermost pole is spontaneous use of sentences with age-appropriate choice of vocabulary and syntactic forms. Within the example activity, making a peanut butter sandwich, the initial level of talk might be the level of highly scaffolded comments, requests, and commands about ongoing actions (i.e., the models, expansions, cloze prompts, preparatory sets) as described in Chapter 7. In this way, the adult provides the child with an ongoing map between events that are seen (as well as felt, heard, and smelled) and the talk used to refer to these events. The concurrence of the talk with the related action allows for the connections from all sensory inputs to enter the system simultaneously. The active connections between visual and other sensory input with auditory word input enable a mapping to occur from one input system to another (Locke, 1995; Pangburn, 2002; Roy, 2000). Thus, the words are attached to their meaning, and the connections to all points along the constellation reorganize and refine to accommodate this new information. The level of the talk shifts along this continuum toward the goal of spontaneous use of referents and developmentally appropriate forms as the child internally reconstructs the event and its related language with greater complexity.

A task such as labeling pictures neither requires nor serves to construct larger units of language, or macrostructures. Macrostructures are coherent episodes of discourse or talk tied together by topic, sequential action, causality, and/or predetermined goals and the resulting plans to achieve them. These macrostructures include culturally determined patterns for ordering information and taking turns in conversation, called *discourse structures*. These same elements also structure nonverbal events, such as enacting the sequence of actions needed to make a peanut butter sandwich. The continuum for examining discourse structures (as well as the underlying nonverbal events) is profiled in the bottom left corner of the model (i.e., the discourse context; Norris, 2000; Norris & Hoffman, 1996, 2001). Within the example activity, making a peanut butter sandwich, the child's expected level of participation might be a temporal sequence or it may be talking about the current action while making the sandwich and verbalizing the next action in the sequence immediately before it is performed. Gradually, subroutines and discourse structures incorporating causality and goals would be incorporated, with the long-term goal of enabling the child to both perform and talk about a relatively complex event independently using language appropriate to the macrostructure (e.g., "first," "next," "because," "will") and social discourse structures. Thus, the child would be able to make and serve peanut butter sandwiches and juice to playmates or dolls, maintaining the social talk ("please," "would you like . . . ") as well as the event-related talk ("I need a better knife").

The final continuum of the model addresses *phonology and motor speech,* or the sound productions used within the discourse (Hoffman & Norris, 1989; Norris, 2000; Norris & Hoffman, 2001). The continuum ranges from developmentally appropriate phonemes that are not produced or stimulable, through spontaneous correct productions in context, indicating that they are integrated with phonemic categories, phonological patterns, words, concepts, sentences, and discourse structures throughout the network. The goals within intervention sessions lie in the middle of the continuum. The expectation is for refinement and reorganization to occur that will be apparent in shifts in productions (Oller, 1975). These shifts could be seen as the production of a sound in which an omission had occurred; a change in any production, although not necessarily to a correct production (e.g., backing to fronting, stopping to affrication); an imitation or approximation of a correct production; the production of phoneme sequences to more closely approximate a word's syllable shape (i.e., reduplication, metathesis, or appearance of medial or final consonants); or production of an unvocalized speech gesture. All productions are evidence that the network is making a change, adding greater complexity, and reorganizing to accommodate new input. Which phonemes are added or which consonants are correctly produced is left to emerge naturally as an outcome of the self-organizing properties of the child's neuro-network.

WHAT TYPES OF MATERIALS (WORD LISTS, PICTURE SETS, TOYS, COMPUTER PROGRAMS) DO YOU RECOMMEND?

Pictures, toys, and other materials must be developmentally appropriate (i.e., within the child's ZPD) and relational (i.e., conducive to forming sequential relationships of meaning between objects and actions). Three general principles guide developmental appropriateness. The first principle is the level of symbolic displacement needed to understand and manipulate the material (Norris, 2000; Norris & Hoffman, 1996). For example, young children require real objects or life-sized toys that look very similar to the actual object in order to recognize and apply play schemes to the material. Pictures must clearly show the objects drawn in an uncomplicated form. Developmentally older children can understand and manipulate increasingly more abstract representations of reality and imagination. Toys become miniature replicas, then represented (e.g., a pencil becomes an airplane just by saying it is so), and eventually invented using words alone (e.g., "Pretend this is my house over here, and I have five horses"). Similarly, pictures for young children should look realistic and capable of being paired with objects to enable the child to understand the representation. For example, a brush, towel, and soap can be used by the child to perform actions on a picture of a dog in a tub.

Developmentally older children can interpret actions, motives, and successive events only suggested by a line drawing. Material that is too displaced (above the child's ZPD) cannot activate existing connections between the constellation units of a neuro-network and thus cannot form new pathways, resulting in an inability of the system to learn. Instead, the system will attend to irrelevant features of the stimuli that can be processed, resulting in a child who appears to be off-task and disengaged. Material that is too simple (i.e., below the child's ZPD) will not provide input that the system can use to add complexity or refinement, resulting in a child who appears bored and inattentive.

The second developmentally appropriate principle is familiarity. Developmentally younger children have a limited number of entities and events represented within their neuro-network. To form and refine connections within their network, the stimuli must involve familiar objects and events (e.g., pictures or toys representing daily routines such as cooking or eating), with less familiar information introduced gradually (e.g., campfires and picnics). Developmentally older children gradually construct scientific and world knowledge (e.g., life cycles of plants and animals, planets, social and cultural experiences of others). Materials must build on knowledge existing within the constellation to add complexity or refine the system.

The third developmentally appropriate principle involves the language used to talk about the stimuli (Norris, 1998b, 2000; Norris & Hoffman, 2001). The same stimuli can be merely named or labeled ("It's a horse") or described by action ("The horse is running"), attribute ("The brown horse is running"), interpretation ("The horse is running fast"), inference ("The brown horse is running fast because it wants to win the race"), evaluation ("The brown horse should win because it tries harder than the other horses"), or analogy ("The brown horse ran faster than the wind"). At the highest level the stimuli can be talked about metalinguistically ("Say the /s/ sound at the end of "horse"). In this case, the neuro-network must use language symbols to consciously isolate and manipulate the language symbols existing within the constellation. That is, "horse" must be activated simultaneously within the system as a concept to be talked about and as a word composed of phonemes. This requires a very complex and integrated network.

Some practices in traditional articulation intervention violate these principles of developmental appropriateness and, as a result, limit or slow progress and generalization of correct sound productions. For example, the displacement principle may be violated by presenting a young child with a series of line drawings of objects that have in common only the same initial phoneme. Toys or full-color storybooks may be processed more easily by a child with a delay. Because the focus is on initial sound, many of the pictured objects also may violate the familiarity principle as picture items are presented for which the child has no knowledge. Thus, these pictures make it difficult for the child to interpret any meaning or action relationships. Furthermore, the talk about these pictures in intervention may violate the third principle, requiring a child to metalinguistically analyze and focus productions on a sound for a picture that the child cannot yet describe at the lower levels of action, attribute, or interpretation. These violations of the developmental appropriateness of the material severely limit the connections that can be formed within and across the constellation. Phonology will refine slowly and generalization will be very poor without these interconnections. An example of this is seen in Phelan (1989), who compared two forms of intervention—traditional and cognitive-communicative—for the speech sound production errors of preschool children. In the former, two children practiced the production of /s/ in isolation, syllables, words, phrases, sentences, and storytelling. In the latter, two children engaged in story construction in which /s/ production was targeted when errors occurred. Both interventions involved explicit modeling of sound production, provision of metalinguistic phonetic cues, and feedback regarding the accuracy of production of /s/. The two children in the story construction intervention reached a 75% correct /s/ production criterion in a conversational speech probe before the two children in the traditional program reached this criterion.

DO YOU INCLUDE PERCEPTUAL (AUDITORY) TRAINING AND/OR ORAL-MOTOR EXERCISES IN YOUR INTERVENTION?

Perception and production of auditory features and motor gestures are elements of the constellation model, as are phonemic categories and canonical structures. Thus, they receive input and are refined when input at any level is provided to the system. The input to the system may be targeted directly at making an auditory distinction or motor gesture, but this is usually done in a context rather than as a series of discrete training trials or exercises. During play or storybook reading, for example, feedback can be given for a word important to the child's message. This may be a request for an auditory discrimination ("Do you mean 'seep' or 'sleep'?"), a production cue ("Watch my mouth, my tongue is going to lick the top of my mouth": /s/–/l/), a visual cue such as *Phonic Faces* ("Make your mouth do the same sounds as the faces"), or a physical prompt. For a child with a very limited sound repertoire, these prompts occur less frequently and focus on any sound important to the message generated by the child. Input instead focuses on higher levels of language with the expectation that the system needs a far greater pool of data (i.e., vocabulary, morphemes, word combinations, event structures) and communicative experience to elaborate and refine phonemic categories and phonological patterns.

Perceptual or motor cues are relatively more frequent and direct for an older child with a specific error, such as a lateralized /s/ or distorted /r/. However, as soon as the sound is stimulable, contexts such as orally reading an age-appropriate book should be used. The student is expected to monitor productions of the sound(s) in words read. The story provides a linguistic context in which the entire constellation of language processes (i.e., words, morphemes, syntax, story structure, as well as phonology) is integrated with the sound production in a meaningful context (Norris, 1998a). The written language provides a scaffold or support for using the sound within these complex contexts. The words, word order, meaning, and story elements are organized by the text so that the child can devote cognitive resources to matching speech productions to the phonemes represented by letters while producing complex sentences.

Monitoring of productions also can easily be facilitated. The SLP can make a running record of correct versus incorrect productions on a printed copy of the text, which can then be examined with the child and the sentence or paragraph reread. The reading can be audiotaped after each sentence and replayed to enable the child to engage in self-monitoring or discriminating correct versus incorrect productions and recasting those with errors. Once the child can maintain correct productions in this structured language context, the difficulty of the task can be increased by asking the child to paraphrase the information immediately following the reading, then to talk inferentially about what could happen next in the story, and finally, to talk about a similar life experience (i.e., spontaneous conversation).

In both situations, the perceptual and motor cues are embedded within communication-based intervention. The sound and production cues given are integrated within the constellation of language processes. Thus, the elaborations and refinements are an integral part of the language used by a child for communication, rather than a skill that the child then must generalize to connected speech.

REFERENCES

Bernthal, J.E., & Bankson, N.W. (2004). *Articulation and phonological disorders* (5th ed.). Boston: Allyn & Bacon.

Blakeley, R.W. (2001). *Screening Test for Developmental Apraxia of Speech Examiner's Manual* (2nd ed.). Austin, TX: PRO-ED.

Bowen, C., & Cupples, L. (1999). Parents and children together (PACT): A collaborative approach to phonological therapy. *International Journal of Language and Communication Disorders, 34,* 35–55.

Carter-Brazier, P.A., Norris, J.A., & Hoffman, P.R. (2003, November). Use of alphabet storybooks to increase print referencing in Head Start reading. Poster session presented at the American Speech-Language-Hearing Association national convention, Chicago.

Conti-Ramsden, G., & Botting, N. (1999). Classification of children with specific language impairment: Longitudinal considerations. *Journal of Speech and Hearing Research, 42*(5), 1195–1204.

Ehri, L.C., Nunes, S.R., Willows, D.M., Schuster, B.V., & Shanahan, T. (2001). Phonemic awareness: Instruction helps children learn to read. Evidence from the National Reading Panel's meta-analysis. *Reading Research Quarterly, 36*(3), 250–287.

Ezell, H.K., & Justice, L.M. (2000). Increasing the print focus of adult-child shared book reading through observational learning. *American Journal of Speech-Language Pathology, 9,* 36–47.

Fry, E.A. (1968). A readability formula that saves time. *Journal of Reading, 11,* 513–516, 575–578.

Hart, B., & Risley, T.R. (1995). *Meaningful differences in the everyday experience of young American children.* Baltimore: Paul H. Brookes Publishing Co.

Hickman, L. (1997). *The Apraxia Profile.* San Antonio, TX: Harcourt Assessment.

Hoffman, P.R., & Norris, J.A. (1989). On the nature of phonological processes: Evidence from normal children's spelling errors. *Journal of Speech and Hearing Research, 32,* 787–794.

Justice, L.M., & Ezell, H.K. (2000). Enhancing children's print and word awareness through home-based parent intervention. *American Journal of Speech-Language Pathology, 9,* 257–269.

Justice, L.M., & Ezell, H.K. (2002). Use of storybook reading to increase the print awareness in at-risk children. *American Journal of Speech-Language Pathology, 11,* 17–29.

Lindblom, B. (1992). Phonological units as adaptive emergents of lexical development. In C.A. Ferguson, L. Menn, & C. Stoel-Gammon (Eds.), *Phonological development: Models, research, implications* (pp. 565–604). Parkton, MD: York Press.

Lindblom, B. (2000). Developmental origins of adult phonology: The interplay between phonetic emergents and evolutionary adaptations of sound patterns. *Phonetica, 57,* 297–314.

Locke, J.L. (1995). *The child's path to spoken language.* Cambridge, MA: Harvard University Press.

Nelson, K. (1985). *Making sense: The development of meaning in early childhood.* New York: Academic Press.

Nelson, K. (1996). *Language in cognitive development: The emergence of the mediated mind.* New York: Cambridge University Press.

Norris, J.A. (1998a). I could read if I just had a little help: Facilitating reading in whole language contexts. In C. Weaver (Ed.), *Practicing what we know: Informed reading instruction* (pp. 513–553). Urbana, IL: NCTE Press.

Norris, J.A. (1998b). Early sentence transformations and the development of complex syntactic structures. In B. Shulman & W. Haynes (Eds.), *Communication development: Foundations, processes and clinical applications* (pp. 293–340). Baltimore: Lippincott Williams & Wilkins.

Norris, J.A. (2000). *SDS-development model: Developmental scales for early childhood.* Criterion Eligibility Project, grant supported by the Louisiana State Department of Education.

Norris, J.A. (2001). *Phonic Faces Manual and Cards.* Baton Rouge, LA: Elementory.

Norris, J.A. (2002). *Icky carrots.* Baton Rouge, LA: Elementory.

Norris, J.A., Healey, E.C., Hoffman, P.R., Blanchet, P., Kaufman, E., & Scott, L. (1998, November). *Approaching fluency treatment from a multifactorial perspective: A changing view.* Seminar presented at the Annual Convention of the American Speech-Language-Hearing Association, Austin, TX.

Norris, J.A., & Hoffman, P.R. (1990). Language intervention within naturalistic environments. *Language, Speech, and Hearing Services in Schools, 21,* 72–84.

Norris, J.A., & Hoffman, P. (1996). Attaining, sustaining, and focusing attention: Intervention for children with ADHD. *Seminars in Speech and Language, 17,* 59–71.

Norris, J.A., & Hoffman, P.R. (2001). Language development and late talkers: A connectionist perspective. In R.G. Daniloff (Ed.), *Connectionist approaches to clinical language problems* (pp. 1–109). Fairfax, VA: TechBooks.

Norris, J.A., & Hoffman, P.R. (2002). Phonemic awareness: A complex developmental process. *Topics in Language Disorders, 22,* 1–34.

Norris, J.A., & Hoffman, P.R. (2003, November). *Use of alphabet storybooks to increase print referencing in parent-child reading.* Poster session presented at the American Speech-Language-Hearing Association national convention, Chicago, IL.

Oller, D.K. (1975). Simplification as the goal of phonological processes in child speech. *Language Learning, 24,* 299–303.

Pangburn, B.E. (2002). *Experience-based language acquisition: A computational model of human language acquisition.* Unpublished doctoral dissertation, Louisiana State University, Baton Rouge.

Phelan, E.L. (1989). *Relative efficacy of treatment strategies for functional misarticulation in preschool children: Sensory-motor and cognitive approaches.* Unpublished doctoral dissertation, Louisiana State University, Baton Rouge.

Piaget, J. (1952). *The origins of intelligence in children.* New York: International Universities Press.

Piaget, J. (1954). *The construction of reality in the child.* New York: Basic Books.

Roy, D.K. (2000). Learning visually grounded words and syntax of natural spoken language. *Evolution of Communication Journal, 4,* 33–57.

Saffran, J.R., Newport, E.L., Aslin, R.N., Tunick, R.A., & Barrueco, S. (1997). Incidental language learning: Listening (and learning) out of the corner of your ear. *Psychological Science, 8,* 101–105.

Seidenberg, M.S., & McClelland, J.L. (1989). A distributed, developmental model of word recognition and naming. *Psychological Review, 96,* 523–568.

Shelton, R.L., Johnson, A.F., Willis, V., & Arndt, W.B. (1975). Monitoring and reinforcement by parents as a means of automating articulatory responses: II. Study of preschool children. *Perceptual and Motor Skills, 40,* 599–610.

Stothard, S.E., Snowling, M.J., Bishop, D.V.M., Chipchase, B.B., & Kaplan, C.A. (1998). Language-impaired preschoolers: A follow-up into adolescence. *Journal of Speech, Language, and Hearing Research, 41,* 407–418.

Van Hattum, R.J. (Ed.). (1969). Program scheduling. In *Clinical speech in schools* (pp. 163–195). Springfield, IL: Charles C Thomas.

van Kleeck, A. (1996). Emphasizing form and meaning separately in prereading and early reading instruction. *Topics in Language Disorders, 7*(2), 27–49.

Vygotsky, L.S. (1978). *Mind in society: The development of higher psychological processes* (M. Cole, V. John-Steiner, S. Scribner, & E. Souberman, Eds.). Cambridge, MA: Harvard University Press.

Chapter 13

Special Considerations in Intervention

SHELLEY VELLEMAN

T he remediation of phonotactic deficits is a critical area of phonological intervention for children who are very young, have very severe impairments, or have childhood apraxia of speech (CAS). This area of intervention has been neglected in the literature (with the exception of Bernhardt, 1994; Bernhardt & Gilbert, 1992; Bernhardt & Stoel-Gammon, 1994; Grunwell, 1982; and Velleman, 2002); most sources focus solely on remediating inappropriate productions of specific sounds or sound classes, whether it be through traditional sound-by-sound, minimal pair, or phonological process therapy. Often, position-specific targeting of particular sounds or classes is recommended (e.g., teaching fricatives in final position), but the structures themselves are not the focus. Yet, children in these groups often lack the critical syllable or word shapes within which sound segments must be produced. Targeting a new sound in a new position may be far too difficult for a child who falls within one of these categories. A child who produces no final consonants, for example, may not be able to master the production of a particular sound (e.g., [s]) or sound class (e.g., fricatives) in that position until he or she has demonstrated some ability to close syllables in general, regardless of the accuracy of the segment that fills that slot.

Common phonotactic goals include

- Initial consonants, for children with severely atypical phonological patterns

- Final consonants

- Two-syllable or longer words

- Consonant clusters in initial, medial, or final position

- Two different syllables within the same word (i.e., suppression of reduplication)

- Two different consonants or vowels within the same word (i.e., suppression of harmony)

When such goals are addressed, the structure, rather than the sound segments or features themselves, is the target. Thus, if the goal is for the child to produce final consonants, any final consonant will do, regardless of the particular consonant that terminates the target word. Of course, it is useful to choose target words that include final consonants that are typically easier for children to learn (e.g., nasals or fricatives) or that might be expected to be easier for that particular child to produce (e.g., they are already present in the child's inventory, the child is stimulable for sounds in that position). However, segmental accuracy should not be the focus. Similarly, if the objective is to reduce reduplication, any production in which the two syllables are different from each other satisfies the objective, regardless of their relationship to the actual target syllables.

Phonotactic considerations are also very important in selecting remediation approaches for other targets. It may be possible in some cases, for example, to "buy two objectives for the price of one" by addressing a new sound or sound class (e.g., fricatives) in a new syllable or word position (e.g., final position). If this is done, however, it should be done with full knowledge of what is being attempted. In general, it is important to carefully consider the phonotactic conditions under which new sounds or sound classes are to be addressed. This is especially critical when treating children with CAS, who often have difficulty generalizing mastered sounds to new contexts or learning new sounds in mastered contexts in any case. Addressing a new sound in a new context is most often out of the question for these children. Other, apparently inconsequential, aspects of the phonotactics of the target word may even have an impact on the child's ability to produce it. For example, a child who already produces both consonant–vowel (CV) and CVC syllables and is learning a new sound in initial position may nonetheless find it more difficult to produce that new sound in a CVC than in a CV. Alternatively, a CVC in which the final consonant harmonizes with the target initial consonant may be facilitory. In fact, the use of simpler phonotactic structures can often spur progress on another goal. These may include

- Using reduplicated targets to introduce two-syllable words

- Using targets with consonant harmony to introduce final consonants, initial or final consonant clusters, or a new feature in final position

- Using onsetless words to introduce final consonants, final consonant clusters, or a new feature in final position

- Using open syllables (with no final consonant) to introduce initial clusters

INTERVENTION FOR CHILDREN WITH CHILDHOOD APRAXIA OF SPEECH

These suggestions apply to young children and children with severe phonological disorders as well as to children with CAS. I use and recommend additional approaches that are tailored specifically to the motor planning/sequencing disorders that characterize CAS (Velleman, 2003). Children with this disorder are often able to produce isolated consonant or vowel sounds but are unable to put them together into a syllable. The difficulty appears to lie in the necessity of planning the articulatory transition from consonant into vowel (for a CV syllable, or vice versa for VC). Traditional apraxia therapy often consisted of repeated drilling of a small set of words. These words became established in the children's repertoires as memorized forms, but the activity did not address the planning problem. Therefore, it is preferable to engage the child in tasks that require on-the-spot planning: determination of the current state of the vocal tract (e.g., tongue placement), recognition of the desired intermediate and end states, and planning for the required articulatory gesture (Velleman, 2003; Velleman & Strand, 1994). One such task is the "ba-ba board," a set of pictures or written syllables that prompt the child to produce a sequence of C–V alternations, with either the consonant or the vowel held constant: [babibobu], [badamana], and so forth. For children who are young or who have severe language CAS, simply repeating the same syllable the same way (e.g., [babababa]) is often a trial. In these cases, the repetitions can be incorporated into pretend play (e.g., pretending to set the table while saying "bowl bowl bowl bowl") or performed by adapting counting books to the purpose (e.g., pointing to cows in a counting book while saying "moo moo moo moo").

To establish new phonemes within the repertoires of children with CAS, the use of visual or tactile cues (e.g., those advocated by Bashir, Grahamjones, & Bostwick, 1984; Chumpelik, 1984; Hayden & Square, 1994; and Square, 1994, 1999) can be helpful. Integral stimulation methods, in which the child rehearses the word or phrase first simultaneously with the therapist, then in imitation, and finally in delayed imitation (Strand, 1995; Strand & Skinder, 1999), have also been shown to be successful for this purpose.

It is important to establish some key words that the child with CAS can produce automatically. Verbal routines are useful for this purpose; they have the advantage of being predictable and, often, of being produced in unison. Thus, very little communicative pressure exists: Everyone knows what will be said, and everyone will say it together so no one person's production will stand out. Useful verbal routines include songs, rhymes, and predictable books (Kehoe & Stoel-Gammon, 2001). Standard routines can be creatively altered to address the target word (e.g., "Old MacDonald had some cheese"; "The bees on the bus go buzz buzz buzz"). For helping children with CAS or other severe speech difficulties to learn popular children's songs, *Time to Sing!* (Center for Creative Play, 2000) is invaluable.

DIALECT CONSIDERATIONS IN INTERVENTION

Providing therapy to a child who speaks a different dialect from the speech-language pathologist (SLP) is even more difficult than assessing such a child (as discussed in Chapter 4), because it requires constant, ongoing self-monitoring and self-education on the part of the therapist. Ideally, a speaker of the child's own dialect should provide treatment (Goldstein, 2000; Seymour & Valles, 1998). When this is not possible (as is, unfortunately, often the case), goals and objectives have to be selected carefully, targeting structures and elements that are dialect-appropriate. Personal experience as a clinician has taught me that it is difficult to suppress corrections based on my own dialect, so it is far better to select target words that are dialect-neutral. For example, when working with a child who speaks African American English (AAE), I would not target iambic weak–strong–weak (wSw) stress patterns, or even medial [l] production, using the word *umbrella* because I pronounce that word as "umBRELLa" but the correct AAE pronunciation is "UMbrella." A clinician can model dialect-neutral words in the same way that they are targeted to be produced by the child. If the SLP has any doubt about the dialect-appropriate pronunciation of a word, it is his or her clinical responsibility to check with a parent or another speaker of that dialect. Even more difficult is targeting phonological goals in a dialect-appropriate order because little information is available about order of acquisition of English structures and elements in dialects other than Mainstream American English. (See Chapter 4 for further discussion of this issue as it relates to AAE.)

Providing phonological therapy to a child whose first language is not one that the SLP speaks fluently is an even greater challenge. In the best of all possible worlds, this would never be necessary. In our current world it is necessary more often than not. The second-choice option is for the SLP to collaborate with or supervise an SLP assistant or other trained (para)professional who does speak the child's language fluently. If this is not possible, then parents or other caregivers must be trained to be active collaborators in the therapy process. Cultural barriers are often massive and sometimes prohibitive; these issues are discussed in other sources (e.g., Goldstein, 2000) and will not be addressed here. Language barriers may crop up in unexpected ways, even when the family members speak English quite well. For example, I worked at one point with a young girl who had been exposed primarily to Russian, although her older school-age siblings had learned some English at school and sometimes used it at home. The father, who was the one to bring the girl to therapy, translated and modeled the correct pronunciations of her word attempts. Occasionally, he said, "I don't know what she's saying. It's English." This mystified me, because the utterances definitely did not sound like English, until I found out that Russians say "She's speaking English" when a child produces jargon, just as Americans tend to say "She's speaking Chinese" or "It's Greek to me" when toddlers produce long strings of sounds with no apparent relationship to real words.

Regardless of who interacts directly with the child, the certified SLP carries the responsibility for the phonological content of the therapeutic process. A thorough review of the sounds, structures, and patterns of the target language must be carried out, as well as of the normal process of phonological development and any information that may be available about phonological delays and disorders in that language. A thorough analysis of the child's use of his or her native language phonology is the next step. Goals and objectives should be selected based on the functional importance in that language of the structures, elements, or patterns that are deficient. For example, producing final consonants is not of critical functional importance for children learning Japanese; it is far more important for them to be able to produce multisyllabic words. As always, several goals and objectives should be developed. Even less is known in other languages than in English about how to determine the direction in which a child's phonological system is ready to expand, so goals should be cycled periodically (Hodson & Paden, 1991), especially if progress is lacking after several weeks of treatment.

Target words should be selected based on their functionality for the child as well as their appropriateness to the objective and the ease with which they can be elicited (through actions, pictures, and so forth). Dictionaries of baby-talk words are sorely lacking, so parents and other speakers of the language should be used as informants when working with young children. Just as a good SLP would refer to a Mainstream American English-speaking toddler's stomach as *tummy* rather than *stomach* or *abdomen,* the baby-talk word *bipa* rather than the formal *estomago* should be used in Spanish. Similarly, sound effect noises, which may be appropriate phonological targets for young or severely phonologically disabled children, must be language specific and may even differ by dialect. Again, cultural barriers may make it more difficult to identify such words. (It has been my experience, for example, that Hispanic mothers are reluctant to provide such "improper" labels to a professional.) Activities should be as similar to those of the child's experience as possible, especially if they are to be carried out by family members.

REFERENCES

Bashir, A., Grahamjones, F., & Bostwick, R. (1984). A touch-cue method of therapy for developmental verbal apraxia. *Seminars in Speech and Language, 5*(2), 127–137.

Bernhardt, B. (1994). Phonological intervention techniques for syllable and word structure development. *Clinics in Communication Disorders, 4*(1), 54–65.

Bernhardt, B.H., & Gilbert, J. (1992). Applying linguistic theory to speech-language pathology: The case for nonlinear phonology. *Clinical Linguistics & Phonetics, 6*(1–2), 123–145.

Bernhardt, B., & Stoel-Gammon, C. (1994). Nonlinear phonology: Introduction and clinical application. *Journal of Speech and Hearing Research, 37,* 123–143.

Center for Creative Play. (2000). *Time to sing!* [audio CD]. Pittsburgh, PA: Author.

Chumpelik, D. (1984). The prompt system of therapy: Theoretical framework and applications for developmental apraxia of speech. *Seminars in Speech and Language, 5,* 139–153.

Goldstein, B. (2000). *Cultural and linguistic diversity resource guide for speech-language pathologists.* San Diego: Singular Publishing Group.

Grunwell, P. (1982). *Clinical phonology.* Rockville, MD: Aspen.

Hayden, D.A., & Square, P.A. (1994). Motor speech treatment hierarchy: A systems approach. *Clinics in Communication Disorders, 5,* 162–175.

Hodson, B.W., & Paden, E.P. (1991). *Targeting intelligible speech: A phonological approach to remediation* (2nd ed.). Austin, TX: PRO-ED.

Kehoe, M.M., & Stoel-Gammon, C. (2001). Development of syllable structure in English-speaking children with particular reference to rhymes. *Journal of Child Language, 28*(2), 393–432.

Seymour, E.H., & Valles, L. (1998). Language intervention for linguistically different learners. In C.M. Seymour & E.H. Nober (Eds.), *Introduction to communication disorders: A multicultural approach* (pp. 89–110). Boston: Butterworth-Heinemann.

Square, P.A. (1994). Treatment approaches for developmental apraxia of speech. *Clinics in Communication Disorders, 4,* 151–161.

Square, P.A. (1999). Treatment of developmental apraxia of speech: Tactile-kinesthetic, rhythmic, and gestural approaches. In A.J. Caruso & E.A. Strand (Eds.), *Clinical management of motor speech disorders in children* (pp. 149–186). New York: Thieme Medical Publishers.

Strand, E.A. (1995). Treatment of motor speech disorders in children. *Seminars in Speech and Language, 16*(2), 126–139.

Strand, E.A., & Skinder, A. (1999). Treatment of developmental apraxia of speech: Integral stimulation methods. In A.J. Caruso & E.A. Strand (Eds.), *Clinical management of motor speech disorders in children* (pp. 109–148). New York: Thieme Medical Publishers.

Velleman, S.L. (2002). Phonotactic therapy. *Seminars in Speech and Language, 23*(1), 43–56.

Velleman, S.L. (2003). *Resource guide for childhood apraxia of speech.* Albany, NY: Delmar Learning.

Velleman, S., & Strand, K. (1994). Developmental verbal dyspraxia. In J.E. Bernthal & N.W. Bankson (Eds.), *Child phonology: Characteristics, assessment, and intervention with special populations* (pp. 110–139). New York: Thieme Medical Publishers.

Chapter 14

A Treatment Program
for Enhancing Stimulability

Adele W. Miccio

timulability, a child's ability to immediately modify speech production errors when presented with a model (Milisen, 1954), is an important diagnostic tool (Carter & Buck, 1958; Diedrich, 1983; Elbert, 1997; Powell & Miccio, 1996; Somers et al., 1967) and is a critical element of many assessment batteries (Hodson, Scherz, & Strattman, 2002; Khan, 2002; Miccio, 2002; Tyler, 1996; Tyler & Tolbert, 2002). The importance of stimulability as a prognostic indicator has been demonstrated by treatment research.

Stimulability has been shown to explain generalization patterns that occur following treatment (Dinnsen & Elbert, 1984; Miccio, Elbert, & Forrest, 1999; Powell, Elbert, & Dinnsen, 1991; Rvachew, Rafaat, & Martin, 1999; Tyler, Edwards, & Saxman, 1987). Stimulability demonstrates that the structure and function of the articulatory mechanism is intact to some degree and the required articulatory movements are produced in more supportive circumstances (Bain, 1994; Turton, 1973). If a child imitates a sound that is not produced in the phonetic inventory, it is conceptually distinct from the sound used in error (Dinnsen & Elbert, 1984; Powell & Miccio, 1996). Stimulable sounds are most likely to be acquired naturally in the absence of treatment (Miccio et al., 1999), and nonstimulable sounds are least likely to change without treatment (Miccio et al., 1999; Powell et al., 1991). Kwiatkowski and Shriberg (1993) suggest that children who are stimulable for production of speech sounds have the ability to focus on speech production and are motivated to change.

Given the positive prognostic factors associated with stimulability, it is a logical treatment priority. A child with a very small phonetic inventory who is not stimulable for production of absent sounds has limited opportunity to produce phonological contrasts and, consequently, is likely to be unintelligible (Kent, Miolo, & Bloedel, 1994). Because a small phonetic inventory limits the number of different utterances a child may produce, homonymy (the use of one form for multiple meanings) results. To increase intelligibility, it is important to increase the size of a child's phonetic inventory as rapidly as possible so that more phonological contrasts can be produced. The more stimulable sounds become, the more rapidly change will occur in the phonological system.

Treatment research suggests that speech-language pathologists may maximize treatment effects by planning for systemwide generalization and strategically teaching the sound(s) that will introduce the most change into the phonological system (see Gierut, 1998, for a review). A number of treatment studies have shown that treating more complex sounds results in greatest systemwide change (see Gierut, 2001, for a review). Dinnsen, Chin, Elbert, and Powell (1990) identified an implicational hierarchy for describing the complexity of phonetic inventories from the least to the most complex. For a child to acquire the features of the most complex inventory (Level E), he or she must first acquire the features of the less complex inventories (Levels A through D). Tyler and Figurski (1994) explored the clinical utility of this implicational hierarchy and found that teaching a more complex phonetic distinction resulted in more sounds being added to the phonetic inventory than did teaching a less complex phonetic distinction. Teaching complex distinctions, however, necessitates targeting sounds with the most elaborate feature structures (Dinnsen, Chin, & Elbert, 1992). These sounds are most likely to be excluded from the inventory (Powell, Elbert, Miccio, Strike-Roussos, & Brasseur, 1998).

CLINICAL APPLICATION OF THE TREATMENT RESEARCH LITERATURE

Although stimulability has been suggested as an important factor in determining treatment targets (Lof, 1996; Miccio et al., 1999; Powell et al., 1991), little discussion has addressed how to treat nonstimulable sounds. In fact, many clinicians avoid direct intervention with nonstimulable sounds. If a major clinical concern is increasing the number of phonological contrasts in an intelligible child's sound system, then the primary goal of a treatment program for a child with an impoverished phonetic inventory is to increase the number of sounds in the inventory as quickly and efficiently as possible. Why, then, are nonstimulable sounds often avoided in favor of stimulable sounds? One rationale for treating stimulable sounds is that nonstimulable sounds are simply too difficult to teach and the cost–benefit ratio is questionable (Fey & Stalker, 1986). Nonstimulable sounds are also more frustrating for small children to master (Hodson & Paden, 1991).

Consequently, stimulable sounds are targeted so that rapid improvement may be achieved despite the fact that limited systemwide change is likely to occur. A stimulable target is often an unmarked, early developing sound such as a bilabial or alveolar stop or nasal. Acquisition of these early developing sounds, however, does not generalize beyond local change (Gierut, Morrisette, Hughes, & Rowland, 1996). If a child has a very small phonetic inventory and the domain of generalization is limited to stimulable sounds, systemwide generalization cannot be predicted and the phonetic inventory will remain relatively small despite extensive treatment (Powell, 1996).

If stimulability is as important a predictor of success following treatment as the treatment itself, a more efficacious treatment program would be one that gives priority to nonstimulable sounds. These sounds are not likely to be acquired without direct treatment (Miccio et al., 1999; Powell et al., 1991). For the results of stimulability research to be applied successfully in the clinic, treatment strategies must be designed to address the problems and frustrations noted by clinicians and researchers.

STIMULABILITY AS THE TREATMENT TARGET

Powell (1996) targeted increasing the phonetic inventory early in the treatment process with a child with a persistent speech sound disorder by encouraging the child to experiment with speech sounds. His modular approach utilizes warm-up activities that encourage the child to imitate English phones as well as establishing new sounds and promoting generalization of newly learned sounds. Rvachew and colleagues (1999) directly targeted stimulability using phonetic placement and speech perception activities directed at target sounds. Rvachew and Nowak (2001) found that teaching both stimulable and nonstimulable sounds increased the rate of progress using a traditional approach.

Enhancing Stimulability for Phonological Acquisition

Emphasis on early intervention has resulted in the identification of children with phonological disorders at younger ages (Stoel-Gammon, 1994). Toddlers, however, do not respond readily to conventional assessment and treatment methodologies (Tyler, 1996). To meet the need for a treatment program designed for use with very young children with very limited phonetic inventories, Miccio and Elbert (1996) designed an approach to increase the number of stimulable sounds in the phonetic inventory by pairing consonants with alliterative characters and motions. To achieve early success as well as target nonstimulable sounds, Miccio and Elbert (1996) taught all consonants at once during every session (both stimulable and nonstimulable) in a broad approach. The most recent version of this approach, its necessary components, and its rationale are described here.

Components of Treatment to Enhance Stimulability

Determine Stimulable and Nonstimulable Sounds

To establish which sounds are stimulable and nonstimulable, a sound-specific stimulability probe is administered for all consonants that are absent from the phonetic inventory as determined by an articulation test that provides an adequate sampling of each consonant in each possible word position. Examples of stimulability probes adapted from the Carter and Buck (1958) Nonsense Syllable Task are available in the literature (Bernthal & Bankson, 2004; Miccio, 2002; Powell & Miccio, 1996). The stimulability probe is administered to assess a client's ability to imitate the examiner's productions in isolation and in syllables. Those sounds that a client cannot imitate in either isolation or in consonant-vowel (CV) syllables are considered nonstimulable and become the primary intervention targets.

Directly Target Nonstimulable Sounds

Teaching nonstimulable sounds results in acquisition of the nonstimulable sound as well as untreated stimulable sounds (Miccio et al., 1999; Powell et al., 1991). As a direct consequence of teaching sounds with more complex phonetic distinctions, more sounds will be added to the phonetic inventory (Gierut, 2001; Tyler & Figurski, 1994). More generalization occurs when unknown aspects of the system are taught (Gierut, 1998).

Make Targets the Focus of Joint Attention

Children are more likely to produce a target sound when they are attending to and interested in its corresponding referent. This literature on semantic development indicates that children spontaneously repeat words when parents have previously labeled the objects that were the focus of joint attention (Baldwin & Markman, 1989; Baldwin et al., 1996). This suggests that speech sounds may be easier to learn when they are associated with interesting objects that have been verbally labeled for them by adults.

Associate Speech Sounds with Hand/Body Motions

Fazio (1997) observed that children with specific language impairment were most likely to remember poems after a 2-day delay when the poem was learned with accompanying hand motions. The hand motions appeared to serve as retrieval cues for remembering the poem. To learn new speech sounds, children not only must learn to articulate the sounds but must also retrieve the new sounds at later dates and learn to use them in lexical items. Multimodal input increases ability to retain newly learned speech sounds (Rauscher, Krauss, & Chen, 1996). Pairing speech sounds with motions may also assist a child with more accurate retrieval of newly learned speech sounds at a later date.

Associate Speech Sounds with Alliterative Character of Interest to the Child

Pairing speech sounds with interesting characters increases interest in the stimulability activities and encourages full participation in activities. In addition, relatively recent attention to the importance of phonology to emerging literacy abilities has shown that the most crucial aspects of early reading are phonological awareness and knowledge of the alphabetic principle (Adams, Treiman, & Pressley, 1998; Lyon, 1995). Associating speech sounds with alliterative characters provides an immediate opportunity for a child to generalize newly learned information to larger linguistic units. It also enhances the opportunity for a child to develop conscious awareness of the newly learned sound segments.

Encourage Vocal Practice

Speech sound production practice is a crucial element for the acquisition of new sounds as well as generalization of those sounds to untreated linguistic units (Powell et al., 1998; Saben & Ingham, 1991). Very young children are unlikely to attend to or respond to drill activities. Enhancing stimulability encourages vocal practice by including sound elicitation activities that involve turn-taking and requesting.

Ensure Early Success

Edwards (1983) suggested that treatment targets should be relatively easy so that immediate success may be obtained. To achieve this, treatment should include sounds that are sometimes produced correctly or already included in the phonetic inventory. An effective strategy that incorporates Edwards's ideas is to teach all sounds concurrently, both stimulable sounds and nonstimulable sounds. The child will achieve immediate success when stimulable sounds are produced but will also receive remediation for more difficult, nonstimulable sounds at the same time.

Ensure Successful Communicative Attempts

During sound elicitation activities, the child is free to choose any sound. When the clinician takes a turn, however, he or she always chooses a nonstimulable sound. Because the child pairs a recognizable motion with the intended sound, the child's communicative intent is successful. If a child produces an unintended sound, the clinician knows the intended sound by its paired motion and turn-taking continues without disruption. The successful communication encourages more verbalization (Rescorla & Ratner, 1996), and the child is more likely to attempt production of nonstimulable sounds.

An Example of Treatment to Enhance Stimulability

As noted previously, the treatment program to enhance stimulability was designed to increase the size of the phonetic inventory by teaching most major consonants at once. Because the primary goal is to enhance stimulability, sounds are taught in isolation (e.g., [z:::::]) or in the case of some sounds, such as stops or glides, in a CV context (e.g., [gʌ]. Each major consonant is associated with a character representing an animal or object. In addition, a characteristic body movement or hand motion is associated with each character and its sound (see Table 14.1 for motions used with stimulus characters to elicit consonant production). The consonants /ð/, /ʒ/, and /ŋ/ are not included because of their low frequency of occurrence in content words or phonotactic constraints against production in syllable onset position. Verbal praise is used to reinforce correct speech production. A typical treatment session begins with elicitation of an abbreviated version of a stimulability probe that elicits one vowel context each session. At the beginning of a session, for example, the client is asked to imitate [f] in isolation and in the contexts [fi], [ifi], and [if]. All other nonstimulable sounds are also elicited in this context. At the beginning of the next session, [f] is again elicited in isolation in the contexts [fa], [afa], and [af]. At the third session, stimulability testing will involve the vowel [u]. In this way, the complete stimulability probe is completed in every session.

To evaluate generalization to real words, we also include a short imitative palindrome probe at the end of each session. In this probe, the child imitates the clinician's production of one palindrome for each target consonant (e.g., *tot, dad, pop, bob*). This probe tests for generalization across syllable positions in a very simple phonotactic environment. No reinforcement is provided during any probe. Probes provide a quick picture of synchronic change during sessions and diachronic change across sessions.

Table 14.1.   Stimulus characters used to elicit consonant production

Consonant		Character	Associated motion
Stops	/p/	Putt-Putt Pig	Glide hands in a skating motion
	/b/	Baby Bear	Pantomime rocking a baby
	/t/	Talkie Turkey	Raise a pretend phone receiver to ear
	/d/	Dirty Dog	Make digging motion with hands
	/k/	Coughing Cow	Place hand near the top of throat
	/g/	Goofy Goat	Roll eyes toward ceiling
Fricatives	/f/	Fussy Fish	Fussily push hand away from body
	/v/	Viney Violet	Move arm up as a winding vine
	/θ/	Thinking Thumb	Move thumb in a circle
	/s/	Silly Snake	Move finger up arm
	/z/	Zippy Zebra	Zip coat
	/ʃ/	Shy Sheepy	Clutch hands together and push down
Affricates	/ʧ/	Cheeky Chick	Move hand sassily toward cheek
	/ʤ/	Giant Giraffe	Move hand upward in stair steps
Nasals	/m/	Munchie Mouse	Push lips together and rub tummy
	/n/	Naughty Newt	Shake finger in scolding motion
Glides	/w/	Wiggly Worm	Shiver
	/j/	Yawning Yoyo	Yawn and move hand as to suppress it
	/h/	Happy Hippo	Laugh and shake shoulders
	/l/	Lazy Lion	Stretch arms in L shape
	/r/	Rowdy Rooster	Rev motorcycle gears

Note: Several motions and characters have been revised since Miccio & Elbert (1996), based on efficacy experiments and feedback from clinicians and clients. (Reprinted from *Journal of Communication Disorders, 29,* Miccio & Elbert, Enhancing stimulability: A treatment program, pp. 335–351; copyright © 1996, with permission from Elsevier.)

Review of Sounds and Their Associated Characters

After a probe is administered, 5- × 7-inch cards with pictures of the characters are reviewed one at a time with the associated sound and motion. The character cards are shown to the client one by one to focus the child's attention on each character. With the clinician and client's attention jointly focused on the character, the clinician models the character's sound and associated movement. This ensures that the client understands the target sounds and their associated motions. The character for /p/, for example, is Putt-Putt Pig, who moves her hooves back and forth in a skating motion. All of the stop consonants are associated with ballistic motions to help the client understand the production characteristics of stops. However, all fricatives are associated with continuous motions to emphasize the continuous quality of fricatives. The character for /z/, for example, is Zippy Zebra, who pantomimes zipping up his coat. All consonants, including those that are present in the child's phonetic inventory, are reviewed in this manner. Associated body movements are always used concurrently with speech production.

Stimulability Activities

Attempts to facilitate speech sound production are embedded in play-like activities that provide the client with multiple opportunities to imitate consonants. Developmentally appropriate activities are designed specifically around the target sound characters. During these activities the client and clinician always take turns so that the clinician is constantly modeling the target sounds and the client has many opportunities to imitate them.

Any number of stimulability activities may be used during the session. A set of character playing cards, for example, may be used to play familiar games such as Go Fish. The client and clinician each hold a group of cards and ask each other in turn for a particular card. Because of the large number of nonstimulable sounds in a client's inventory, a client may fail to produce the intended sound when making a request. The associated movement, however, cues the clinician as to which card the client is requesting. When a client fails to say [s:] but mimes zipping up her coat, for example, the clinician knows the intended sound was [s]. Consequently, the clinician may provide appropriate feedback about how to correctly produce [s] without a conversational breakdown occurring. The clinician may say, "So, do I have Silly Snake? Let me see. Silly Snake says [s::::]. Oh yes, here's Silly Snake. He says [s:::]." In this way, a multimodality, auditory-visual-tactile cue is provided. If the child imitates the sound correctly, positive verbal feedback is given. In this way, stimulability tasks are incorporated into games and activities designed to draw attention to speech sounds without resorting to drill-like activities. To elicit speech production, the child is given an assertive role involving communicative functions of requesting actions and objects or directing attention to sounds of interest.

To ensure that a client achieves success while producing speech sounds, all conso-nants, even those in the inventory, are included. If a child does not successfully imitate a nonstimulable sound, she may next request a character with a stimulable sound. If, for example, the early developing bilabial stops are present in the inventory, a child will receive positive feedback when requesting Putt-Putt Pig and producing [p] correctly. In addition, including alliterative characters provides multiple opportunities to indirectly target generalization of newly learned sounds to larger lexical items and to connected speech by using character names. A clinician may ask the client if they like to play with

Putt-Putt Pig or what is special about Putt-Putt Pig, for example. Often, children tell the clinician that Putt-Putt Pig is pink and wears a purple dress and has purple ribbons. The clinician uses this opportunity to comment positively on the use of [p] in connected speech or to demonstrate [p] for the child. In this way, stimulable sounds are reinforced and stabilized in the sound system, and nonstimulable sounds receive direct intervention.

Although the child is free to request any card during an activity, the clinician's role is to redirect attention to nonstimulable sounds by modeling a nonstimulable sound as she makes a request during her turn. The child is encouraged but not required to imitate the sound along with the clinician. When the child takes his or her next turn, he or she may request any character, either one that is associated with a stimulable sound or one that is nonstimulable. Because both stimulable and nonstimulable sounds are targeted to expand the phonetic inventory, the child is successful and frustration is kept to a minimum.

Two or three activities are used each session to maintain joint attention and interest. Many activities have been used successfully. Some favorite activities include using lotto boards with the alliterative characters, playing character card games, mailing the character cards, sending the characters to space, and so forth. Simple games that provide multiple opportunities to practice speech sounds are most successful. Another favorite activity consists of placing all the cards face down in a basket so the clinician and child may take turns picking a card. When the child picks a card, the clinician must guess the name of the character. The child gives a clue by making the associated motion and attempting to produce the target sound. As with the other activities, the clinician identifies the intended target sound by the associated motion and either reinforces the correct production or draws attention to the correct production through modeling and phonetic placement cues. For the youngest children, cards may be used in more active play such as a fishing game. Many experiential play activities are appropriate for use with the sound–character cards. Spinner games are popular with slightly older children. The client and clinician take turns with the spinner and when the spinner lands on a character, the sounds and their associated motions are produced. For older children, the cards are incorporated into board games.

In summary, characters are introduced and associated with their sounds and motions at the beginning of the session. Throughout the session, the clinician and child take turns and the clinician is fully involved in the activities so that modeling and speech production are the integral parts of the treatment. Motions are only elicited when paired with speech sounds. In our experience, children who do not respond to conventional treatment approaches such as traditional therapy (Van Riper & Erickson, 1996) or minimal pair treatment (Weiner, 1981) readily imitate the movements and, with very little encouragement, try to imitate the sounds. As children become more successful in their communicative attempts, they also become more receptive to the speech production tasks. When children are comfortable with speech production and imitating the clinician, instructions to listen and watch the clinician say the sound or phonetic placement cues are occasionally used to shape more precise articulation. All treatment activities provide a supportive framework that encourages the development of stimulability skills and enhances the awareness of sound properties.

This treatment program can also be adapted to small groups and the character cards may be used for sound awareness activities in classroom circle time. Siblings and parents have also participated in stimulability treatment. Parents have reported calling attention to their children's target sounds by using the sounds with their corresponding motions at home. Feedback from parents is positive because generalization is encouraged while maintaining a pleasant, nonthreatening atmosphere that encourages speech production.

SUMMARY

The purpose of this treatment program is to enhance stimulability for speech production. It is most appropriate for young children with multiple sounds in error and for whom those sounds are absent from the phonetic inventory. Once a child is stimulable for production of the majority of speech sounds, the clinician may provide more intensive treatment for those sounds that are most resistant to change and provide opportunity for stimulable sounds to generalize across the phonological system. Once a child has a large phonetic inventory, he or she is likely to benefit from treatment programs that address directly the phonemic aspects of the target phonological sound system or correct production of any residual speech errors.

Both anecdotal comments from parents and a social validity measure (Powell, 1989) showed that parents were very satisfied with the treatment program, particularly at the rapid rate at which children became more vocal and used new speech sounds. This is consistent with the work of Rvachew and Nowak (2001), who reported that parental satisfaction was greater when children showed greater progress toward acquisition earlier in a treatment program.

This treatment program is based on the prediction that nonstimulable sounds will not be acquired without direct treatment and stimulable sounds are likely to undergo change in the absence of treatment or be acquired during treatment of nonstimulable sounds (Miccio et al., 1999; Powell et al., 1991). The program incorporates a horizontal goal attack strategy (Fey, 1986; Williams, 2000) that targets multiple sounds at once. In addition, it follows several principles from the research literature on phonological treatment and early language learning. The efficiency and effectiveness of our treatment programs are enhanced by the addition of principles tested in the research literature.

Although this treatment may be characterized as a phonetic approach to treatment, attention is also drawn to the phonological system. As children become stimulable for production of sounds, they also begin to learn the relationships between different speech sounds. Increased understanding of a feature leads to further acquisition of other sounds that share that feature (McReynolds & Bennett, 1972; Powell, Miccio, Elbert, Brasseur, & Strike-Roussos, 1999). Locke (1983) argued that all things phonologic are phonetic. Attention to the physical aspects of sound production assists with the organization of the sound system and the interaction among subsystems (Ferguson & Farwell, 1975).

REFERENCES

Adams, M.J., Treiman, R., & Pressley, M. (1998). Reading, writing, and literacy. In I. Sigel & A. Renninger (Eds.), *Handbook of child psychology: Vol. 4. Child psychology in practice* (pp. 275–355). New York: John Wiley & Sons.

Bain, B.A. (1994). A framework for dynamic assessment in phonology: Stimulability revisited. *Clinics in Communication Disorders, 4,* 12–22.

Baldwin, D.A., & Markman, E.M. (1989). Establishing word–object relations: A first step. *Child Development, 60,* 381–398.

Baldwin, D.A., Markman, E.M., Bill, B., Desjardins, R.N., Irwin, J.M., & Tidball, G. (1996). Infants' reliance on a social criterion for establishing word–object relations. *Child Development, 67,* 3135–3153.

Bernthal, J.E., & Bankson, N.W. (2004). *Articulation and phonological disorders* (5th ed.). Boston: Allyn & Bacon.

Carter, E.T., & Buck, M.W. (1958). Prognostic testing for functional articulation disorders among children in the first grade. *Journal of Speech and Hearing Disorders, 23,* 124–133.

Diedrich, W. (1983). Stimulability and articulation disorders. *Seminars in Speech and Language, 4,* 297–311.

Dinnsen, D.A., Chin, S.B., & Elbert, M. (1992). On the lawfulness of change in phonetic inventories. *Lingua, 86,* 207–222.

Dinnsen, D.A., Chin, S.B., Elbert, M., & Powell, T.W. (1990). Some constraints on functionally disordered phonologies: Phonetic inventories and phonotactics. *Journal of Speech and Hearing Research, 33,* 28–37.

Dinnsen, D.A., & Elbert, M. (1984). On the relationship between phonology and learning. In M. Elbert, D.A. Dinnsen, & G. Weismer (Eds.), *Phonological theory and the misarticulating child* (ASHA Monographs No. 22; pp. 59–68). Rockville, MD: American Speech-Language-Hearing Association.

Edwards, M.L. (1983). Selection criteria for developing therapy goals. *Journal of Childhood Communication Disorders, 7,* 36–45.

Elbert, M. (1997). From articulation to phonology: The challenge of change. In B. Hodson & M.L. Edwards (Eds.), *Perspectives in applied phonology* (pp. 43–60). Gaithersburg, MD: Aspen Publishers.

Fazio, B.B. (1997). Learning a new poem: Memory for connected speech and phonological awareness in low-income children with and without specific language impairment. *Journal of Speech, Language, and Hearing Research, 40,* 1285–1297.

Ferguson, C., & Farwell, C. (1975). Words and sounds in early language acquisition. *Language, 51,* 419–439.

Fey, M.E. (1986). *Language intervention with young children.* San Diego: College-Hill Press.

Fey, M.E., & Stalker, C. (1986). A hypothesis testing approach to treatment of a child with an idiosyncratic morphophonological system. *Journal of Speech and Hearing Disorders, 41,* 324–336.

Gierut, J.A. (1998). Treatment efficacy: Functional phonological disorders in children. *Journal of Speech, Language, and Hearing Research, 41,* S85–S100.

Gierut, J.A. (2001). Complexity in phonological treatment: Clinical factors. *Language, Speech, and Hearing Services in Schools, 32,* 229–241.

Gierut, J.A., Morrisette, M., Hughes, M.T., & Rowland, S. (1996). Phonological treatment efficacy and developmental norms. *Language, Speech, and Hearing Services in Schools, 27,* 215–230.

Hodson, B.W., & Paden, E.E. (1991). *Targeting intelligible speech: A phonological approach to remediation.* Austin, TX: PRO-ED.

Hodson, B.W., Scherz, J.A., & Strattman, K.H. (2002). Evaluating communicative abilities of a highly unintelligible preschooler. *American Journal of Speech-Language Pathology, 11,* 236–242.

Kent, R.D., Miolo, G., & Bloedel, S. (1994). The intelligibility of children's speech: A review of evaluation procedures. *American Journal of Speech-Language Pathology, 3,* 81–95.

Khan, L.M. (2002). The sixth view: Assessing preschoolers' articulation and phonology from the trenches. *American Journal of Speech-Language Pathology, 11,* 250–254.

Kwiatkowski, J., & Shriberg, L.D. (1993). Speech normalization in developmental phonological disorders: A retrospective study of capability-focus theory. *Language, Speech, and Hearing Services in Schools, 24,* 10–18.

Locke, J.L. (1983). Clinical phonology: The explanation and treatment of speech sound disorders. *Journal of Speech and Hearing Disorders, 48,* 339–341.

Lof, G.L. (1996). Factors associated with speech-sound stimulability. *Journal of Communication Disorders, 29,* 255–278.

Lyon, G.R. (1995). Toward a definition of dyslexia. *Annals of Dyslexia, 45,* 3–27.

McReynolds, L.J., & Bennett, S. (1972). Distinctive feature generalization in articulation training. *Journal of Speech and Hearing Disorders, 37,* 462–470.

Miccio, A.W. (2002). Clinical problem solving: Assessment of phonological disorders. *American Journal of Speech-Language Pathology, 11,* 221–229.

Miccio, A.W., & Elbert, M. (1996). Enhancing stimulability: A treatment program. *Journal of Communication Disorders, 29,* 335–352.

Miccio, A.W., Elbert, M., & Forrest, K. (1999). The relationship between stimulability and phonological acquisition in children with normally developing and disordered phonologies. *American Journal of Speech-Language Pathology, 8,* 347–363.

Milisen, R. (1954). The disorder of articulation: A systematic clinical and experimental approach. *Journal of Speech and Hearing Disorders, Monograph Supplement 4,* p. 38.

Powell, T.W. (1989). *Stimulability as a factor in the phonologic generalization of misarticulating preschool children.* Unpublished doctoral dissertation, Indiana University, Bloomington.

Powell, T.W. (1996). Stimulability considerations in the treatment of a child with a persistent disorder of speech sound production. *Journal of Communication Disorders, 29,* 315–333.

Powell, T.W., Elbert, M., & Dinnsen, D.A. (1991). Stimulability as a factor in the phonological generalization of misarticulating preschool children. *Journal of Speech and Hearing Research, 34,* 1318–1328.

Powell, T.W., Elbert, M., Miccio, A.W., Strike-Roussos, C., & Brasseur, J. (1998). Facilitating [s] production in young children: An experimental evaluation of motoric and conceptual treatment approaches. *Clinical Linguistics & Phonetics, 12,* 127–146.

Powell, T.W., & Miccio, A.W. (1996). Stimulability: A useful clinical tool. *Journal of Communication Disorders, 29,* 237–254.

Powell, T.W., Miccio, A.W., Elbert, M., Brasseur, J., & Strike-Roussos, C. (1999). Patterns of sound change in children with phonological disorders. *Clinical Linguistics & Phonetics, 13,* 163–182.

Rauscher, F., Krauss, R.M., & Chen, Y. (1996). Gesture, speech and lexical access: The role of lexical movements in speech production. *Psychological Science, 7,* 226–231.

Rescorla, L., & Ratner, N.B. (1996). Phonetic profiles of toddlers with specific expressive language impairment. *Journal of Speech and Hearing Research, 39,* 153–165.

Rvachew, S., & Nowak, M. (2001). The effect of target-selection strategy on phonological learning. *Journal of Speech, Language, and Hearing Research, 44,* 610–623.

Rvachew, S., Rafaat, S., & Martin, M. (1999). Stimulability, speech perception skills, and the treatment of phonological disorders. *American Journal of Speech-Language Pathology, 8,* 33–43.

Saben, C., & Ingham, J.C. (1991). The effects of minimal pairs treatment on the speech sound production of children with phonological disorders. *Journal of Speech and Hearing Research, 34,* 1023–1040.

Somers, R.K., Leiss, R.H., Delp, M., Gerber, A., Fundrella, D., Smith, R., et al. (1967). Factors related to the effectiveness of articulation therapy for kindergarten, first and second grade children. *Journal of Speech and Hearing Research, 13,* 428–437.

Stoel-Gammon, C. (1994). Measuring phonology in babble and speech. *Clinics in Communication Disorders, 4,* 1–11.

Turton, L.J. (1973). Diagnostic implications of articulation testing. In W. Wolfe & D. Goulding (Eds.), *Articulation and learning* (pp. 195–218). Springfield, IL: Charles C. Thomas.

Tyler, A.A. (1996). Assessing stimulability in toddlers. *Journal of Communication Disorders, 29,* 279–298.

Tyler, A.A., Edwards, M.L., & Saxman, J.H. (1987). Clinical application of two phonologically based treatment procedures. *Journal of Speech and Hearing Disorders, 53,* 393–409.

Tyler, A.A., & Figurski, G.R. (1994). Phonetic inventory changes after treating distinctions along an implicational hierarchy. *Clinical Linguistics & Phonetics, 8,* 91–108.

Tyler, A.A., & Tolbert, L. (2002). Speech-language assessment in the clinical setting. *American Journal of Speech-Language Pathology, 11,* 215–220.

Van Riper, C., & Erickson, R.L. (1996). *Speech correction: An introduction to speech pathology and audiology* (9th ed.). Boston: Allyn & Bacon.

Weiner, F. (1981). Treatment of phonological disability using the method of meaningful minimal contrasts: Two case studies. *Journal of Speech and Hearing Disorders, 46,* 97–103.

Williams, A.L. (2000). Multiple oppositions: Theoretical foundations for an alternative approach. *American Journal of Speech-Language Pathology, 9,* 282–288.

Chapter 15

The Importance of Phonetic Factors in Phonological Intervention

SUSAN RVACHEW

E very clinician possesses a set of theoretical assumptions or beliefs that have an implicit or explicit impact on his or her clinical practice. Schwartz (1992) discussed the way in which a clinician's theoretical assumptions play a role in every aspect of the clinical process from the characterization of the child's error patterns to the choice of treatment procedures. It is important for the clinician to bring these sets of beliefs to conscious awareness in order to ensure consistency and coherence among them (e.g., one's beliefs about how phonology develops under normal circumstances should be consistent with one's beliefs about why some children fail to develop intelligible speech at the typical rate). Furthermore, research in other domains has shown that consistency between a clinician's theoretical assumptions and the choice of procedures and activities is also important to clinical efficacy (Weisz, Donenberg, Han, & Kauneckis, 1995).

This chapter outlines my approach to the treatment of phonological disorders. Throughout, I link the recommended treatment procedures and activities to the representation-based theoretical perspective articulated by Edwards, Fourakis, Beckman, and Fox (1999). Links to published treatment efficacy data are also made explicit. The examples that I present focus on phoneme level errors, although I typically target error patterns at the phoneme and syllable structure levels simultaneously, following Bernhardt and Gilbert (1992). I will focus on activities that can be implemented on a computer, although I am not suggesting that computer-based activities are inherently more effective than traditional activities. Rather, I find it easier to integrate all of my assessment, documentation, and treatment tasks into one 5-pound laptop than to carry around bags of files and tests and boxes of picture cards and toys

REPRESENTATION-BASED APPROACH

The intervention that I will be describing follows from a theoretical perspective in which the child's phonological knowledge is derived from the gradual accumulation of knowledge about the acoustic/phonetic and articulatory/phonetic characteristics of syllables and words. It is assumed that this learning process begins before the emergence of first words when the infant is learning to attend selectively to native-language phonetic contrasts. The process of mapping between the child's perceptual knowledge of the native language sound system and articulatory knowledge of that system also begins prelinguistically with the emergence of babbling at around 7 months of age. Although babbling behavior is necessarily constrained by the limitations of an infant's articulatory system (Davis & MacNeilage, 1995), it is reasonable to assume that the infant is actively attempting to reproduce sound categories that are learned as a consequence of listening to speech input (e.g., see Guenther, 1995; Plaut & Kello, 1999). The development of infant babble is significantly disrupted by any processes that degrade the auditory input, such as sensori-neural (Oller, 2000) or conductive hearing loss (Rvachew, Slawinski, Williams, & Green, 1999). Furthermore, these developments during the prelinguistic period are intimately connected to later speech and language development. The ability of the infant to encode the fine phonetic detail of speech is correlated with receptive and expressive vocabulary skills during the toddler period (Werker, Fennell, Corcoran, & Stager, 2002), as is an infant's ability to produce good quality babble comprising a variety of consonant-vowel combinations (McCune & Vihman, 2001).

When a toddler begins to understand and use meaningful words, underlying representations for individual words are derived from all of the exemplars of that word that are stored in memory (Pierrehumbert, 2002). The quality of the representations depends on the existence of a large store of detailed exemplars for each given word. More abstract knowledge of the native language phonological system is derived from the developing set of connections among underlying representations for words based on similarities at all levels of the phonological system, including featural, segmental, and prosodic (cf. Bernhardt & Stoel-Gammon, 1994). Initially the child's phonological system will be quite primitive, reflecting a toddler's tendency to encode only gross acoustic/phonetic details about heard words and the limitations of his or her articulatory system. Consider, for example, Waterson's (1971) son, who produced a large number of words with a small set of word shapes. All two-syllable words containing a bilabial consonant were produced as a form similar to [bebe] and single-syllable words containing a sibilant were produced as a form similar to [ɪʃ]. Over time, more and more acoustic details will be stored regarding each word as the child's experience with these words increases. Gradually the underlying representations of these words will become more distinct at each level of the phonology. Pressure to develop more distinctive underlying representations will come from sources external to the child, such as increased experience with speech input and the consequences of communicative breakdown, and from internal sources such as his or her developing cognitive, attentional, and memory capacities and the need to organize a lexicon that is growing rapidly.

The implication of this model of the developmental process is that phonological disorders may arise from disruptions in input processes (insufficient input or difficulties with the processing and encoding of that input), output processes (planning and execution of articulatory movements), or the organizational processes whereby phonological knowledge is derived from the mapping between input and output. Recently a great deal of effort has been directed at the task of identifying different subtypes of phonological disorder with the implication being that breakdowns at different levels of the system will require a different treatment approach (e.g., Dodd, Leahy, & Hambly, 1989). Reciprocal relationships exist among all levels of the system, however, and in fact it has been shown that children with phonological disorders demonstrate deficits in their ability to encode and reproduce the phonetic characteristics of speech sound categories in addition to deficiencies in their phonological knowledge (Edwards et al., 1999; Munson, Beckman, & Edwards, in press; Stackhouse & Wells, 1997). A child with a motor speech disorder such as childhood apraxia of speech will benefit from intervention procedures that directly target motor planning for different syllable structures (see Chapter 2) but may also require specific attention to his or her perceptual and phonological knowledge. A child who has poor perceptual knowledge of the acoustic characteristics of the sound contrasts of the native language due to chronic otitis media can also be expected to have imprecise underlying representations and phonological knowledge, leading in turn to an impaired ability to articulate words consistently and precisely.

The treatment program that follows from this theoretical perspective has three phases. During the first phase, a child is exposed to a variety of exemplars of the target phoneme and contrasting phonemes in order to ensure categorical perception of the target phoneme. Phonetic placement, visual feedback, and shaping techniques are used simultaneously to ensure that the child is able to articulate the phoneme in a variety of phonetic contexts. During the second phase, minimal pair production activities are introduced for a brief period to stabilize the child's phonological knowledge of the new phoneme contrast. During the final phase, the child is provided with plenty of opportunity to practice using the phoneme in communicative contexts. Other goals such as improved syntax or phonological awareness can be integrated with phonology intervention during this third phase.

PHASE I: ACOUSTIC/PHONETIC AND ARTICULATORY/PHONETIC KNOWLEDGE

Phonemic Perception Training

Children with speech delay are likely to have difficulty with the categorical perception of difficult phoneme contrasts such as those involving liquids and fricatives. These perceptual difficulties are most likely to manifest themselves when the children are asked to categorize suboptimal stimuli, such as synthetic speech (Broen, Strange, Doyle, & Heller, 1983; Hoffman et al., 1985; Rvachew & Jamieson, 1989), words recorded from children (Chaney, 1988; Hoffman, Stager, & Daniloff, 1983), or speech that has been digitized and electronically altered to remove cue redundancy (Edwards, Fox, & Rogers, 2002; Monnin & Huntington, 1974).

Rvachew and Jamieson (1995) concluded that these children's perceptual and productive errors reflect a mismatch between the child's phonological knowledge and the adult's system of underlying phonological contrasts. For example, some children appear to be unaware of /ʃ/ as a phoneme and, therefore, stimuli containing [ʃ] are assimilated to the /s/ phoneme category during perception and production tasks involving these fricatives (Rvachew & Jamieson, 1989). Other children demonstrate knowledge of a given phoneme contrast but define it in terms of nonstandard acoustic cues. For example, Hoffman et al. (1983) found that children who misarticulated /ɹ/ produced target /ɹ/ with a second formant frequency that was midway between the value appropriate for /w/ and the value appropriate for /ɹ/. These same children were apt to categorize words produced with this aberrant second formant frequency as exemplars of the /ɹ/ category, whereas children who are typically developing perceived these words to be exemplars of the /w/ category. This example shows that a child's pattern of articulation errors can be based on knowledge deficits at the level of the phonetic details as well as at the level of abstract phonemic contrast.

These problems with categorical perception of misarticulated phonemes can be remediated quickly in most cases using a very simple computer game called the *Speech Assessment and Interactive Learning System* (SAILS; Avaaz Innovations, 1994). This game teaches children to identify words that are pronounced correctly and words that are pronounced incorrectly. The program consists of a number of modules, each targeting a different word that begins or ends with a commonly misarticulated phoneme. Each module consists of 10–30 tokens recorded from children and adults, in which half are articulated correctly (e.g., *rat* → [ɹæt]) and half are articulated incorrectly (e.g., *lake* → [wæt] or [jæt]).The stimuli that are presented are drawn from a continuum that includes prototypical exemplars, correct but not prototypical exemplars, mildly distorted exemplars, and clearly incorrect exemplars of the target word. This kind of stimulus variability is necessary in order to help the child develop a clear sense of the range of acoustic characteristics that are appropriate to the target phoneme category as well as a sharply demarcated boundary between the target and the contrasting categories. The recorded words are presented to the child one at a time in random order. The child is also presented with two response alternatives on the computer monitor, a picture of the target word, and a picture of a large X. Using the *rat* module as an example, I instruct the child to point to the picture of the rat if they hear the word *rat* and to point to the X if they hear a word that is "not *rat*." The child could play this game independently because the program provides feedback about the correctness of the child's responses. However, I prefer to sit with the child in order to provide more detailed corrective feedback. I control the mouse and ask the child to point to the appropriate response alternative on the monitor so that I can prevent the child from clicking the wrong response alternative. When providing feedback I call attention to both the sound of the words and the articulatory gestures used to produce them (e.g., "Yes, that boy said 'rat'; I heard the growly 'rrr' at the beginning of the word" or "No, that didn't sound like the word 'rrrat'—he used his lips to say the word so it sounded like 'wwwat'"). Then, if the child's initial choice was incorrect, I represent the speech stimulus and give the child a second chance to identify the word as a well-produced version of *rat* or a misarticulated version of *rat*.

This program can be effective for a given phoneme with as few as three 10- to 20-minute sessions provided over 3 consecutive weeks (Rvachew, Rafaat, & Martin, 1999). Typically, I present only those modules that correspond to the phoneme that I am targeting at the time. However, my colleagues at the Alberta Children's Hospital and I have recently shown that this approach can be effective when a standard version of the program is provided to all children receiving phonology intervention (Rvachew, Nowak, & Cloutier, in press). In this randomized control study, student research assistants provided the SAILS program to children with moderate or severe phonological disorders for 16 consecutive weeks. Each child experienced the same modules in the same order, targeting commonly misarticulated phonemes in both the onset and coda positions of single-syllable words. Simultaneously, the children received speech therapy from speech-language pathologists (SLPs) on a weekly basis. The children's regular speech therapy program was not controlled in any way. Each child's SLP chose the treatment targets and implemented the treatment approach that he or she felt was most appropriate for that child. The gains in articulatory accuracy that were observed for the experimental group were more than twice those observed for the control group that received their regular speech therapy program without the addition of the SAILS program.

Readers with long memories will recognize some similarity between the SAILS program and the ear training procedures recommended by Van Riper (e.g., see Van Riper & Emerick, 1984). However, the use of multiple talkers and a range of stimuli representing both prototypical and less prototypical exemplars of the target category is absolutely crucial to the effectiveness of the SAILS program. Guenther and colleagues (1999) showed that using only perfect examples of a given category is actually detrimental to the induction of categorical perception. Lively, Logan, and Pisoni (1993) demonstrated that the use of stimuli recorded from multiple talkers during training is essential for successful generalization of new perceptual knowledge to untrained words produced by unfamiliar talkers. The clinician using his or her own voice alone cannot accomplish optimal assessment and treatment of difficulties with phonemic perception.

Stimulability

Many recent publications have focused attention on phonetic factors in the motor domain. Electropalatography (EPG) studies, for example, have shown that children with phonological disorders often produce lingual consonants with "undifferentiated lingual gestures" (Gibbon, 1999), and EPG is showing promise as a treatment tool (e.g., Dent, Gibbon, & Hardcastle, 1995). Other researchers have shown that stimulability is a reliable predictor of phoneme acquisition in spontaneous speech (Miccio, Elbert, & Forrest, 1999). Furthermore, the use of phonetic placement to ensure stimulability for target phonemes improves the success of phonological interventions (Powell, Elbert, Miccio, Strike-Roussos, & Brasseur, 1998; Rvachew, Rafaat, et al., 1999). Typically, the "low-tech" procedures described by Secord (1981) will be adequate to ensure that the child can produce the target phoneme in the onset and coda position of syllables. I never use nonspeech oral-motor exercises in isolation from speech practice (see Forrest, 2002). I will, if necessary, shape from a nonspeech movement to a speech movement and I will use a nonspeech activity to help the child understand the meaning of my instructions regarding articulatory placement. For example, blowing bubbles at a mirror can be a fun way to help the child understand what I mean by "rounded lips" and can be a useful prelude to teaching the child to round the lips for the production of [w] or to inhibit rounding of the lips for the production of [ɹ].

When a child is having extraordinary difficulty achieving the correct articulatory placement, visual feedback can be very helpful. EPG is not readily available, but speech analyzers that provide waveform and spectrographic feedback can be obtained for relatively low cost and implemented on any desktop or laptop computer with a sound card, microphone, and speakers. *ProTrain 2000* (Avaaz Innovations, Inc., 1999), for example, displays two spectrograms at once: the clinician's model of a correct production and the child's attempt to match the clinician's model. A spectrogram is a visual display depicting formant frequencies over time. Formant frequencies reflect the shape of the vocal tract, and changes in formant frequencies over time reflect changes in vocal tract shapes as speech is articulated. Demonstrations of the use of spectrographic feedback to teach [ɹ] production have been published (Masterson & Rvachew, 1999; Shuster, Ruscello, & Toth, 1995), and I have made one available on-line (see http://www.medicine.mcgill.ca/microp). The advantage of using this sort of visual feedback is that a child can receive reinforcement for making improvements toward accurate production of a phoneme, even when those improvements are not perceptible to the ear of the clinician or the child. Furthermore, the child's task is to reproduce a particular pattern of formant movements rather than to produce a particular phoneme. This allows the child to discover his or her own articulatory solution to the problem of producing a sound that will be perceived as the target phoneme.

PHASE II: PHONOLOGICAL KNOWLEDGE

During this phase the child is given an opportunity to use the new speech sound to communicate meaning in the context of meaningful minimal pair activities that are conducted at the single word or short phrase levels. Weiner (1981) demonstrated the effectiveness of a very simple procedure in which pairs of picture cards representing meaningful minimal pairs (e.g., rock, walk; write, white; red, wed) are laid out on the table top. The child instructs the clinician to pick up the cards one at a time and the clinician picks up the card corresponding to what the child said (rather than what the child might have meant). The object of the game is to get the clinician to remove all of the cards from the table. Howell and Dean (1994) recommend other equally simple games that they implement within the context of the Metaphon approach. If a child has learned to perform the SAILS task and stimulability was achieved during the first phase of the treatment program, the child should achieve success at a rate of 80% correct or better with only one session of meaningful minimal pair activities. Diedrich and Bangert (1980) suggested that effective clinicians move from the single-word to the sentence and narrative levels very quickly, and thus I try to move onto Phase III as soon as possible. However, sometimes the child will demonstrate overgeneralization of the new phoneme (e.g., producing the word *walk* as "rock"). In this case I continue with the meaningful minimal pair activities for a session or two and reintroduce the SAILS game. Another possibility is that the child will produce a meaningful contrast between the target sound and the error sound, but the child's production of the target phoneme will be distorted. In this case I combine Phase I and Phase II activities within the same sessions for another week or two, conducting the SAILS phonemic perception training procedure, phonetic placement procedures, and the meaningful minimal pair procedure within the same session.

PHASE III: PHONETIC MAPPING

During the final phase, the child is given opportunities to practice correct articulation of the target phoneme in sentence, conversation, and narrative contexts to ensure a consistent phonetic mapping (Masterson & Rvachew, 1999). During this phase, underlying representations for lexical items containing the new phoneme are restructured to incorporate new phonological knowledge and the child acquires the habit of producing the new phoneme consistently in the appropriate contexts. Many software tools are available for implementing the necessary drill activities without requiring any preparation on the part of the clinician. The best products that have been developed specifically for clinical use are the

LocuTour Multimedia products such as *Articulation I: Consonant Phonemes* (Scarry-Larkin, 1994). This program presents the child with photographs of objects that were selected to target a specific phoneme in a given word position. The program then presents an auditory model of a single word, short phrase, or long sentence containing one or more exemplars of the target phoneme. The program records the child's imitation of the model. Both the model and the child's response can be replayed and compared.

Other commercially available programs provide more fun and more opportunities for authentic communication between child and clinician. The Disney Baby and Disney Toddler products, for example, are terrific for young children right through the preschool period (e.g., *Winnie the Pooh Baby;* Disney Learning, 2001), and the Living Books series of computerized books (e.g., *Arthur's Birthday;* Living Books, 1994) is excellent for younger and older children. The trick to using this kind of software for clinical purposes is to maintain control of the mouse so that the child must tell the clinician what to do in order to witness the desired effect on the computer monitor. *Arthur's Birthday* obviously offers many opportunities for the child to practice /ɝ/ production, at the level of patterned sentences (e.g., "Click Arthur," "Click the birthday cake," "Click the ribbon") and the level of spontaneous conversation ("If you click Arthur, I think he will blow out the candles on the birthday cake"). A currently popular game is *The Sims* (Electronic Arts, 2003) in which the player can create and name characters and then help them through their daily lives. The game offers endless opportunities to instruct multiple characters to produce certain activities. It can be used for almost any treatment target at the segmental or syllable structure level because each character can be given a name having the desired phonetic characteristics. The child can then give instructions as simple or as complex as is appropriate for his or her level of ability (e.g., "Make Roger go the bathroom, and Randy clean up the water, and Rebecca serve dinner"). After the child produces the commands correctly, you can execute them and watch the characters accomplish the tasks. Finally, a number of children's word processors integrate text and drawing tools so that children can create their own books. These programs offer many opportunities to practice the production of target structures while constructing narratives and illustrations.

Of course, I wouldn't design a treatment program designed solely around software-based activities, because the child must be able to cut and color and walk and jump while holding a conversation or constructing a narrative, all the while producing the target sound consistently. Activities in which the child is sitting still in front of a computer monitor may give an inflated impression of the child's ability to produce the target phoneme consistently under natural speaking conditions.

It is during the phonetic mapping phase of the treatment program that phonological goals can be targeted simultaneously with attention to the child's morphology, syntax, or narrative skills. Rvachew, Gaines, Cloutier, and Blanchet (in press) found that children with moderate and severe phonological disorders omit bound morphemes more frequently than would be predicted from the child's use of the relevant phonemes in uninflected words. The findings of this descriptive study suggested that effective remediation of the children's phonological errors will not necessarily lead to spontaneous resolution of difficulties with expressive morphology. Tyler, Lewis, Haskill, and Tolbert (2002) have demonstrated that targeting morphology can lead to spontaneous improvements in phonology, at least in some cases. They have also developed materials for the effective remediation of the common morpheme errors produced by young children (Haskill, Tyler, & Tolbert,

2001). The software packages mentioned earlier also provide opportunities to practice the production of many different morphemes. They are particularly valuable for teaching verb tenses. With *The Sims* software, for example, the child can describe what happened and the characters' states with respect to their basic needs, and then he or she can indicate what will happen next next (e.g., "Roger clean<u>ed</u> up the bathroom"; "Now he feel<u>s</u> tired"; "Next, he <u>will</u> read a book").

Phonological awareness can also be targeted during this phase of the intervention. Phonological awareness refers to the knowledge that spoken words can be segmented into smaller abstract units such as syllables or phonemes. It is an important preliteracy skill and one of the best predictors of success in the acquisition of reading (Torgesen, Wagner, & Rashotte, 1994). During the preschool period children become aware of the phonetic similarities and differences among words on the basis of large units such syllables and rimes. Awareness of these larger units appears to occur as a natural consequence of language development during this period. After school entry, children learn to segment words on the basis of each individual phoneme, even those associated with complex onsets or codas (e.g., the word *splint* is comprised of the sounds [s], [p], [l] [ɪ], [n], and [t]). Children with moderate or severe phonological delay are at significant risk of delayed acquisition of phonological awareness, even when their language skills are age appropriate (e.g., Bird, Bishop, & Freeman, 1995; Larrivee & Catts, 1999; Rvachew, Ohberg, Grawburg, & Heyding, 2003). Remediation of the child's expressive phonological errors does not lead to spontaneous resolution of the child's difficulties with phonological awareness (Gillon, 2000, 2002; Rvachew, Nowak, et al., in press). Recently one of my graduate students developed an intervention program that proved successful in the remediation of delayed onset and rime awareness (Grawburg, 2004). The participants were 4-year-old children who had moderately or severely delayed expressive phonological skills. Each child received eight treatment sessions lasting approximately 45 minutes at once weekly intervals. During these sessions the children received the SAILS phonemic perception intervention described previously and learned to sort objects and pictures on the basis of shared onsets (pictures of *sun* and *sand* were matched to the letter *s* while pictures of *boat* and *bean* were matched to the letter *b*) or shared rimes (pictures of *fan* and *ran* were sorted into a *can* while pictures of *men* and *ten* were sorted into a *hen*). Although these activities were implemented in the context of table top games and gross motor activities, computer software tools such as children's word processors can also be used to teach children to match or sort words on the basis of shared onsets, rimes, or phonemes. A large number of commercially available programs target phonological awareness and/or phonics but they must be used with caution. The activities are often characterized by mismatches between the goal of the program and the fine motor or cognitive capacities required to be successful. For example, activities that involve rime matching are most appropriate for younger preschool-age children. If the child must shoot down rapidly moving targets or remember which of many frogs said what in order to demonstrate their knowledge of rime, he or she will become frustrated and refuse to play the game. Computer books and children's word processors allow the clinician more flexibility in the design of appropriate phonological awareness activities that are well integrated with the child's speech therapy goals.

PROGRESS MONITORING AND DISCHARGE CRITERIA

Continuous monitoring of response accuracy throughout the child's treatment program is necessary in order to decide when to progress from one phase of the intervention program to the next, when to introduce new targets, or when to discontinue treatment. I tend to persist with the first phase until a high level of accuracy is achieved for both phonemic perception and stimulability. The child should be able to imitate the target phoneme at the syllable or word level in a variety of phonetic contexts with 80%–90% accuracy before moving to the second and third phases. If the first phase of the program is completed successfully, the child should be able to rapidly achieve a similarly high level of accuracy with the minimal pair activities at the single-word level. The decision to discontinue the third phase should be made on the basis of the child's performance during probes that comprise words that represent the child's segment and syllable structure targets but that are not specifically taught during treatment sessions. Inclusion of stimuli that target the child's initial error is also valuable in order to be sure that contrastive use of a new phoneme has been established. I find the *Picture Gallery* series of computer-based pictures to be very convenient for creating customized probes for each client that can be saved under the client's name and thus easily retrieved for administration at regular intervals. I require the child to both name and describe the pictures contained in the probe and score the child's production of the target structures for both phonemic and phonetic accuracy. If the child begins the treatment program with a complete absence of a phonemic contrast between /ɹ/ and /w/, for example, I want to be able to document the child's progress toward the acquisition of a contrast even in the absence of full phonetic accuracy for production of the /ɹ/ phoneme. I would be reluctant to recommend discharge, however, if the contrast manifested itself as a consistent distortion of the target phoneme.

Many studies have shown that the phonetic mapping phase of the intervention program can be discontinued before full mastery of the target phonemes has been achieved. McKercher, McFarlane, and Schneider (1995) described changes in production accuracy during periods of active treatment and during treatment rest and recommended the following decision rules: 1) discontinue treatment on the target phoneme when production accuracy exceeds 40% correct and introduce a new treatment target; 2) if all potential treatment targets are produced with greater than 40% accuracy, reduce the intensity of the treatment program, or discontinue treatment but monitor the child's performance frequently; and 3) if the child's production accuracy exceeds 75% for all potential treatment targets, discharge the child from treatment but review the child's progress periodically until mastery is achieved.

It is relatively easy to make the decision to discontinue treatment when the child is progressing toward mastery of the targeted phonemes and syllable structures. However, deciding how to proceed when the child is not responding positively to the intervention is more difficult given the paucity of research that identifies the causes of treatment failure or assesses the efficacy of the various ways in which one might respond. Kwiatkowski and Shriberg (1993) reported that *child focus* was a variable closely associated with treatment failure. However, an apparent lack of motivation on the part of the child may be the result rather than the cause of a failure to progress at the expected rate, and for this reason I avoid giving treatment breaks to uncooperative or marginally cooperative children. In my experience, a thorough reanalysis of the child's phonological system followed by the selection of a more appropriate treatment goal or treatment approach can lead to marked improvements in the child's focus during treatment sessions. Many years ago I was treating a child who was making no progress toward suppression of the process of stopping fricatives. I was prompted to reexamine the child's error patterns by the publication of Bernhardt and Stoel-Gammon (1994). The nonlinear analysis revealed that the child had difficulty with all of the features associated with the glottal node in addition to the obvious problem with continuancy. He produced neither continuants nor voiceless aspirated stop consonants. I discontinued my focus on /f/ and /s/ and proceeded to teach him to produce /h/+vowel syllables so that he could learn to control the initiation and cessation of vocal fold vibration. I then reintroduced the supralaryngeal fricative /s/ using a chaining procedure (he, sss+he, sssee), and all the other fricatives and the aspirated stops emerged spontaneously shortly thereafter. (This is an interesting case in which a thorough phonological analysis led me to recognize a problem that was essentially phonetic in nature—the child had difficulty coordinating articulatory events at the laryngeal and supralaryngeal levels.) In another case, a clinician consulted with me just as she was planning to discharge a child who was not cooperating with speech therapy activities in the clinic or at home. A nonlinear analysis revealed a number of very unusual error patterns involving syllable structure, despite a complete repertoire of English consonants. For example, all unstressed syllables were omitted or replaced by [ɪn] (e.g., magic → mædʒɪn, pocket → patɪn). Refocusing the intervention on syllable structure and away from segment level errors resulted in a marked change in the child's demeanor as well as an improved rate of progress.

SUMMARY

The past quarter century has seen many significant advances in our understanding of the nature of children's developing phonological knowledge as well as an explosion of technical innovations that allow us to more effectively address children's phonetic knowledge of the acoustic and articulatory properties of the native language sound system. The increasing number of randomized control studies of the efficacy of specific treatment practices also contributes to the confidence with which we can approach our clinical practice. SLPs who take advantage of this knowledge base can be sure of providing phonology intervention that is effective, efficient, and fun.

REFERENCES

Avaaz Innovations. (1994). SAILS: Speech Assessment and Interactive Learning System (Version 1.2) [Computer software]. London, Ontario, Canada: Author.

Avaaz Innovations. (1999). ProTrain 2000 [Computer software]. London, Ontario, Canada: Author.

Bernhardt, B., & Gilbert, J. (1992). Applying linguistic theory to speech-language pathology: The case for nonlinear phonology. *Clinical Linguistics & Phonetics, 6,* 123–145.

Bernhardt, B., & Stoel-Gammon, C. (1994). Nonlinear phonology: Introduction and clinical application. *Journal of Speech and Hearing Research, 37,* 123–143.

Bird, J., Bishop, D.V.M., & Freeman, N.H. (1995). Phonological awareness and literacy development in children with expressive phonological impairments. *Journal of Speech and Hearing Research, 38*(2), 446–462.

Broen, P.A., Strange, W., Doyle, S.S., & Heller, J.H. (1983). Perception and production of approximant consonants by normal and articulation-delayed preschool children. *Journal of Speech and Hearing Research, 26*(4), 601–608.

Chaney, C. (1988). Identification of correct and misarticulated semivowels. *Journal of Speech and Hearing Disorders, 53*(3), 252–261.

Davis, B.L., & MacNeilage, P.F. (1995). The articulatory basis of babbling. *Journal of Speech and Hearing Research, 38,* 1199–1211.

Dent, H., Gibbon, F., & Hardcastle, B. (1995). The application of electropalatography (EPG) to the remediation of speech disorders in school-age children and young adults. *European Journal of Disorders of Communication, 30,* 264–277.

Diedrich, W., & Bangert, J. (1980). *Articulation learning.* Houston, TX: College-Hill Press.

Disney Interactive. (2001). Winnie the Pooh Baby [CD-ROM]. Burbank, CA: Author.

Dodd, B., Leahy, J., & Hambly, G. (1989). Phonological disorders in children: Underlying cognitive deficits. *British Journal of Developmental Psychology, 7,* 55–71.

Edwards, J., Beckman, M.E., & Munson, B. (2004). The interaction between vocabulary size and phonotactic probability effects on children's production accuracy and fluency in nonword repetition. *Journal of Speech, Language, and Hearing Research, 47,* 421–436.

Edwards, J., Fourakis, M., Beckman, M.E., & Fox, R.A. (1999). Characterizing knowledge deficits in phonological disorders. *Journal of Speech, Language, and Hearing Research, 42,* 169–186.

Edwards, J., Fox, R.A., & Rogers, C.L. (2002). Final consonant descrimination in children: Effects of phonological disorder, vocabulary size, and articulatory accuracy. *Journal of Speech, Language, and Hearing Research, 45,* 231–242.

Electronic Arts, Inc. (2003). The Sims Double Deluxe [CD-ROM]. Redwood City, CA: Author.

Forrest, K. (2002). Are oral-motor exercises useful in the treatment of phonological/articulatory disorders? *Seminars in Speech and Language, 23,* 15–25.

Gibbon, F.E. (1999). Undifferentiated lingual gestures in children with articulation/phonological disorders. *Journal of Speech, Language, and Hearing Research, 42,* 382–397.

Gillon, G.T. (2000). The efficacy of phonological awareness intervention for children with spoken language impairment. *Language, Speech, and Hearing Services in Schools, 31*(2), 126–141.

Gillon, G.T. (2002). Follow-up study investigating the benefits of phonological awareness intervention for children with spoken language impairment. *International Journal of Language and Communication Disorders, 37*(4), 381–400.

Grawburg, M. (2004). *A perception based phonological awareness training program for preschoolers with articulation disorders.* Unpublished master's thesis. McGill University, Montréal, Québec.

Guenther, F.H. (1995). Speech sound acquisition, coarticulation, and rate effects in a neural network model of speech production. *Psychological Review, 102*(3), 594–621.

Guenther, F.H., Husain, F.T., Cohen, M.A., & Shinn-Cunningham, B.G. (1999). Effects of categorization and discrimination training on auditory perceptual space. *Journal of the Acoustic Society of America, 106*(5), 2900–2912.

Haskill, A., Tyler, A., & Tolbert, L. (2001). *Months of morphemes.* Eau Claire, WI: Thinking Publications.

Hoffman, P.R., Daniloff, R.G., Bengoa, D., & Schuckers, G.H. (1985). Misarticulating and normally articulating children's identification and discrimination of synthetic [r] and [w]. *Journal of Speech & Hearing Disorders, 50*(1), 46–53.

Hoffman P.R., Stager, S., & Daniloff, R.G. (1983). Perception and production of misarticulated /r/ . *Journal of Speech and Hearing Disorders, 48*(2), 210–215.

Howell, J., & Dean, E. (1994). *Treating phonological disorders in children. Metaphon: Theory to practice* (2nd ed.). London: Whurr Publishers.

Kwiatkowski, J., & Shriberg, L.D. (1993). Speech normalization in developmental phonological disorders: A retrospective study of capability-focus theory. *Language, Speech, and Hearing Services in Schools, 24,* 10–18.

Larrivee, L.S., & Catts, H.W. (1999). Early reading achievement in children with expressive phonological disorders. *American Journal of Speech-Language Pathology, 8,* 118–128.

Lively, S.E., Logan, J.S., & Pisoni, D.B. (1993). Training Japanese listeners to identify English /r/ and /l/. II: The role of phonetic environment and talker variability in learning new perceptual categories. *Journal of the Acoustical Society of America, 94*(3, Pt. 1), 1242–1255.

Living Books. (1994). Arthur's birthday [CD-ROM]. Based on the book *Arthur's Birthday* by M. Brown (1986). Novato, CA: Broderbund.

Masterson, J.J., & Rvachew, S. (1999). Use of technology in phonology intervention. *Seminars in Speech and Language 20*(3), 233–250.

McCune, L., & Vihman, M.M. (2001). Early phonetic and lexical development: A productivity approach. *Journal of Speech-Language and Hearing Research, 44,* 760–684.

McKercher, M., McFarlane, L., & Schneider, P. (1995). Phonological treatment dismissal: Optimal criteria. *Journal of Speech-Language Pathology and Audiology, 19,* 115–123.

Miccio, A.W., Elbert, M., & Forrest, K. (1999). The relationship between stimulability and phonological acquisition in children with normally developing and disordered phonologies. *American Journal of Speech-Language Pathology, 8*(4), 347–363.

Monnin, L., & Huntington, D. (1974). Relationship of articulatory defects to speech sound discrimination. *Journal of Speech and Hearing Research, 17*(3), 352–366.

Munson, B., Edwards, J., & Beckman, M.E. (in press). Relationships between nonword repetition accuracy and other measures of linguistic development in children with phonological disorders. *Journal of Speech, Language, and Hearing Research.*

Oller, D.K. (2000). *The emergence of the speech capacity.* Mahwah, NJ: Lawrence Erlbaum Associates.

Pierrehumbert, J.B. (2002). Word-specific phonetics. In C. Gussenhoven & N. Warner (Eds.), *Proceedings of the seventh conference on laboratory phonology* (pp. 101–139). Berlin: Mouton de Gruyter.

Plaut, D.C., & Kello, C.T. (1999). The emergence of phonology from the interplay of speech comprehension and production: A distributed connectionist approach. In B. MacWhinney (Ed.), *The emergence of language* (pp. 381–415). Mahwah, NJ: Lawrence Erlbaum Associates.

Powell, T.W., Elbert, M., Miccio, A.W., Strike-Roussos, C., & Brasseur, J. (1998). Facilitating [s] production in young children: An experimental evaluation of motoric and conceptual treatment approaches. *Clinical Linguistics & Phonetics, 12*(2), 127–146.

Rvachew, S., Gaines, B.R., & Cloutier, G., & Blanchet, N. (in press). Productive morphology skills of children with speech delay. *Journal of Speech-Language Pathology and Audiology.*

Rvachew, S., & Jamieson, D.G. (1989). Perception of voiceless fricatives by children with a functional articulation disorder. *Journal of Speech & Hearing Disorders, 54*(2), 193–208.

Rvachew, S., & Jamieson, D.G. (1995). Learning new speech contrasts: Evidence from adults learning a second language and children with speech disorders. In W. Strange (Ed.), *Speech perception and linguistic experience: Issues in cross-language research* (pp. 411–432). Timonium, MD: York Press.

Rvachew, S., Nowak, M., & Cloutier, G. (2004). Effect of phonemic perception training on the speech production and phonological awareness skills of children with expressive phonological delay. *American Journal of Speech-Language Pathology, 13,* 250–263.

Rvachew, S., Ohberg, A., Grawburg, M., & Heyding, J. (2003). Phonological awareness and phone-mic perception in 4-year-old children with delayed expressive phonology skills. *American Journal of Speech-Language Pathology, 12,* 463–471.

Rvachew, S., Rafaat, S., & Martin, M. (1999). Stimulability, speech perception skills, and the treatment of phonological disorders. *American Journal of Speech-Language Pathology, 8,* 33–43.

Rvachew, S., Slawinski, E.B., Williams, M., & Green, C. (1999). The impact of early onset otitis media on babbling and early language development. *Journal of the Acoustic Society of America, 105,* 467–475.

Scarry-Larkin, M. (1994). Articulation I: Consonant phonemes [CD-ROM]. San Luis Obispo, CA: LocuTour Multimedia.

Schwartz, R.G. (1992). Clinical applications of recent advances in phonological theory. *Language, Speech, and Hearing Services in Schools, 23,* 269–276.

Secord, W. (1981). *Eliciting sounds: Techniques for clinicians.* San Antonio, TX: Harcourt Assess-ment.

Shuster, L.I., Ruscello, D.M., & Toth, A.R. (1995). The use of visual feedback to elicit correct /r/. *American Journal of Speech-Language Pathology, 4,* 37–44.

Stackhouse, J., & Wells, B. (1997). *Children's speech and literacy difficulties: A psycholinguistic framework.* London: Whurr Publishers.

Torgeson, J.K., Wagner, R.K., & Rashotte, C.A. (1994). Longitudinal studies of phonological processing and reading. *Journal of Learning Disabilities, 27*(5), 276–286.

Tyler, A.A., Lewis, K.E., Haskill, A., & Tolbert, L.C. (2002). Efficacy and cross-domain effects of a morphosyntax and a phonology intervention. *Language, Speech, and Hearing Services in Schools, 33,* 52–66.

Van Riper, C., & Emerick, L. (1984). *Speech correction: An introduction to speech-pathology and audiology.* Englewood-Cliffs, NJ: Prentice Hall.

Waterson, N. (1971). Child phonology: A prosodic view. *Journal of Linguistics, 7,* 179–211.

Weiner, F. (1981). Treatment of phonological disability using the method of meaningful minimal contrast: Two case studies. *Journal of Speech and Hearing Disorders, 46,* 97–103.

Weisz, J.R., Donenberg, G.R., Han, S.S., & Kauneckis, D. (1995). Child and adolescent psychother-apy outcomes in experiments versus clinics: Why the disparity? *Journal of Abnormal Child Psychology, 23,* 83–106.

Werker, J.F., Fennell, C.T., Corcoran, K.M., & Stager, C.L. (2002). Infants' ability to learn phoneti-cally similar words: Effects of age and vocabulary size. *Infancy, 3*(1), 1–3.

Chapter 16

A Model and Structure
for Phonological Intervention

A. Lynn Williams

I entered the field of speech-language pathology during the 1980s—a dynamic period of change, particularly in the area of speech disorders in children. As a hospital-based speech-language pathologist (SLP) during that time, I used minimal pair therapy as one of the only phonological options available to address error patterns identified in the sound systems of children with speech disorders. Intuitively, minimal pair therapy made sense to contrast child error with the target sound in order to confront them with the homonymy that resulted from their collapse of an adult phonemic contrast. I continued to use this approach for the next decade, through my doctoral studies at Indiana University and into my first academic position in teaching and training graduate students in clinical phonology. Minimal pair therapy was effective and efficient in treating speech sound disorders in children and was flexible enough to be used within a variety of assessment frameworks, including phonological process analysis, place–voice–manner analysis, and assessment of productive phonological knowledge.

During my supervision of one client in my early academic career in California, however, I noticed little to no progress had been achieved in a 5-week intervention period in which minimal pairs were being used. This child (age 3;5) exhibited an unusual error pattern in which she substituted [l] for /w/, /s/, and /ʃ/ word-initially (Williams, 2000b). We used minimal pairs to develop contrastive word pairs for [l] ~ [w], [l] ~ [s], and [l] ~ [ʃ]. Five contrastive word pairs were used to train each of the three targets in separate treatment sets, and one treatment set of 20 responses was completed on each minimal contrast for a total of 60 responses per treatment session. The following are some examples of some of the minimal pair treatment exemplars for each sound contrast:

[l] ~ [w]	[l] ~ [s]	[l] ~ [ʃ]
Lee ~ we	Lou ~ Sue	lip ~ ship
lake ~ wake	lay ~ say	lock ~ shock
light ~ white	leap ~ seep	line ~ shine

After 5 weeks of limited progress, the clinician and the child were becoming discouraged and frustrated. In reviewing the clinician's lesson plans and trying to determine what therapeutic changes needed to be made, I noticed the fairly obvious fact that rather than the child's exhibiting three separate, idiosyncratic errors involving target /w/, /s/, and

189

/ʃ/, all of the errors were related to a single rule in which the child collapsed all of these continuants to [l], which was also a continuant. Although we had provided intervention separately to each of the individual sounds that comprised the child's rule, it apparently had not been sufficient for the child to make the connection that all of her target sounds were related to the same rule. After this discovery, I questioned whether integrating her targets into a single treatment set of multiple sound contrasts would facilitate her learning the new rule in a more focused manner than was provided to her with the individual and separate minimal pairs. For the child's next therapy session, we developed multiple oppositions that contrasted all of her targets simultaneously in larger, integrated contrastive word pairs. The resulting treatment exemplars included some of the following:

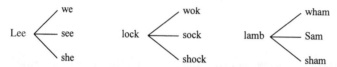

We were amazed, thrilled, and elated that in the first session, the child achieved 90%–100% accuracy on all three target sounds! She met both treatment and generalization criteria by the third treatment session, and treatment was terminated on those target sounds. Widespread phonological change was noted in her posttreatment phonological analysis in that her improvement also extended to the target sounds in untrained positions and to untrained sounds. Readers are referred to Williams (2000b) for detailed data on the child's treatment and generalization performance. Although the results were remarkable, the fact that the child had received 5 weeks of minimal pair therapy certainly contributed to the significant change that occurred in one treatment session with multiple oppositions. However, it seemed evident that the multiple oppositions provided input that was more focused across a rule set, making it more learnable, and that it was not solely the priming of the minimal pair therapy that was responsible for obtaining the dramatic treatment outcomes.

I have devoted a good deal of my career since the 1990s to understanding how children's sound systems are structured and the manner in which multiple oppositions appear to facilitate phonological restructuring. I have examined the multiple oppositions approach in intervention studies with a number of children who exhibit moderate to profound phonological impairments and have found that this approach is effective in restructuring children's sound systems in a short period of time (Williams, 2000a; Williams & Kalbfleisch, 2001).

For the remainder of this chapter, I discuss the theoretical foundations of the multiple oppositions approach, particularly in relation to the minimal pair approach. I then present a structure, or treatment paradigm, for implementing the multiple oppositions approach, or any of the contrastive approaches, in treating speech sound disorders in children. Finally, I discuss some new developments in software programs that will make the use of multiple oppositions or any contrastive approach more accessible to SLPs.

THE MODEL OF MULTIPLE OPPOSITIONS

The multiple oppositions approach addresses the extensive absence of adult sounds that commonly occurs in children with severe speech disorders by utilizing multiple contrastive sound pairs. It is not unusual for children with multiple sound errors to produce one sound for several adult phonemes. For example, a child who says [tu] for "two," "Sue," "shoe," "coo," "chew," "stew," and "true" has collapsed the phonemic contrast involving /t/, /s/, /ʃ/, /k/, /tʃ/, /st/, and /tr/. In this example, the child's intelligibility will be significantly affected by the 1:7 phoneme collapse that exists. The goal of phonological intervention, then, is to teach the child these contrasts using contrastive sound pairs by incorporating a conceptual approach that relies on attaching meaning to what the child says and what he or she has to learn to disambiguate his or her utterances.

The multiple oppositions model of phonological intervention is directed at addressing these larger collapses in a structured and systemic way. Multiple oppositions (Williams, 2000a, 2000b, 2003) provide focused intervention *across* a child's entire rule set by using larger, integrated contrastive sound pairs. The multiple oppositions approach uses a functional/systemic approach to select a maximum of four target sounds from a given rule set (see previous section on Target Selection). In the 1:7 phoneme collapse mentioned previously, the child's error, [t], would be contrasted with /s/, /tʃ/, /k/, and /tr/ in multiple contrastive word pairs. The word pairs might include the following:

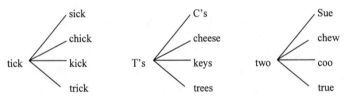

The larger, integrated treatment sets of multiple oppositions address several error sounds from one rule set. This model of intervention, then, is based on holistic, systemic sound learning that can be accounted for by principles of distributed learning. It is hypothesized that differences in learning that may result from the implementation of different intervention models may relate to differences in the size of the linguistic "chunks" that are presented to children in treatment. The larger, integrated treatment sets of multiple oppositions involve intervention across a child's entire rule set rather than to an isolated aspect of the child's system or rule. In addition, the larger, integrated treatment sets take into account the unique sound system and phonological organization that each child creates to accommodate his or her limited system relative to the full adult sound system. As a consequence, not only are more sounds trained (i.e., larger treatment sets) but also the integrated treatment sets comprise target sounds from across the child's error rule. Focusing the child's attention on the error pattern in this manner confronts him or her with the extent of phonologic change that must be achieved while exposing the child to the relatedness of all of the target sounds to the error pattern. The distributed input of the larger, integrated treatment sets therefore enlarges the frame of relevant learning that is needed. Thus, the larger, integrated treatment input represents the gestalt of the learning that needs to occur. The assumption is that the whole of the learning task is greater than the sum of its parts.

I have proposed in an earlier work (Williams, 2000b) that the complexity of the treatment input presented to the child with regard to the size and nature of the treatment sets poses an interesting question of learnability. In particular, is it easier for a child to learn new sound contrasts and reorganize his or her sound system when intervention is provided using the more complex input of larger, integrated treatment sets of the multiple oppositions approach or the less complex input of smaller, nonintegrated treatment sets of the minimal pair approach?

Two possible hypotheses are associated with each intervention model. First, it could be hypothesized that the smaller, nonintegrated treatment sets of minimal pairs would be easier to learn because a child has to learn only a single contrast, which results in a greater focus in treatment, less semantic load with regard to the number of treatment exemplars, and fewer demands placed on the child's attention and memory. Alternatively, the second hypothesis suggests that although the smaller, nonintegrated treatment sets are less complex, the input would be relatively more difficult for the child to learn and integrate phonemically. Based on the second hypothesis, the fact that the single contrast is fragmented from a larger, more diverse rule pattern makes it more difficult for the child to integrate the input into a new rule set. Therefore, the larger, integrated treatment sets of multiple oppositions would actually make it easier for the child to systematically reorganize his or her sound system because the distributed input enlarges the frame of relevant learning and presents the child with the range and diversity of the new contrasts to be learned, which does not occur when intervention is provided on a single contrast that is isolated from the entire rule set.

When considering these two possible hypotheses, it appears that the integration of the treatment input across an entire rule set accounts for the different learning outcomes of the child who achieved limited progress in 5 weeks using the isolated treatment input of minimal pairs that individually incorporated each of the three target sounds /w/, /s/, and /ʃ/. Immediate and significant changes occurred, however, when those same target sounds were incorporated into the larger and integrated treatment sets of multiple oppositions. Although these data do not represent an empirical comparison of the two intervention approaches, they do suggest that the input facilitated different learning outcomes.

A comparison of the models of multiple oppositions and minimal pairs for contrastive word pairs, assumptions, and rationale is provided in Table 16.1. This comparison was taken from Williams (2002) and is based on a phonological analysis completed for a child who had an extensive phoneme collapse in which 17 obstruents and clusters were collapsed to [g] word-initially.

A STRUCTURE FOR PHONOLOGICAL INTERVENTION

I believe that treatment has a structure to it that is important in helping to navigate a child's learning during intervention. If we have a clear idea of the intervention steps, we can more effectively guide the child through the treatment process. With our treatment paradigm, we let the child determine the pace of intervention and even the need for supplemental steps or procedures. In other words, matriculation in treatment is data-driven by the child's performance throughout all phases of the intervention.

Before I describe the treatment paradigm, I believe it is important to know an individual clinician's perspective on speech disorders in order to understand his or her approach to phonological intervention. I consider speech disorders to be an integration of phonetic and phonemic competence. Specifically, the child must learn the articulatory gestures (phonetic) to produce a new sound contrast as well as the linguistic rules (phonemic) to use the new contrast appropriately. Consequently, I view speech disorders as occurring along a phonetic–phonemic continuum. Although I believe that the majority of

Table 16.1. Comparison of multiple oppositions and minimal pairs contrastive treatment approaches

	Multiple oppositions (Williams, 2000)	Minimal pairs (Weiner, 1981)
Contrastive pairs	Multiple contrastive word pairs of child's error with several target sounds selected from a rule set	Single contrastive word pairs of child's error with one target sound
Example of contrastive sounds	$g \Leftarrow \begin{matrix} d \\ f \\ t\int \\ st \end{matrix}$	g ~ d/ # ____
Examples of contrastive treatment exemplars	$goo \Leftarrow \begin{matrix} dew \\ food \\ chew \\ stew \end{matrix}$ $Gore \Leftarrow \begin{matrix} door \\ four \\ chore \\ store \end{matrix}$	go ~ doe gate ~ date gown ~ down
Assumptions	Learning is facilitated by the size and nature of linguistic "chunks" presented to child (learning of the whole is greater than the sum of its parts). Learning is a dynamic interaction between child's unique sound system and intervention.	Child will fill in the gap between what is trained and what still needs to be learned across the rule set. Adult-based categories (e.g., backing) are the basis for the child's error and sound organization.
Predictions	Learning will be generalized across a rule set (i.e., learning will generalize to the obstruents and clusters that are collapsed to [g] in the 1:17 phoneme collapse) and result in systemwide restructuring	The target contrast (g ~ d) will generalize to other phonetically similar sounds affected by the child's error pattern.

Source: Williams (2002).

speech disorders lie closer to the phonemic end of the continuum, some speech disorders have a strong phonetic component. Regardless of the placement on the phonetic–phonemic continuum, children with speech disorders require aspects of each in remediating their sound disorders. The focus on either the phonetic or phonemic aspects of sound production will vary depending on the child's learning needs. I believe that intervention that focuses on one aspect to the exclusion of the other will be limited in terms of longer intervention periods and/or in failure to generalize.

This perspective of duality in speech disorders requires phonological intervention to be structured in a manner that facilitates both types of learning. Consequently, I believe that any phonological intervention program should be structured to include the following goals:

1. Provide opportunities for the child to discover the rule(s) that are being trained.

2. Provide focused practice on the new target(s) in order for them to become automatic.

3. Provide the child with linguistic/communicative feedback with regard to the semantic meaning of the child's production.

4. Provide opportunities to practice the new target(s) in naturalistic play activities.

To meet these goals, I described a treatment paradigm (Williams, 2000a, 2003) that attempts to combine focused practice within a communicative context that is supplemented with naturalistic play activities. A diagram of the treatment paradigm is illustrated in

Figure 16.1. The initial phase of treatment relies more heavily on focused practice with the use of imitation (phonetic learning). Once the phonetic aspects of the new contrast are established, the remainder of the intervention phases use communicative contexts at a spontaneous level of production (phonemic learning). This treatment paradigm can be used with any of the contrastive approaches. It provides a basic structure for matriculation through intervention using the four goals listed previously. The next sections describe the rationale underlying the treatment paradigm and the general principles that are considered within this paradigm.

Treatment Paradigm: Rationale and General Principles

The rationale underlying the treatment paradigm that I use in phonological intervention is based on similar psycholinguistic principles outlined by Johnston (1984) in her FAAcTual approach for language intervention. The acronym for FAAcTual represents intervention that is *functional* or meaningful and communicative, provides linguistic input that is *appropriate* to the child's developmental level and interests, allows for *active* rule discovery, and provides input that is *therapeutic*. These principles are incorporated into the intervention paradigm through the following activities:

- Opportunities for the child to discover the rule being trained in a meaningful manner are provided through the use of Metaphon activities that occur in Phase 1. These activities introduce the child to the new rule in a manner that makes the abstract concept of the rule more concrete and meaningful for the child.

- Unusually focused therapeutic input is provided that reduces the child's search for the new contrast and therefore reduces the demands on attention and memory. This occurs through a high proportional frequency of occurrence of the target contrast(s) that are provided in salient contexts using stress and intonation paired with physical prompts of the new contrast to be learned; for example, contrasting long and short arm movements that correspond with production of the fricative and stop phonemes (Phases 2 and 3).

- The new contrast is incorporated in both focused and naturalistic play activities in order to expose the child to the range and application of the new rule. Opportunities are provided to the child to use the new contrast(s) in meaningful and naturalistic play activities (Phases 2 and 3).

- Linguistic/communicative feedback is provided regarding the semantic meaning of the child's productions.

In addition to these psycholinguistic principles, an additional principle is incorporated to address the dual nature of phonologic learning that includes learning the appropriate application of the new linguistic rule (phonemic) *and* the new articulatory pattern (phonetic). Specifically, the activities that address this principle include the following:

- Focused practice is provided on the new contrast(s) to be learned in order for the sound(s) to become automatic.

- Generally, five contrastive sound pairs are incorporated in intervention with a dense response rate of around 60–100 responses per session (Phases 2 and 3).

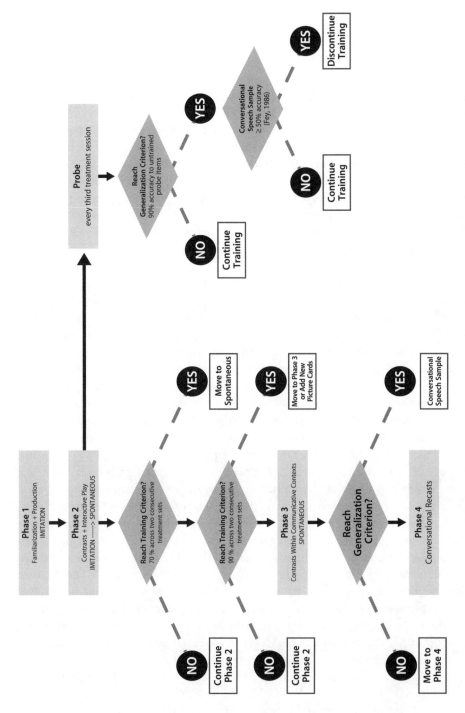

Figure 16.1. Treatment paradigm for contrastive intervention. (From *Speech Disorders Research Guide for Preschool Children, First Edition*, by WILLIAMS. Copyright © 2003. Reprinted with permission of Delmar Learning, a division of Thomson Learning: www.thomsonrights.com. Fax 800-730-2215.)

With the exception of Phase 1, which is a familiarization phase, movement to all subsequent phases or steps within a phase is data-based and driven by the child's performance. Two different criteria (treatment and generalization) are incorporated within the paradigm that govern the child's matriculation throughout intervention and determine the ultimate termination of intervention on a particular target.

Treatment criteria are specified for Phases 2 and 3 and for steps within Phase 2. The treatment criteria guide the SLP in making treatment decisions regarding when to move from imitative to spontaneous production and when to add additional treatment exemplars or move to more communicative contexts in treatment. There are two treatment criteria: one for switching from imitative to spontaneous production in Phase 2, and one for moving from Phase 2 to Phase 3. The first criterion (imitation to spontaneous production) is 70% accuracy across two consecutive training sets. A training set consists of 20 responses for minimal pair therapy and 20–40 responses for multiple oppositions depending on the number of target contrasts that are being trained (i.e., two, three, or four target sounds). If five contrastive exemplars are used, a training set of 20 responses would require four presentations (or repetitions) of the five minimal pair word sets or two presentations of five multiple opposition word sets that include two target sounds (e.g., t ~ [s, k]). Once the treatment criterion is achieved at this level, intervention switches to a spontaneous level of production. The new treatment criterion is set at 90% accuracy across two consecutive training sets. The difference in criterion levels (i.e., 70% versus 90% accuracy) reflects the initial focus of intervention at the phonetic level with imitative productions. I have found over the years that it is not necessary to require a more stringent mastery level of production at this imitative step, which would retain the child longer within the phonetic stage. Once the phonetic aspects of producing the new sound contrast are relatively established at a 70% accuracy level, the focus of intervention can shift to a more phonemic level of treatment involving spontaneous production. The higher criterion level of 90% accuracy addresses the level of performance that is frequently required for the child to learn and integrate the phonemic aspects of the new contrast within his or her sound system.

The generalization criterion specifies a predetermined level of performance that is required in order to judge that adequate phonologic learning has occurred and no further intervention is required. Two different generalization criteria are specified within the treatment paradigm. The first generalization criterion (90% accuracy) is based on the child's performance on a generalization probe that includes the target sound in untrained words and serves as a gateway to the second generalization criterion. If the first generalization criterion is achieved on the probe, then the SLP would check the child's production of the target sound at a conversational level. This second generalization criterion (50% accuracy in conversational speech) is a discontinuation criterion that functions as a safety net in making the clinical determination of "when enough is enough." The second generalization criterion is based on Fey's (1986) recommendation that if the child produces a target sound with at least 50% accuracy in spontaneous connected speech, the sound will continue to emerge on its own without further direct intervention. Thus, when this criterion is met, treatment is discontinued for that sound.

Intervention Materials: It's About Time

I use pictures of meaningful words to develop contrastive word sets, either within a multiple opposition or minimal pair intervention approach. This is frequently difficult and time consuming, especially when constructing contrastive word pairs for idiosyncratic errors such as the [l] ~ [s] contrast, and multiple contrastive treatment sets such as [t] ~ [s, k, ʧ, tr]. Although several commercial picture files are available (e.g., *Contrast Pairs for Phonological Training* [Palin, 1992]; *Remediation of Common Phonological Processes* [Monahan Broudy, 1993]), they do not include all possible contrasts that might be selected for treatment and, in fact, typically only include contrasts for common phonological processes (e.g., fronting, stopping, final consonant deletion, cluster reduction). Furthermore, none of the available commercial materials are designed for the newer models of phonological intervention, such as multiple oppositions or maximal oppositions.

The time required to collect, copy, cut, and paste pictured stimuli for the contrastive treatment materials that are needed to make individualized materials for each child is often beyond the time that SLPs have available. In fact, Long (2001) reported that time management is a significant issue in the daily lives of SLPs. McKinley and Williams (2003) completed a feasibility study that compared the time it took experienced SLPs in three regional test sites to develop contrastive treatment materials for multiple oppositions using a traditional card file method versus a computerized method, *Sound Contrasts in Phonology* (SCIP). The results indicated that it took almost three times longer to develop treatment materials using the traditional method (average time = 20.2 minutes) compared with SCIP software (average time = 6.9 minutes). SCIP addresses the significant issue of time and access for SLPs to implement contrastive models of phonological intervention with children. It will include an extensive database of picture illustrations for 2,000 words and more than 2,000 nonsense words, which will allow SLPs to develop and store a large number of individualized treatment sets for each child. SCIP will incorporate contrastive word pairs for word-initial substitution and omission patterns and word-final substitution and omission patterns by searching through the database and finding words that match the appropriate target phoneme(s). It can be used to develop contrastive treatment materials for all the contrastive phonological approaches, including multiple oppositions, minimal pairs, and maximal oppositions. A sample screen display of multiple oppositions contrasts is shown in Figure 16.2 (McKinley & Williams, 2003). In this example, a contrastive word set for the error pattern of final consonant deletion (Ø ~ /ʧ, f, z, t/) is shown.

SCIP is currently being developed in collaboration with Thinking Publications, with funding support from the National Institutes of Health, National Institute on Deafness and Other Communication Disorders. The projected date for commercial availability is late 2005.

SUMMARY

I have described a relatively new model of phonological intervention, multiple oppositions, and a treatment paradigm that can be incorporated for structuring the implementation of any contrastive intervention model. Although I do not believe that one particular treatment approach fits all children or is appropriate for one child throughout treatment, I do believe that a general model of phonological intervention can be suitable for the majority of children with speech disorders. To elaborate on this seemingly contradictory statement, I believe a treatment approach such as multiple oppositions is appropriate for children who are at a rule-based stage in their phonological development and who have severe speech disorders that are characterized by large gaps in their sound system and reflected

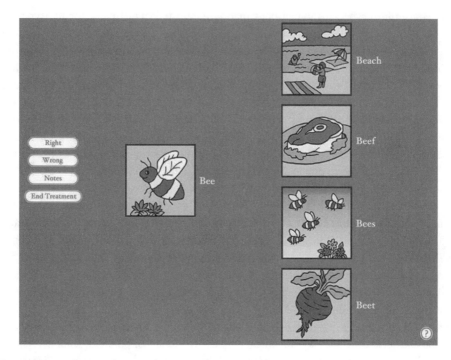

Figure 16.2. Sample screen display from *Sound Contrasts in Phonology* (SCIP) software (*Source:* McKinley & Williams, 2003).

in extensive phoneme collapses. The use of larger, integrated contrastive treatment sets provides focused intervention across an entire rule and facilitates learning in a systemic and holistic manner. This approach would not be appropriate for children who have a few sounds in error, or who are at the whole-word stage of phonological acquisition. For these children, a minimal pair approach that addresses individual sound errors within single contrastive word pairs would be indicated, or the cycles approach (Hodson & Paden, 1991) might be appropriate for younger children who are at an earlier stage of phonological development. Similarly, as children progress in treatment with multiple oppositions and they expand and reorganize their sound systems, a minimal pair approach might be more appropriate (see Williams, 2000a, for further discussion).

Conversely, a general model of phonological treatment that addresses the homonymy that occurs when ambient phonemic contrasts are absent provides a universal framework from which to view phonological intervention. That is, the construct of inducing phonemic splits to eliminate homonymy and increase speech intelligibility is general enough to fit the majority of children with speech disorders. In this manner, intervention does not need to be prescribed according to the type of speech disability, such as articulation impairment, phonological impairment, or childhood apraxia of speech. Such an etiology-based approach assumes that children in different groups learn a sound system differently and that difficulties observed in one group, such as inconsistencies, omissions, substitutions, vowel distortions, and so forth, are specific to a particular subgroup and are not seen in other groups. This perspective further assumes that SLPs have a variety of therapeutic options tailored to treat each of these disorders. In contrast, a general model of phonological intervention, which embraces the dual phonetic/phonemic aspects involved in phonologic learning, allows flexibility for SLPs to modify and adapt the procedures to meet the needs of each child. As Johnston (1984) suggested, all we can do is control the input we provide to the children. We engineer the input we present to the child and it is the child who ultimately puts it all together.

REFERENCES

Fey, M.E. (1986). *Language intervention with young children.* Boston: Allyn & Bacon.

Hodson, B.W., & Paden, E. (1991). *Targeting intelligible speech: A phonological approach to remediation* (2nd ed.). Austin, TX: PRO-ED.

Johnston, J.R. (1984). Fit, focus, and functionality: An essay on early language intervention. *Child Language Teaching and Therapy, 1,* 125–134.

Long, S. (2001). About time: A comparison of computerized and manual procedures for grammatical and phonological analysis. *Clinical Linguistics & Phonetics, 15*(5), 399–426.

McKinley, N., & Williams, A.L. (2003). Sound contrasts in phonology (SCIP) [Computer software]. Phase II Small Business Innovative Research (SBIR) grant (R43) proposal funded by the National Institutes of Health, National Institute on Deafness and Other Communication Disorders, awarded to Thinking Publications, Eau Claire, WI.

Monahan Broudy, D. (1993). *Remediation of common phonological processes* (2nd ed.). Austin, TX: PRO-ED.

Palin, M.W. (1992). *Contrast pairs for phonological training.* Chicago: Riverside.

Weiner, F.F. (1981). Treatment of phonological disability using the method of meaningful minimal contrast: Two case studies. *Journal of Speech and Hearing Disorders, 46,* 97–103.

Williams, A.L. (2000a). Multiple oppositions: Case studies of variables in phonological intervention. *American Journal of Speech-Language Pathology, 9,* 289–299.

Williams, A.L. (2000b). Multiple oppositions: Theoretical foundations for an alternative contrastive intervention approach. *American Journal of Speech-Language Pathology, 9,* 282–288.

Williams, A.L. (2002, November). Models of assessment and intervention: Phonology in clinical settings. Short course presented at the annual convention of the American Speech-Language-Hearing Association, Atlanta, GA.

Williams, A.L. (2003). *Speech disorders resource guide for preschool children.* Clifton Park, NY: Thomson Delmar Learning.

Williams, A.L., & Kalbfleisch, J. (2001, August). Phonological intervention using a multiple opposition approach. Poster session presented at the 25th World Congress of the International Association of Logopedics and Phoniatrics, Montreal, Canada.

Chapter 17

Phonological Intervention

The How or the What?

JUDITH A. GIERUT

W hen asked clinical questions about my views on phonological intervention, the most appropriate place to begin the discussion is with an examination of the desired goals of treatment. A clear understanding of what is to be ultimately accomplished in treatment will directly inform the structure and course of such treatment. That is to say, the end serves to define the means. In this regard, the primary goal of phonological treatment is to induce change in a child's presenting knowledge of the sound system of the surrounding speech community. The aim is for *normalization* by way of inducing changes in a child's linguistic knowledge (Gierut, Elbert, & Dinnsen, 1987; Shriberg & Kwiatkowski, 1994). Given the known critical period for phonological learning (Shriberg, Gruber, & Kwiatkowski, 1994), this must be achieved in the most efficient and expedient way possible. Thus, two key questions emerge: What does it mean to change linguistic knowledge, and how can change be induced efficaciously in treatment? The answers to these questions will lead us in a straight path to the plan and delivery of phonological intervention.

Before answering these questions, it is necessary to place my remarks within the larger context of the conduct of clinical research. We have been engaged on the Learnability Project (http://www.indiana.edu/~sndlrng) in treatment efficacy research that is designed to evaluate the impact of linguistic and psycholinguistic variables on children's phonological learning for purposes of informing evidence-based clinical practice. The research setting affords the unique opportunity to systematically vary aspects of treatment and to measure the nature and extent of change in children's sound systems in rich detail. While this environment closely resembles the clinic and our results have direct bearing on service delivery, it is imperative that experimental control be maintained. The protocol followed in clinical research must be pre-scripted in order for the treatment results to be reliable, valid, and replicable. Therefore, children enrolled in the Learnability Project are exposed to the same type and amount of treatment, with little room for variation. Treatment procedures and stimulus materials are fixed a priori to align with the research question being addressed, and greater attention is paid to measurement. These details notwithstanding, the

Preparation of this manuscript was supported by the National Institutes of Health (Grant DC01694 to Indiana University, Bloomington). I would like to thank Jessica Barlow, Michele Morrisette, Holly Storkel, and members of the Learnability Project for their input.

principles employed in treatment research are actually drawn from those used in the clinical setting including, for example, obtaining baseline measures, providing models, delivering corrective feedback, capitalizing on successive approximations, and incorporating branching as needed. Olswang (1998) outlined the relevant components of treatment that are common to both research and clinical settings, and underscores the continuity between treatment efficacy research and efficacious clinical treatment. These recommended components have been adopted and incorporated into our own research. With this harmony between treatment research and clinical treatment in mind, we now turn to the key questions of change in knowledge and change with treatment as the fundamentals of phonological intervention.

CHANGE IN KNOWLEDGE WITH TREATMENT

Change essentially translates to generalization and its potential effect on treated and/or untreated sounds that a child produces in error. Change in sound production, however, does not necessarily imply change in linguistic knowledge. In a seminal clinical exchange on the construct of generalization, Johnston (1988) made this important distinction between *underlying change in linguistic knowledge* versus *surface change in behavior.* Change in knowledge includes, for example, an increase in the membership of a linguistic category, expansion of the scope of a linguistic category, or insight into the constituent structure of a linguistic category. According to Johnston, change in knowledge is associated with an elaboration, modification, or restructuring of the inherent linguistic categories of a child's internal grammar. As applied to the sound system, change in linguistic knowledge translates to a change in the phonotactics of the child's grammar. *Phonotactics* are generally defined as the permissible sounds and sound sequences of a language. Change may therefore include an elaboration of new manners or places of articulation, an extension of sounds to new contexts or syllable shapes, or an implementation of new phonemic distinctions or contrasts, as a few examples. Thus far, these types of gains have been documented across various levels of the phonological hierarchy, thereby affecting a child's knowledge of the feature, segment, syllable, foot, or prosodic word (e.g., Elbert & McReynolds, 1979; Gierut, 1999; Kehoe, 1997; Tyler & Figurski, 1994).

Change in knowledge contrasts with change in behavior, which is described as automatization or consistent use of language structures (Johnston, 1988). As applied to the sound system, change in behavior may be associated with gains in production accuracy of sounds that are already being used by a child but that are used inconsistently. As another example, behavior changes may be associated with improved self-monitoring skills. Changes in behavior have also been documented (e.g., Koegel, Koegel, Voy, & Ingham, 1988), but as Johnston acknowledges, the latter are quantitative improvements; they do not also reflect qualitative advances in the state of a child's linguistic knowledge. Thus, the desired goal of phonological intervention is to alter the child's underlying knowledge of the ambient sound system.

Considering how change in knowledge can best be triggered in clinical treatment, an obvious answer may be found in the particular methods, approaches, or paradigms that are employed in teaching. Many documented and widely used methods of phonological intervention are available. Some available options include traditional (Van Riper, 1963), cycles (Hodson & Paden, 1983), conventional minimal pair (Weiner, 1981), whole language (Norris & Hoffman, 1990), or Metaphon approaches to intervention (Howell & Dean, 1994). These differ in their implementation and goal attack strategy and vary in their emphasis on perception, production and/or metalinguistic skills, and focused and/or distributed practice in treatment. Despite these differences, numerous comprehensive reviews attest to the effectiveness of these methods in inducing change in a child's knowledge of the sound system (for a summary, see Bernthal & Bankson, 2004).

Although it appears that the available treatment paradigms have strong merit, the choice among treatments is less clear. That is, which treatment method should be used with which child? This bears on the topic of *treatment efficiency,* or whether one teaching approach is better than another in inducing generalization and change. To date, only a handful of clinical investigations have ventured to ask this question. Specifically, the efficiency of the traditional method has been tested relative to conventional minimal pair (Ward & Bankson, 1989) and (modified) Metaphon procedures (Powell, Elbert, Miccio, Strike-Roussos, & Brasseur, 1998). Likewise, the conventional minimal pair approach has been evaluated relative to (modified) cycles (Tyler, Edwards, & Saxman, 1987) and whole language (Hoffman, Norris, & Monjure, 1990) paradigms. These are landmark studies; yet, a number of gaps remain. The full complement of methodological comparisons has not yet been explored, and systematic replications are lacking. Also, in some cases, a treatment approach may have been altered from its original conceptualization (e.g., Powell et al., 1998; Tyler et al., 1987); consequently, the reported efficiency may not be the same as when the method is implemented in its original format. These limitations notwithstanding, a common theme has emerged from these comparisons of treatment efficiency; namely, the different teaching approaches have been shown to be on par with each other in affecting change in a child's linguistic knowledge, such that no single treatment method has surfaced as being better than another. This observation has led to the suggestion that the method of treatment may be secondary to promoting change in a child's linguistic knowledge of the sound system (Gierut, 1998c). This poses a clinical dilemma, however. If our teaching method is of secondary importance, then which elements of intervention are most essential? Following from typical language development, an alternate solution is that the input of treatment may serve instead as the primary trigger of linguistic change (e.g., Connell, 1988; Gleitman & Newport, 2000; Johnston, 1988). For clinical purposes, this means that the target sounds and phonological structures to which we expose a child in treatment may be crucial to generalization. The implication is that *what* is treated may be more important than *how* it is taught (Gierut, 2001, 2003). By way of analogy, think about this relative to standard educational practices. Federal and state governments and local school corporations set curricular goals for given grade levels (i.e., the "what to teach"), but individual classroom teachers are afforded the flexibility to use methods, strategies, and approaches to teaching that best match their own educational philosophies and the children they are instructing (i.e., the "how to teach"). My suggestion then is that establishing the phonological curriculum may be the real key to motivating linguistic change, with the methods to be used in teaching that curriculum being open to vary by clinician and child. Thus, in my view, the three most important elements in the implementation of phonological intervention are the nature of the input, the predicted generalization that derives from that input, and the measurement of change in linguistic knowledge that follows from that input.

INPUT, PREDICTIONS, AND MEASUREMENT

One consistent outcome of recent treatment efficacy research conducted in our lab and others is that more complex linguistic input promotes the greatest change in a child's overall sound system (for review, see Gierut, 1998c, 2001, 2003; Gierut, Morrisette, Hughes, & Rowland, 1996). The effects of a complex treatment target have been shown to have a positive impact on the treated sound in untreated contexts, in addition to other untreated sounds. Change in untreated sounds includes within-class generalization or generalization to sounds that share the same manner of articulation as the treated sound (e.g., treat a fricative, learn other untreated fricatives). It also includes across-class general-ization, or generalization to sounds that differ in manner from the treated sound (e.g., treat a liquid, learn other untreated nasals). Thus, the end result is that systemwide changes in the phonotactics of a child's grammar take place following treatment of a complex target. Notably, this accords with Johnston's (1988) description of change in linguistic knowledge.

At first glance, treatment of a complex phonological target may seem to be at odds with the expected course of typical development as defined by normative scales. However, on close inspection, the construct of complexity is wholly consistent with principles of language learnability that have been shown to cut across modules of grammar—that is, syntax, semantics, and phonology (Pinker, 1995; Tesar & Smolensky, 1998; Wexler, 1982; cf. Gierut, 2003, for review). In other words, the way in which typical language acquisition proceeds is by exposure to more complex components of grammar. This is termed *positive evidence;* namely, it is input that illustrates for the child the full range of advanced constructions, categories, and structures that are permissible in the target language. It seems then that the current findings of treatment efficacy research are actually mirroring what takes place and has long been known about typical language development.

Thus far, treatment effects following exposure to complex phonological targets have been reported for different levels of the phonological hierarchy including, for example, the phonetic (Tyler & Figurski, 1994), phonemic (Gierut, 1992), and syllabic (Gierut & Champion, 2001) levels of structure. In addition, complexity has been evaluated with respect to clinical considerations in sound selection including developmental norms (Gierut et al., 1996), stimulability (Powell, Elbert, & Dinnsen, 1991), and consistency (Gierut et al., 1987), to name a few. Complexity has even been tested relative to the words that are used as input in treatment (Morrisette & Gierut, 2002). That is, when a sound is taught in high-frequency words that have few rhyming counterparts, this leads to greater systemwide generalization and change. Table 17.1 provides a representative listing of some of the treatment targets that have been identified from investigations of phonological complexity. The changes that are expected to occur following treatment of such targets are also shown.

By examining these factors relative to a child's presenting sound system, the treatment target and the words to be presented in treatment can be identified directly, thus informing one of three critical components of intervention. We briefly illustrate this approach to intervention with a focus on the segmental level; a more detailed clinical case application

Table 17.1. Representative examples of treatment targets that are based on phonological complexity, and corresponding changes that are predicted in other aspects of the phonological system

Complex treatment targets	Predicted changes
Affricates	Fricatives
Clusters	Singletons, specifically affricates
Consonants	Vowels
Fricatives	Stops
Fricative + liquid clusters	Stop + liquid clusters
Late acquired sounds	Early acquired sounds
Liquids	Nasals
Consonant + liquid clusters in onset position	Occurrence of liquids in coda position
Nonstimulable sounds	Stimulable sounds
Stridency contrast between [s] and θ	One liquid, either [l] or [r]
Velars	Coronals
Voiced stops, fricatives, or affricates	Voiceless stops, fricatives, or affricates

Note: For more complete listings with corresponding references, see Gierut (2001, 2003).

is reported in Gierut (2004). Comparable steps may be taken when treatment is to be directed at the featural, syllabic, or other levels of the phonological hierarchy. A first step is to identify those sounds that are produced with 0% accuracy across all contexts, because these are phonotactically excluded from a child's grammar. This defines the initial pool of potential targets for treatment. Next in the process is to eliminate from the pool any sounds that are predicted to be learned from treatment of another target. For example, if a child produces both stops and fricatives in error, stops would be removed as a potential treatment target. As shown in Table 17.1, the reason is that treatment of fricatives predictably enhances the learnability of stops. Continuing in this way, additional sounds that are removed from the pool may be those that are stimulable or acquired early relative to normative scales. This process of whittling the pool of potential target sounds continues, allowing a clinician to hone in on the optimal complex input for each child. Sounds eliminated from the pool, however, should not be disregarded. These are central to the remaining two elements that are essential to intervention because they predict generalization and, consequently, they must be monitored to confirm (or refute) those predictions.

In terms of monitoring change, it is possible to document generalization through formal diagnostic testing; however, the inherent limitations of such tests result in somewhat shallow phonological samples. Consider, for example, that conventional phonological tests elicit a given target sound just once in each relevant word position. This gives the child a limited opportunity to demonstrate his or her range of phonological abilities. Informal probe measures designed specific to an individual child's sound system may be more informative. A number of word lists are readily available, which sample the phonological properties of English at phonetic, phonemic, and morphological levels across word positions and in multiple exemplars, while taking into account a word's frequency and its rhyming counterparts (e.g., Gierut, 1998a; Gierut et al., 1987). In our research, we administer such probes in measurement of change in the treated complex target and other untreated sounds, all of which were part of the initial pool of potential treatment targets. (For research purposes, we do sample all sounds of English whether correct or incorrect in production, in addition to onset and coda clusters.) This more extensive sample provides a measure of treated sound accuracy in untreated words and untreated positions, as well as untreated sound production within and across classes. It is necessary to underscore that an evaluation of change in linguistic knowledge must extend the probe sample beyond the treated sound. Often in clinical settings, only the treated sound is probed for generalization and change, with the expectation that what is treated is what will change. Following from treatment of complex linguistic input, however, other broader possibilities for change arise. Consequently, probe measures must be structured to monitor systemwide improvements that encompass treated and also untreated aspects of a child's presenting sound system.

On the Learnability Project, we administer such detailed probes using a spontaneous picture-naming task, with samples obtained at five points over the course of treatment. The format is that a child sees a picture and is asked to name it. Feedback is provided in the form of general encouragement to attend to the task, but there is no commentary about the (in)accuracy of responding. Multiple versions of the probe have been developed so that a child's responses do not become stimulus bound. That is, the words remain the same on each probe, but the order of administration and stimulus pictures vary at each sampling point. To illustrate, the word *red* in the first sample might be the second item of the probe, elicited by a picture of a red wagon. In the second sample, it might be the fifteenth item presented, being elicited by a red balloon. In the third sample, it might be the 29th, elicited by a red fire engine, and so forth. On each probe, the child is producing the word "red," but the corresponding picture is varied. These different versions of the probe are then randomized across children of a given study. The resulting probe data are phonetically transcribed for descriptive purposes, and accuracy of sound production is computed to obtain a quantitative evaluation of the amount and extent of change in treated and untreated sounds as a measure of generalization. It should be noted that the words of the probe are reserved specifically for purposes of documenting generalization. Probe items are never introduced in treatment.

The time course of probing is in sync with the treatment sequence that is used on the Learnability Project. Given the need to maintain experimental control in clinical research, there is procedural consistency across children. Every child goes through a baseline phase. During baseline, an extensive probe sample (described previously) is obtained and repeated depending on a child's order of enrollment. That is, the number of baselines increases as successive children are enrolled. Following baseline, children then receive a phase of imitation treatment whereby a target sound (or sounds, depending on the experimental question) is elicited following the clinician's model. The target sound occupies the initial position of either real words or nonwords, with the latter being specific to an experiment. Also, depending on the experiment, the target sound may either be presented autonomously or in contrast to another sound (Barlow & Gierut, 2002). Treatment always begins at the level of the sound in a real word and/or nonword. Following from the literature (Elbert, Dinnsen, Swartzlander, & Chin, 1990; Weiner, 1981), isolated sound production is not part of our protocol, nor is treatment in connected speech. The real/nonwords used in treatment correspond to visual referents that are presented either in paper or digital format, again particular to an experiment. The number of stimuli is also experiment specific, with the range of items being 6 to 16 (Elbert, Powell, & Swartzlander, 1991). In the imitation phase of treatment, drill play is used because this has been shown to be most effective (Shriberg & Kwiatkowski, 1982). Children are provided with feedback about the accuracy of each production. This takes the form of praise and encouragement for correct outputs and an additional input model for errored outputs following a fixed feedback loop. The fixed feedback loop works like this: Following an errored response, the clinician provides corrective feedback about placement, then repeats the model of the target word for a second production attempt by the child. If a child's second attempt is correct, positive remarks are made; if it is incorrect, treatment advances to the next trial and next item. Thus, for every errored response, a child is given corrective feedback with one and only one additional opportunity to incorporate this feedback before moving on. We recognize that, at first, treatment of complex targets may appear to be a daunting task because it may seem that a child is being set up to fail given the nature of the input. However, all of the conventional supporting methods that are used clinically to stabilize a child's response are employed. Successive approximations are accepted along the way (cf. Gierut & Champion, 2001, for illustration in treatment of three-element clusters) and placement cues are provided (cf. Shriberg, 1980, for illustration of evocation of /r/). The fixed feedback loop also ensures that a child receives appropriate encouragement for outputs that are correct and an added model for those that are incorrect. Treatment continues in the imitation phase for a maximum of seven sessions or until a child achieves 75% accuracy of production over two consecutive treatment sessions, whichever of these comes first. Following this, the probe (as in baseline) is again adminis-tered. Treatment then shifts to a spontaneous mode of responding, whereby a child produces the target sound in the stimulus words without a preceding model. The visual displays remain the same as in imitation, as does the drill play procedure with corrective feedback and feedback loop. Treatment in the spontaneous phase continues for a maximum of 12 sessions or until a child achieves 90% accuracy over three consecutive treatment sessions, whichever of these comes first.

At the completion of treatment, the probe is again repeated. The child receives no further intervention, but the sound system continues to be monitored in a posttreatment period of follow-up. At 2 weeks and 2 months following the completion of treatment, the probe measure is administered.

Thus, all children participate in a maximum of 19 treatment sessions, with these being scheduled three times per week in 1-hour blocks (i.e., 19 hours of individualized intervention). Throughout, there are five sampling points: baseline, phase shift, posttreat-ment, 2 weeks posttreatment, and 2 months posttreatment. At each sample, generalization data are collected to evaluate the treated target in untreated words and contexts, as well as all other untreated sounds in error. We should point out that these procedural details were established by consulting the prior treatment efficacy literature, and reflect average or typical sequences reported by others. It is also the case that the experimental design of given studies may necessitate slight departures from what we have described herein.

Given the necessity to maintain experimental control, demonstrate reliability and validity, and ensure replicability, no supplementary or complementary treatment is provided for other linguistic, motoric, or other nonlinguistic limitations; also, no home program is provided. These are areas in which a clinical setting may afford some more flexibility. For the most part, our clinical treatment research has emphasized the role of complex input on children's production as the mode of response. The reason relates to observed precedence relationships between perception and production (Williams & McReynolds,

1975), and metalinguistic abilities and production (Gierut, 1998b). Likewise, however, a child's response mode in treatment is driven by the experimental question being raised and by documented deficits. That is to say, perceptual and/or metalinguistic treatment may not be warranted unless diagnostic testing demonstrates that a child's performance in these domains is affected.

SUMMARY

We have been using these laboratory procedures with an emphasis on input complexity in the clinical treatment of preschool children who are preliterate with functional phonological delays. However, emerging evidence suggests that the same intervention approach may assist a range of populations and disorder types. Some examples of the populations that have been reported as benefiting from a complexity approach to treatment include toddlers (Tyler & Figurski, 1994); bilinguals (Anderson, 2002) and second language learners of English (Eckman & Iverson, 1993); children with developmental apraxia (Colone & Forrest, 2000) and hearing impairment (McReynolds & Jetzke, 1986); and those evidencing cognitive impairments (Dyer, Santarcangelo, & Luce, 1987) and nonfunctional (i.e., organic) disorders (Ballard & Thompson, 1999). This intervention approach not only appears to be relevant to phonology but also to syntax and semantics (Kiran & Thompson, 2003; Thompson, Shapiro, Kiran, & Sobecks, 2003). Although far more treatment efficacy research remains to be done, the construct of input complexity may hold promise as a general strategy that defines the structure, course, and ultimate outcome of clinical intervention.

REFERENCES

Anderson, R.T. (2002). Onset clusters and the sonority sequencing principle in Spanish: A treatment efficacy study. In F. Windsor, M.L. Kelly, & N. Hewitt (Eds.), *Investigations in clinical phonetics and linguistics* (pp. 213–224). Mahwah, NJ: Lawrence Erlbaum Associates.

Ballard, K.J., & Thompson, C.K. (1999). Treatment and generalization of complex sentence production in agrammatism. *Journal of Speech, Language, and Hearing Research, 42,* 690–707.

Barlow, J.A., & Gierut, J.A. (2002). Minimal pair approaches to phonological remediation. *Seminars in Speech and Language, 23,* 57–68.

Bernthal, J.E., & Bankson, N.W. (2004). *Articulation and phonological disorders* (5th ed.). Boston: Allyn & Bacon.

Colone, E., & Forrest, K. (2000, November). *Comparison of treatment efficacy for children with persistent speech sound disorders.* Poster presented at the American Speech-Language-Hearing Association meeting, Washington, DC.

Connell, P.J. (1988). Induction, generalization and deduction: Models for defining language generalization. *Language, Speech and Hearing Services in Schools, 19,* 282–291.

Dyer, K., Santarcangelo, S., & Luce, S.C. (1987). Developmental influences in teaching language forms to individuals with developmental disabilities. *Journal of Speech and Hearing Disorders, 52,* 335–347.

Eckman, F.R., & Iverson, G.K. (1993). Sonority and markedness among onset clusters in the interlanguage of ESL learners. *Second Language Research, 9,* 234–252.

Elbert, M., Dinnsen, D.A., Swartzlander, P., & Chin, S.B. (1990). Generalization to conversational speech. *Journal of Speech and Hearing Disorders, 55,* 694–699.

Elbert, M., & McReynolds, L.V. (1979). Aspects of phonological acquisition during articulation training. *Journal of Speech and Hearing Disorders, 44,* 459–471.

Elbert, M., Powell, T.W., & Swartzlander, P. (1991). Toward a technology of generalization: How many exemplars are sufficient? *Journal of Speech and Hearing Research, 34,* 81–87.

Gierut, J.A. (1992). The conditions and course of clinically induced phonological change. *Journal of Speech and Hearing Research, 35,* 1049–1063.

Gierut, J.A. (1998a). Natural domains of cyclicity in phonological acquisition. *Clinical Linguistics & Phonetics, 12,* 481–499.

Gierut, J.A. (1998b). Production, conceptualization and change in distinctive featural categories. *Journal of Child Language, 25,* 321–342.

Gierut, J.A. (1998c). Treatment efficacy: Functional phonological disorders in children. *Journal of Speech, Language, and Hearing Research, 41,* S85–S100.

Gierut, J.A. (1999). Syllable onsets: Clusters and adjuncts in acquisition. *Journal of Speech, Language, and Hearing Research, 42,* 708–726.

Gierut, J.A. (2001). Complexity in phonological treatment: Clinical factors. *Language, Speech and Hearing Services in Schools, 32,* 229–241.

Gierut, J.A. (2003). *Phonological complexity and language learnability.* Manuscript submitted for publication.

Gierut, J.A. (2004). Clinical application of phonological complexity. *CSHA Magazine, 34,* 6–16.

Gierut, J.A., & Champion, A.H. (2001). Syllable onsets II: Three-element clusters in phonological treatment. *Journal of Speech, Language, and Hearing Research, 44,* 886–904.

Gierut, J.A., Elbert, M., & Dinnsen, D.A. (1987). A functional analysis of phonological knowledge and generalization learning in misarticulating children. *Journal of Speech and Hearing Research, 30,* 462–479.

Gierut, J.A., Morrisette, M.L., Hughes, M.T., & Rowland, S. (1996). Phonological treatment efficacy and developmental norms. *Language, Speech, and Hearing Services in Schools, 27,* 215–230.

Gleitman, L.R., & Newport, E.L. (2000). The invention of language by children: Environmental and biological influences on the acquisition of language. In L.R. Gleitman & M. Liberman (Eds.), *Language: An invitation to cognitive science* (pp. 1–24). Cambridge, MA: MIT Press.

Hodson, B.W., & Paden, E.P. (1983). *Targeting intelligible speech: A phonological approach to remediation.* San Diego: College-Hill Press.

Hoffman, P.R., Norris, J.A., & Monjure, J. (1990). Comparison of process targeting and whole language treatments for phonologically delayed preschool children. *Language, Speech and Hearing Services in Schools, 21,* 102–109.

Howell, J., & Dean, E. (1994). *Treating phonological disorders in children. Metaphon: Theory to practice* (2nd ed.). London: Whurr Publishers.

Johnston, J.R. (1988). Generalization: The nature of change. *Language, Speech, and Hearing Services in Schools, 19,* 314–329.

Kehoe, M. (1997). Stress error patterns in English-speaking children's word productions. *Clinical Linguistics & Phonetics, 11,* 389–409.

Kiran, S., & Thompson, C.K. (2003). The role of semantic complexity in treatment of naming deficits: Training semantic categories in fluent aphasia by controlling exemplar typicality. *Journal of Speech, Language, and Hearing Research, 46,* 608–622.

Koegel, R.L., Koegel, L.K., Voy, K.V., & Ingham, J.C. (1988). Within-clinic versus outside-of-clinic self-monitoring of articulation to promote generalization. *Journal of Speech and Hearing Disorders, 53,* 392–399.

McReynolds, L.V., & Jetzke, E. (1986). Articulation generalization of voiced-voiceless sounds in hearing–impaired children. *Journal of Speech and Hearing Disorders, 51,* 348–355.

Morrisette, M.L., & Gierut, J.A. (2002). Lexical organization and phonological change in treatment. *Journal of Speech, Language, and Hearing Research, 45,* 143–159.

Norris, J.A., & Hoffman, P.R. (1990). Language intervention within naturalistic environments. *Language, Speech and Hearing Services in Schools, 21,* 72–84.

Olswang, L.B. (1998). Treatment efficacy research. In C.M. Frattali (Ed.), *Measuring outcomes in speech-language pathology* (pp. 134–150). New York: Thieme.

Pinker, S. (1995). Language acquisition. In L.R. Gleitman & M. Liberman (Eds.), *Language: An invitation to cognitive science* (pp. 135–182). Cambridge, MA: MIT Press.

Powell, T.W., Elbert, M., & Dinnsen, D.A. (1991). Stimulability as a factor in the phonologic generalization of misarticulating preschool children. *Journal of Speech and Hearing Research, 34,* 1318–1328.

Powell, T.W., Elbert, M., Miccio, A.W., Strike-Roussos, C., & Brasseur, J. (1998). Facilitating [s] production in young children: An experimental evaluation of motoric and conceptual treatment approaches. *Clinical Linguistics & Phonetics, 12,* 127–146.

Shriberg, L.D. (1980). An intervention procedure for children with persistent /r/ errors. *Language, Speech and Hearing Services in Schools, 11,* 102–110.

Shriberg, L.D., & Kwiatkowski, J. (1982). Phonological disorders II: A conceptual framework for management. *Journal of Speech and Hearing Disorders, 47,* 242–256.

Shriberg, L.D., & Kwiatkowski, J. (1994). Developmental phonological disorders I: A clinical profile. *Journal of Speech and Hearing Research, 37,* 1100–1126.

Shriberg, L.D., Gruber, F.A., & Kwiatkowski, J. (1994). Developmental phonological disorders III: Long-term speech-sound normalization. *Journal of Speech and Hearing Research, 37,* 1151–1177.

Tesar, B., & Smolensky, P. (1998). Learnability in optimality theory. *Linguistic Inquiry, 29,* 229–268.

Thompson, C.K., Shapiro, L.P., Kiran, S., & Sobecks, J. (2003). The role of syntactic complexity in treatment of sentence deficits in agrammatic aphasia: The complexity account of treatment efficacy (CATE). *Journal of Speech, Language, and Hearing Research, 46,* 591–607.

Tyler, A.A., & Figurski, G.R. (1994). Phonetic inventory changes after treating distinctions along an implicational hierarchy. *Clinical Linguistics & Phonetics, 8,* 91–108.

Tyler, A.A., Edwards, M.L., & Saxman, J.H. (1987). Clinical application of two phonologically-based treatment procedures. *Journal of Speech and Hearing Disorders, 52,* 393–409.

Van Riper, C. (1963). *Speech correction: Principles and methods* (4th ed.). Englewood Cliffs, NJ: Prentice Hall.

Ward, J.M., & Bankson, N.W. (1989, November). *Phonological generalization associated with the traditional and minimal contrast approaches.* Paper presented at the annual meeting of the American Speech-Language-Hearing Association, St. Louis, MO.

Weiner, F.F. (1981). Treatment of phonological disability using the method of meaningful minimal contrast: Two case studies. *Journal of Speech and Hearing Disorders, 46,* 97–103.

Wexler, K. (1982). A principle theory for language acquisition. In E. Wanner & L.R. Gleitman (Eds.), *Language acquisition: The state of the art* (pp. 288–315). Cambridge, UK: Cambridge University Press.

Williams, G.C., & McReynolds, L.V. (1975). The relationship between discrimination and articulation training in children with misarticulations. *Journal of Speech and Hearing Research, 18,* 401–412.

Chapter 18

Summary, Reflections, and Future Directions

ALAN G. KAMHI

How does one conclude a book with so many different perspectives on assessment, classification, goal selection, and treatment? Readers may hope that Karen or I will provide some guidance in sifting through the different perspectives. Readers may justifiably wish to know what we think of the different perspectives. I would like to think that our opinion does not matter—that students and clinicians reading this book will form their own opinions about the different approaches to the questions raised. To help form these opinions, the first part of this chapter highlights some of the major points from each of the chapters in the book. This is followed by some of my own views and thoughts on diagnosis, classification, target selection, and treatment approaches. I found it difficult to comment separately on target selection and treatment approaches, so my comments for these two sections appear after the treatment section.

In some instances, my views may be consistent with one contributor; in other instances, I may prefer the view of a different contributor. In some cases, my view may seem unique, but its uniqueness is probably more in the way I combine different views rather than the novelty of a particular idea. This is what most experienced clinicians do: take what they like, ignore what they don't like, and try to get children's speech normalized as quickly as possible.

ASSESSMENT AND CLASSIFICATION

The five contributors to the first section of the book took somewhat different approaches in presenting their views about assessment, diagnosis, and classification. The chapters by Davis (Chapter 1), Miccio (Chapter 3), and Tyler (Chapter 4) present general approaches to assessment, classification, and diagnosis. The chapters by Velleman (Chapter 2) and Goffman (Chapter 5) focus more specifically on the special populations of children with developmental apraxia of speech (DAS) and children who speak a nonstandard dialect of English.

Davis begins in Chapter 1 by presenting her unique classification of developmental speech disorders. She classifies primary developmental speech disorders into two broad categories, functional and etiological, and further divides etiological into peripheral, neural, and developmental. Peripheral factors include respiratory, phonatory, and articulatory subsystems of the speech production system and auditory subsystems of the perceptual system. The neural factors Davis considers, such as motor control, are central rather than peripheral. Developmental factors include general cognitive delays. The functional category, in which the underlying cause of the speech delay is not known, contains the largest group of children with speech disorders.

Davis's assessment protocol is designed to identify phonetic and phonological patterns in children's speech. An independent analysis that examines production patterns for consonants, vowels, syllable structure, and prosodic factors is used to assess phonetic abilities, whereas a relational analysis that compares child productions with adult target forms addresses the phonological system. The second component of Davis's assessment protocol focuses on the child's overall language system. Like the other contributors, she uses a conversational sample to assess language abilities. The third component of her assessment protocol addresses the larger context of the child's communication abilities, including intelligibility, communicative effectiveness, and family factors. An important principle of Davis's assessment approach is that the specific evaluation procedures will differ according to the child's age and developmental abilities. In the last part of her chapter, she discusses how the assessment framework changes for different ages. Consistent with her chapter on goal selection in the next section, Davis clearly embraces a developmental approach.

Velleman also takes a broad-based approach to assessment, noting that phonology not only includes phonetic and phonemic factors but also cognitive and language factors. She describes her approach as one that is "pragmatic, eclectic, and individual-focused." The first question she asks in assessment is "What is not working here?" Like some of the approaches to target selection in the next section (e.g., Tyler [Chapter 6] and Williams [Chapter 9]), Velleman wants to know what aspect of the child's phonology is interfering the most with successful communication. Is it too much homonymy, too much variability, or unexpected (idiosyncratic) patterns? Like most contributors, Velleman uses both independent and relational analyses to assess a child's phonological system. She goes on to tackle the difficult issue of differentiating childhood apraxia of speech (CAS) from other phonological disorders. Vowel deviations and abnormal prosody are two symptoms that she finds useful in identifying children with CAS.

In the second part of her chapter, Velleman provides an excellent discussion of the phonological features that differentiate mainstream English from African American English. She concludes by reminding clinicians that it is important for them to learn as much as possible about the language or dialect a child speaks. Performing thorough, independent analyses and using reports and observations of the children's communicative abilities is particularly important in assessing children from different linguistic backgrounds.

Miccio begins her chapter by noting that it is relatively easy to identify unintelligible preschool children with phonological disorders. The challenge of assessment is to determine the nature of the disordered sound system and the severity of the problem. Miccio believes that the underlying cause or contributing factors must be determined in order to make treatment recommendations. She supplements standardized speech and language assessments with a picture-naming probe to elicit multiple examples of late-emerging sounds and any sounds found to be in error from previous testing. She also obtains a connected speech sample and administers a stimulability probe for consonants that are not present in the child's phonetic inventory.

Like Miccio, Tyler's assessment approach consists of both standardized and nonstandardized analyses. Her protocol is similar to Miccio's with the exception of the supplemental probe. She describes in some detail her analysis of the conversational sample. When time permits, she uses PROPH (Computerized Profiling) to analyze a 100-word sample from the standardized articulation test and the speech sample. If a cursory analysis of the sample reveals expressive language difficulties, she uses Systematic Analysis of Language Transcripts (SALT) to further analyze the sample. In addition, if 5- to 6-year-old children have severe phonological disorders or associated language deficits, Tyler uses the Test of Phonological Awareness (Torgesen & Bryant, 1994) or the Comprehensive Test of Phonological Processing (Wagner, Torgesen, & Rashotte, 1999) to assess phonological awareness. Finally, although she does not routinely evaluate perceptual skills, if she suspects a perceptual deficit, Tyler recommends using Locke's (1980) Speech Production-Perception Task (SPPT). The SPPT provides information about phonemic identification abilities.

Goffman's chapter provides an interesting theoretical discussion about whether speech production is a motor or linguistic process. Her major conclusion is that speech production is both a motor *and* a linguistic process. She supports this conclusion by showing how children with DAS and children with specific language impairments (SLI) both have difficulties on many motor tasks. It is no surprise that children with DAS have motor difficulties, but it is generally not well known that children with SLI also have problems in this area. Some interesting clinical implications derive from this conclusion. Goffman suggests that intervention approaches often are based on a particular aspect of a child's profile rather than on a more general diagnostic classification. The assessment process needs to go beyond existing measures of segmental repertoires, syllable shapes, and error patterns to include more elaborated and integrated measures of language and motor development. The interactive model that Goffman advocates appears to have some things in common with Norris and Hoffman's interactive constellation model (see Chapter 7) that is presented in the next section.

REFLECTIONS ON ASSESSMENT AND CLASSIFICATION

The most interesting questions about assessment for me are those that affect classification and diagnosis. This is not to say that questions about which tests or procedures to use are unimportant. I find the answers to these questions rather straightforward, however, and, perhaps more important, my colleagues in this book have done such an excellent job answering these questions that there doesn't seem to be anything more to say. For example, Tyler, Miccio, and Davis provide clear descriptions of a broad-based assessment approach that combines standardized and nonstandardized procedures to evaluate speech, language, cognitive, and psychosocial abilities. The chapters in the next section on goal selection also provide some guidance for assessment. Williams, for example, describes the kind of assessment information needed to select maximally distinct sounds (see Chapter 9), whereas Bernhardt offers the reader a taste of what is involved in performing a constraints-based analysis (see Chapter 10).

Classification and diagnostic issues in phonology are much more controversial than assessment issues. For example, despite the numerous studies supporting Shriberg's framework for speech sound disorders (e.g., Shriberg, Lewis, Tomblin, McSweeny, Karlsson, &

Scheer, in press), it is still common practice to differentiate phonological (phonemic based) disorders from articulation (phonetic based) disorders (e.g., Bauman-Waengler, 2004; Bernthal & Bankson, 2004). Reflecting this distinction, the two books just cited are entitled *Articulatory and Phonological Impairments and Articulation and Phonological Disorders,* respectively. Several problems occur, however, in using the distinction between phonemic and phonetic problems to differentially diagnose children with speech sound disorders.

The first problem is how one actually differentiates between phonemic and phonetic problems. It is generally agreed that phonetic errors involve peripheral motor processes, whereas phonemic errors are those "in which the organization and function of the phoneme system is impaired" (Bauman-Waengler, 2004, p. 8). The confusion occurs in determining what a phoneme-based error is. Most phonologists take a narrow view of phoneme errors, restricting them to instances in which the child demonstrates the ability to produce a sound, but does not produce the sound for the appropriate sound class. For example, a child says [su] for *shoe,* but [ti] for *see.* The child can produce an /s/, so the difficulty is not with speech production but with the organization of the phonological system. Although these types of errors are commonly cited in the phonological literature, they represent a very small proportion of the errors most children make.

In contrast to this narrow view of phoneme-based disorders, in clinical practice, the occurrence of phonological simplification patterns and/or processes are often assumed to reflect a phonological or phonemic disorder. Difficulty producing late-emerging sounds ([s], [l], [r]) would reflect an articulation disorder. Unfortunately, the assumption that phonological processes (fronting, stopping, or cluster reduction) reflect phoneme-based organizational difficulties is not true. Phonological processes are simply descriptive labels; they do not indicate the cause of the error pattern. Phonological processes are just as likely (some would say more likely) to be caused by speech production (phonetic) limitations as by organizational or phonemic problems. In other words, many children exhibit velar fronting because they cannot produce /k/ and /g/, not because they have some difficulty organizing their phonological system. It is also possible that the initial cause of the error pattern is no longer present, and the continued substitution of t/k is maintained by habit. After producing t/k for several months or years, it may be difficult for some children to change a habitual motor pattern. Importantly, the continued substitution of t/k would reflect neither a phonemic nor a phonetic problem. Modifying a habitual motor pattern is not easy, as anyone knows who has ever tried to change a golf swing, tennis stroke, or dialectal speech pattern. The important point here is that several different causes can be found for speech sound error patterns. A diagnostic classification that assumes that all errors are phonemic or phonetic does not accurately reflect this multiple causation view.

Another problem with the phonological-articulation distinction is that many children will show a developmental progression from a phonological to an articulation disorder. For example, the 3-year-old child who exhibits widespread stopping, velar fronting, and cluster reduction would be considered to have a phonological disorder. However, when the child is 5 years old and still has difficulty producing /s/, /r/, and /l/, the child would be considered to have an articulation disorder. At some point between age 3 and 5 years, the disorder changes from a phonological problem to an articulation problem, suggesting that the disorder at age 3 is different from the one at age 5. Manifestations of disorders clearly change with age. The 4-year-old child with dyslexia or autism exhibits behaviors that are different from those of the 6-, 10-, or 14-year-old with these disorders, but these differences do not change the nature (phenotype) of the disorder. The same should be true for children with speech sound disorders. Speech normalization follows a predictable path, with fewer phonemic, systemwide errors as the child gets older.

There is one more problem with the distinction between phonological and articulation disorders. When a child is diagnosed with a phonological disorder, it is often assumed that the primary cause of the disorder is linguistic rather than phonetic. Many young children, however, clearly have phonetic problems. Because *articulation disorder* is typically used to describe speech difficulties in older children, clinicians need another term for young children with obvious motor problems. The term used, of course, is developmental apraxia of speech. The increase in children with DAS in recent years is thus due in part to the inherent problems with the distinction between phonological and articulation disorders.

Is there a solution to the confusion created by phonological-articulation distinction? My preference would be to use one term for the general population of children with developmental phonological disorders. I prefer the generic term *speech delay* or *speech sound disorder*. The term *phonological disorder* has not worked as a broad-based term that includes speech production. It is too linked with language and reading and has had difficulty spreading to the community at large (Kamhi, 2004). The term *articulation disorder* also does not work for young children with significant speech sound disorders because it is too narrow, although it may be appropriate for school-age children who do not normalize speech and continue to have residual errors, such as speech distortions of fricatives/affricates and liquids. Shriberg et al. (in press) classifies these children as having *residual errors–speech delay,* a term that works for research but is probably too cumbersome for clinical practice.

Differentiating children with DAS from the larger group of children with developmental speech delays is another difficult diagnostic problem. As Velleman notes in Chapter 2, no one behavior or symptom defines DAS. Like others, she looks for a pattern of difficulty with sequencing sounds, coordinating different levels of language, volitional movements, and nonspeech oral-motor abilities. One characteristic of DAS that emerges from the literature is that affected children do not respond to treatment in the same way as other children with a speech delay. Campbell (1999) found, for example, that children with DAS required almost twice as many treatment sessions to achieve the same results as age-matched children with speech delay.

My preference is to restrict the use of the term DAS to the relatively small group of children who have speech, language, and learning difficulties as well as a positive family history (cf. Shriberg, Aram, & Kwiatkowski, 1997). Having said this, it is important to note that all of the research on DAS is with children with *suspected* DAS because there is no clear diagnostic or phenotypic marker for the disorder (Shriberg et al., 1997).

GOAL AND TARGET SELECTION

As several of the contributors to this section (e.g., Tyler, Williams, and Bernhardt) note, target selection approaches can be broadly classified as developmental or complexity based. Adherents to a developmental approach base decisions for target selection on the normative data for speech development. The specific targets selected will depend on the theoretical framework used for development. Williams, for example, talks about how, early in her career, she listed children's sound errors by word position and classified errors as substitutions, omissions, distortions, or additions (see Chapter 9). Targets were chosen primarily based on developmental norms, with some consideration given to stimulability and consistency of errors. When it became apparent that children's speech development was influenced by sound classes, Williams shifted her selection of targets to focus on the elimination of persistent phonological simplification processes. Her approach to target selection was still developmentally based, but the relevant data were the suppression of processes rather than the age of speech sound acquisition.

Adherents to a complexity approach target the more complex speech or language form. As discussed by Williams, a series of studies in the 1980s and 1990s by Gierut and her colleagues found that greater systemwide change occurred when more phonologically complex sounds were targeted (see Chapter 9). For example, targeting /v/ led to more systemwide change than did targeting the less complex and developmentally earlier emerging sound /f/.

Of the five chapters in this section, the one by Davis best reflects the developmental approach. Davis begins Chapter 8 by noting that valid and appropriate choices about intervention goals require a comprehensive assessment of a child's speech and language behaviors. Such an assessment allows the clinician to make normative comparisons that can be used to determine specific intervention targets and set expectations for the child. Davis does not select goals based solely on normative speech and language data. Information about the child's perceptual, cognitive, psychosocial, and structural abilities is also used to select the most appropriate goals. Davis's flexible and broad-based developmental approach to target selection should be quite appealing to many clinicians.

Tyler, like Davis, emphasizes the necessity of a comprehensive assessment of a child's phonological system in order to determine treatment goals. Indeed, it is hard to imagine any of the contributors to this volume not agreeing with this point. For Tyler, the ultimate goal of a phonological intervention program is generalization, both stimulus generalization (learning untreated sounds) and context generalization (using the newly learned sounds in conversation outside the therapy context). She identifies three major steps to target selection:

1. Choose error patterns that have a major impact on the system in terms of severity and intelligibility.

2. Choose target sounds that affect these error patterns and/or expand the inventory.

3. Select a goal attack strategy.

By first addressing phonological patterns and then choosing targets that result in the most systemwide change, Tyler's approach is both developmental and complexity based. She used a case study of a child who had a very restricted phonetic inventory to illustrate the goal selection process. Despite the evidence in support of targeting nonstimulable sounds, Tyler is concerned that targeting only nonstimulable sounds might be frustrating for a child who is beginning therapy. For this reason, she suggests targeting the stimulable sound /s/ for a new word shape (final position). The other sounds targeted would be /k/

and /t/, which are both nonstimulable. If targeting two nonstimulable sounds proves too difficult, she would replace initial /k/ with /g/. For a goal attack strategy, Tyler prefers the cycle approach because it is brief and has multiple intervention targets. It is clear in reading Tyler's approach to target selection that she is not attached to one particular theory. In some cases, her approach is based on previous research studies, but as with Davis, she will modify targets based on the child's response to treatment.

Williams begins her chapter with a personal history of how her approach to target selection has changed over the years. After years of using dichotomous categorizations (stimulable–nonstimulable, most knowledge–least knowledge) to determine target selection, she came to realize that these categorizations were not capturing the unique phonological systems or specific learning needs of individual children. Her disenchantment led her to focus on children's sound systems to select treatment targets rather than on characteristics of individual sounds. Like Tyler, she realized that a priority in target selection should be the potential a sound has for restructuring the child's phonological system. Sounds that have the most potential for restructuring the system should receive priority in intervention. Where Williams differs from Tyler is in her selection of specific targets. To select a target, Williams uses a distance metric that is based on the classification of sounds (i.e., place, voice, manner) and how distinct the target sound is from the child's error sound.

The remaining two chapters in this section, by Norris and Hoffman and Bernhardt, reflect two different theoretical orientations. Norris and Hoffman's constellation model (see Chapter 7) is based on a connectionist, neural network approach to language learning. Phonology in this model is viewed as an integral and inseparable part of the language system; it is not a distinct system. Specific phonological goals are rarely selected for treatment because Norris and Hoffman believe that the most effective way to facilitate phonological development is to increase a child's vocabulary and language structures. Norris and Hoffman have general, rather than specific, phonological goals, such as adding six new phonemes or increasing the percentage of consonants correct by 40% in spontaneous speech. The specific sounds added or correctly produced depend on the self-organizing principles of the child's system. One clear advantage of Norris and Hoffman's approach is that they never have to consider whether to target phonological or language goals. Phonological goals are always targeted within the general language system using storybooks. When phonology is directly targeted, it is done so from multiple perspectives, including phoneme awareness, print awareness, and sound production.

Bernhardt's approach to goal and target selection is founded on a constraints-based nonlinear phonological analysis and the influence of other client-based factors such as cognitive, motor, perceptual, and environmental factors. In the first part of Chapter 10, Bernhardt explains the three major concepts of the constraints-based nonlinear theory: phonological constraints, hierarchical structure, and the independence of phonological units. Goals are targeted within and across hierarchical levels. For example, possible goals at the phrase and word levels include new phrasal stress and intonation as well as new word lengths, stress, and shapes. Potential segmental targets might include manner, place, and laryngeal features.

Although Bernhardt's approach to target selection may seem very different from the other ones in this section, she makes the point that the process she uses to select specific goals is consistent with the developmental approach as opposed to the complexity (markedness) approach. In the final sections of her chapter, she discusses the importance of cognitive-linguistic, personal-social, and articulatory competence for making decisions about target selection. Although Bernhardt has a unique theoretical orientation, her broad-based approach to target selection is not so different from those of some of the other contributors to this section.

INTERVENTION

There seem to be at least four general types of treatment approaches (Kamhi, 2003):

1. Phonetic based

2. Phonemic based

3. Language-communication based

4. Broad based

Of the seven contributors to this section, Velleman, Miccio, and Rvachew focus on phonetic factors; Williams and Gierut emphasize phonemic factors; Norris and Hoffman present their language–communication-based approach; and Tyler presents her eclectic, broad-based approach. In some cases, the focus an author takes in these chapters might not reflect his or her general approach to treatment. Most of the contributors would probably describe their general approach to treatment as being broad-based because they would consider targeting perceptual, phonemic, and language abilities as well as phonetic ones depending on the needs of the client. Even the most language-oriented authors (Norris and Hoffman) advocate the use of a phonetic approach to help facilitate speech sound productions. A brief summary of the seven chapters is provided below.

Velleman's contribution focuses on young children with severe speech delays and children with CAS. Velleman feels that the remediation of phonotactic (syllable structure) deficits has been a neglected area in the literature. For children with severe speech problems and CAS, targeting a new sound in a new position will often be too difficult. Some common syllable structure goals include initial consonants, final consonants, two-syllable words, and consonant clusters. Sound accuracy is not the goal when targeting syllable structure. In the main part of her chapter, Velleman provides a number of techniques to facilitate phonotactic development.

Miccio's chapter focuses on stimulability (see Chapter 14). She cites a variety of studies that show the importance of stimulability as a prognostic indicator. For example, Gierut and her colleagues have shown that the treatment of more complex sounds results in the greatest systemwide change (see Chapter 17). Despite these findings, few clinicians target complex sounds because they are usually nonstimulable, and there has been little discussion in the literature about how to actually get children to produce nonstimulable sounds. Because clinicians are interested in increasing the number of sounds in a child's inventory as quickly as possible, stimulable sounds are usually targeted despite the fact that systemwide change is not likely to occur. The solution to this problem, according to Miccio, is to make stimulability the treatment target. A large portion of her chapter describes specific procedures to facilitate production of nonstimulable sounds. Although her treatment approach is primarily phonetic in nature, she recognizes the close link between phonetics and the phonological system. Indeed, she concludes the chapter with a quote from Locke (1983), stating that "all things phonologic are phonetic."

Rvachew, like Miccio, also focuses on the importance of phonetic factors in phonological intervention. She begins her chapter by emphasizing the importance of theory for clinical practice. Rvachew's theoretical perspective is the representation-based approach of Edwards, Fourakis, Beckman, and Fox (1999). The central tenet of the approach is that "the child's phonological knowledge is derived from the gradual accumulation of knowledge about the acoustic/phonetic . . . characteristics of syllables and words" (see Chapter 15). The treatment program that follows from this perspective has three phases. In Phase I, the child is exposed to a variety of exemplars of target and contrasting phonemes and provided with a variety of phonetic placement and shaping techniques to facilitate production of the phoneme in a variety of phonetic contexts. In Phase II, minimal pair activities are used to stabilize the child's knowledge of the new phoneme contrast. In Phase III, opportunities are provided to practice the phoneme in communicative contexts. Other goals such as improving syntax or phonological awareness would be targeted in this phase. In the remainder of the chapter, Rvachew describes the three phases in more detail, providing sample activities and case examples that illustrate how to implement each phase. For example, for the first phase, she recommends using a simple computer game called the *Speech Assessment and Interactive Learning System* (SAILS) to teach children to identify words pronounced correctly and incorrectly. In the second phase, Rvachew recommends using speech analyzers that provide waveform and spectrographic feedback for children who are having difficulty with correct articulatory placement. For facilitating correct production in communicative contexts, she suggests using LocuTour Multimedia products such as *Articulation I: Learning Fundamentals*. This program shows children photographs of objects that target a specific phoneme in a particular word position. Rvachew provides a list of several other commercially available programs.

Although Rvachew emphasizes the importance of phonetic factors, it is clear in reading her chapter that she places equal importance on phonemic and language-based factors. Her therapy approach, as with many of the other contributors, is motivated not just by theory but by evidence of change and a willingness to modify the approach and treatment targets when the child is not making progress.

Williams, like many of the other contributors in this volume, views speech disorders as occurring along a phonetic–phonemic continuum, but she believes that the majority of speech disorders lie closer to the phonemic end. She bases this belief on her clinical experience that children are often stimulable for sounds not in their phonetic inventory or can easily produce the new sound with limited auditory, visual, and tactile cues. Regardless of where children fall on the phonetic–phonemic continuum, therapy needs to target both phonetic and phonemic aspects to remediate the overall speech sound disorder.

In the initial phase of treatment, Williams advocates using imitation to practice new sounds. Once the phonetic aspects of the contrast are established, opportunities are provided to practice the new target in a variety of communicative contexts. Meaningful and nonmeaningful words are used to develop the speech sound contrasts. Williams does not think it is appropriate to use a multiple opposition approach with all children. The approach is most appropriate for children with severe delays who are at a rule-based stage in their phonological development. She does not recommend using multiple oppositions with children who have only a few error sounds or with children who are still at an early whole-word stage of development.

Norris and Hoffman were the first to suggest using a language–communication-based approach to improve speech. They view phonology as an integral and inseparable part of the language system, so for them the question about whether to target speech or language is not an issue. Speech is always targeted in conjunction with language and communication. Because their approach to treatment involves using stories, all treatment is intrinsically language and communication based. Norris and Hoffman will, as noted earlier, provide instruction to facilitate individual speech sound production if they feel the child needs this level of support.

Tyler characterizes her approach to intervention as a hybrid that has an auditory-perceptual component, a conceptual component, production training, and phonological awareness activities. Natural conversational interactions are a part of every therapy session. The second part of her chapter describes in some detail the various activities that can be used to target perception, phonemic contrasts, speech production, and phonemic awareness. Tyler's approach is clearly the most broad-based of the contributors in this volume.

Gierut's approach to treatment should be familiar to most speech-language pathologists (SLPs). In the last 15 years, she and her colleagues have published more treatment efficacy studies than any other research group in phonology. Her research group is best known for the finding that more complex linguistic input promotes the greatest change in the child's overall sound system. For example, targeting /v/ will have more of an effect on untreated sounds than targeting /f/. The importance of the target sound is the foundation of Gierut's clinical philosophy. As she says in the first sentence of her chapter, any discussion of phonological intervention must begin by considering the desired goals of treatment. Having a clear understanding of what is to be ultimately accomplished in treatment will directly inform the structure and course of treatment. In other words, "the end serves to define the means" (see Chapter 17).

So what is the goal of treatment according to Gierut? The goal is to normalize a child's linguistic knowledge as efficiently and expediently as possible. Change in knowledge involves more than just a change in sound production; it involves an elaboration, modification, or restructuring of the inherent linguistic categories. Reflecting her linguistic background, Gierut emphasizes the difference between changing knowledge and changing behavior. As applied to the sound system, a change in behavior would be reflected in improvements in production accuracy. Behavioral changes are viewed as quantitative improvements because they may not reflect qualitative changes in a child's linguistic knowledge.

Gierut goes on to note that many of the widely used approaches to phonological intervention (traditional Van Riper, cycles, minimal pair, whole language, Metaphon) have all been shown to be effective in changing a child's knowledge of the sound system. This conclusion leads Gierut to question how important a particular treatment approach is for promoting change. For Gierut the answer is clear: Selecting what to treat is more important than how it is taught. The goals of treatment are the real key for changing linguistic knowledge, not the particular treatment approach used. In the remainder of her chapter, Gierut elaborates on the three central elements of her treatment approach: 1) the goals of treatment, 2) the predicted generalizations that derive from the goals, and 3) the measurement of change.

Accurate monitoring of change is a particularly important aspect of Gierut's intervention. She feels strongly that it is necessary to develop and administer probes that sample target sound production in different word positions with multiple exemplars. Probes must also sample untreated aspects of the child's sound system. These probes have been discussed in detail in Gierut's previous work. Gierut concludes by noting that the complexity approach may be appropriate for treating a range of populations and disorder types. She cites research showing that this approach has been effective in working with populations of children who have cognitive impairments, developmental apraxia, or hearing impairments.

REFLECTIONS ON GOAL SELECTION AND INTERVENTION

Gierut's chapter was reviewed last because the question she asks about which treatment approach to use is one that I have grappled with in the past. In a recent presentation at the annual convention of the American Speech-Language-Hearing Association (Kamhi, 2003), I unknowingly made some of the same points as Gierut. For example, I noted that the problem in speech therapy is not that we do not know how to improve speech abilities. The problem is that there are too many ways to improve speech, and these approaches are often theoretically incompatible with one another. This causes a lot of heated debate about which approach is best. Oral-motor therapy, Van Riper's hierarchical approach (i.e., sound to syllable to word), Hodson's cycle training, minimal/maximal contrast, multiple oppositions, and language-based approaches all have advocates and evidence in support of their effectiveness. There is evidence that all of these approaches are effective in modifying a child's phonological system, which leads Gierut to argue that treatment goals are more important than the approach used (see Chapter 17). I agree. The question, then, is how to decide which goals to target. Should one target oral-motor proficiency, phonological contrasts, specific sound and/or word productions, syllable structure complexity (i.e., phonotactics), intelligibility, phonological awareness, language abilities, or communication effectiveness?

The theory of phonological development or disorders that one embraces determines in large part the goals one chooses to target. There are at least five theoretical orientations that influence target selection:

1. Normal development model

2. Bottom-up model—starting with oral-motor or isolated speech segments

3. Top-down model—language-communication based

4. Broad-based (eclectic) approach

5. Complexity approach

After presenting the treatment goals or principles associated with each perspective, I offer some caveats and potential problems with each of these perspectives.

Typical Development

Treatment that is compatible with typical development would not target any unit smaller than the syllable. Children who are typically developing do not acquire individual speech sounds. The smallest unit of speech production is the canonical CV and VC syllable in babbling. Although young children may develop implicit knowledge of sounds and pho-nemes, explicit awareness of sounds and phonemes often does not develop until children are approximately 5 years of age. Given that typically developing children acquire words, not sounds (Velleman & Vihman, 2002), speech analyses would be word based and treatment would focus on developing word contrasts (e.g., Ingram & Ingram, 2001; Williams, 2000; Chapter 9).

One caveat for this perspective is that there are different views of normal development. Although I find Velleman and Vihman's view of speech development compelling, others may not. Another caveat often voiced about developmental models is that the children we are concerned with are not developing normally, so following the normal developmental model may not be the best way to help these children achieve normal speech. These children may require a different approach to facilitate accurate production of individual speech segments.

Bottom-Up Model: Oral-Motor Approach

The bottom-up model is associated with a discrete skill view of speech learning. Speech development and proficiency require strength, speed, accuracy, awareness of oral move-ments, and the production of individual sound segments. The concern typically raised with this view is that there is little evidence that practicing isolated oral movements facilitates speech production (see Chapter 11). In addition, better communication is usually not a short-term goal with this approach, which means that language and communication abilities may not receive adequate attention in therapy.

Bottom-Up Model: Sounds, Syllables, and Words

Speech learning proceeds in a hierarchical manner from sounds to syllables to words to phrases and so forth (e.g., Van Riper, 1978). In its traditional form, this view is associated with a vertical goal attack strategy in which high criterion levels of accuracy must be reached before moving to the next level. The caveats with this approach are that one may spend a long time working on accurate production of one or two sounds that have little impact on intelligibility or communication. Speech normalization may take a long time if sounds are particularly resistant to change, and, as with the previous bottom-up model, better communication is not a short-term goal of this approach.

Communication and Language Focus

The use of this approach requires a theoretical framework that emphasizes the interactive, interdependent nature of speech and language, such as the one embraced by Norris and Hoffman (see Chapter 7). In the strong version of this approach, language and communica-tion goals will be the sole targets of intervention; speech will not be targeted directly. Camarata (1993), for example, finds that recasting speech errors is sufficient for speech to normalize. Hoffman and Norris (2002) use narrative recall tasks to target speech and language and will provide speech cueing if needed. The strong version of this approach (Camarata, 1993) requires a lot of faith that children's speech will improve without any direct instruction or speech practice. It is difficult to envision this approach being effective with children with severe delays or school-age children who have distortion or residual errors (e.g., /s/, /l/, /r/). With the Norris and Hoffman approach, the concern remains that there may not be sufficient speech practice for children with severe delays or for those with residual and distortion errors.

Broad-Based (Eclectic) Approach

Many clinicians are not wedded to a particular theoretical orientation or they indicate that they are eclectic and use whatever works. These clinicians use a variety of techniques, strategies, and approaches. The most broad-based approach would target everything from oral-motor movements to conversational discourse and use different goal attack strategies depending on the child's developing phonological system. Hodson and Paden's (1991) phonological approach is broad based because it combines elements of traditional speech therapy (motor placement) with a perceptual component, an efficient goal attack strategy (cycling), and phonological assessment. The use of a broad-based approach requires a knowledgeable, flexible clinician who is able to plan and modify treatment according to the needs of the client. Because this approach draws from many theoretical orientations, it may not be easy to teach to new clinicians or anyone else.

Complexity Approach

The basic principle of this approach is that more complex linguistic input promotes the greatest change in a child's overall sound system (see Chapter 17). Choosing to focus on a complex treatment target, such as an unstimulable sound, has been shown to have a positive impact on the treated sound in untreated contexts as well as on untreated sounds (cf. Chapter 17). Changes in untreated sounds include within-class generalization (treat a fricative, learn other fricatives) as well as across-class generalization (e.g., treat a liquid, learn untreated nasals). The caveats with this approach are discussed in the next section on treatment efficiency.

TREATMENT EFFICIENCY AND CLIENT-BASED FACTORS

Two other general factors influence the selection of a treatment approach, treatment efficiency and client-based factors. Treatment that has efficiency as a guiding principle promises the quickest path to speech normalization. The most efficient treatments are those that get something for free. Gierut's complexity approach is efficient because targeting difficult sounds (e.g., /v/) leads to better generalization of untreated sounds than targeting easier sounds such as /f/ (cf. Miccio & Ingrisano, 2000). Focusing on conversation or narratives (Camarata, 1993; Hoffman & Norris, 2002) and getting accurate speech production for free would be the most efficient approach.

As with the other theoretical perspectives, one based on efficiency is not without some concerns. One of the problems often raised about efficiency is that quicker may not always be better. For example, a child may learn to produce a sound quickly in target words and sentences using a particular approach, but the sound is not widely used in conversational speech. One caveat often raised about Gierut's complexity approach is that more time is spent in acquiring unstimulable sounds, and these unstimulable sounds (e.g.,

/v/) have less impact on intelligibility and communication than stimulable ones (e.g., /f/). In other words, although the approach is more efficient, there is a price to pay in how long it takes for generalization to occur to untreated sounds. Another potential caveat is that there is increasing evidence that giving children breaks from treatment may be beneficial for ultimate speech normalization (e.g., Kamhi, 2000). I got to see firsthand how treatment breaks benefited my daughter Franne. Her speech normalized by age 5 with repeated treatment breaks of 1–4 months during the 2 years she received therapy.

The client-based factors that influence treatment decisions include the following:

1. Nature and severity of the speech delay

2. Age of the child

3. Success of previous therapy

4. Child's motivation, attention, and effort

5. Associated problems (mechanism, cognitive-linguistic, and psychosocial)

Shriberg and Kwiatkowski's capability-focus framework (cf. Shriberg, 1997) provides a way to use some of these factors to make treatment decisions. *Capability* refers to the child's current phonological abilities and risk factors (mechanism, cognitive-linguistic, and psychosocial). *Focus* refers to the amount of motivational support a child needs to persist at a difficult task. Shriberg (1997) found that pretreatment capability is the best predictor of normalization rate. Lack of focus is associated with minimal progress even in children with high capability scores. These are important considerations in deciding which approach to use for children with low focus.

Other factors that will affect treatment decisions are the setting (clinic, school, home), participants (individual, group), model of service delivery (pull-out, classroom based), level of family support and involvement, schedule of treatment, and the clinician's experience and confidence in remediating phonological disorders. All but the last one have been addressed in several of the chapters in Part III. The relationship of clinician confidence and treatment efficacy has not been specifically addressed in research with phonological disorders, but clinician attitudes and beliefs are known to play an important role in the therapeutic process (cf. Kamhi, 1994).

A personal example of a clinician attitude is that I am not a very patient clinician. I often change goals or treatment methods if I feel the child is not making sufficient progress. I prefer working simultaneously at several different linguistic levels and targeting a combination of speech, language, conversational, and behavioral goals. My concern with using therapy time efficiently overrides the possibility that I have changed goals or methods too soon.

MATCHING GOALS AND APPROACHES TO CLIENTS

I concluded my 2003 ASHA presentation with suggestions about how to treat different types of children with speech sound disorders. Quite frankly, I didn't know how to end the session. It was much easier discussing the different factors that affect treatment decisions and the various problems with each of the different treatment approaches. Prescribing what to do is much more difficult, especially for someone who agrees with

Stanovich that teachers and scientists are both "committed pragmatists [who] single-mindedly pursue 'what works'—ignoring philosophical strictures along the way" (Stanovich, 2000, p. 416). Like Gierut, I would rather talk about the goals that should be targeted in therapy because goals, more so than methods, do reflect philosophical strictures (i.e., theory).

In thinking about the goals I would target, I begin with the common distinction between long- and short-term goals. Although long-term goals of speech normalization or effective communication are routinely provided in clinic reports, it is easy to lose sight of these goals as one works on the various short-term goals that need immediate attention. A central principle of goal selection is thus: "Keep the long-term goal in mind." The way to do this is to make the long-term goal a short-term goal as well. For example, a preschool child with a severe speech sound disorder needs to be taught ways to communicate intents and meanings despite having a limited phonological system. A short-term goal would be to develop a core lexicon that can be used in short phrases, clauses, and larger discourse forms (i.e., conversations, narratives, descriptions, and event recall). Numerous opportunities for speech motor and phoneme-based learning need to be integrated into these language and communicative activities. Early literacy skills should also be targeted because many children with speech sound disorders are at risk for subsequent reading difficulties (e.g., Bird, Bishop, & Freeman, 1995). A school-age child with a speech sound disorder would benefit from specific instruction in phonological awareness, letter recognition, and linking sounds to letters (e.g., Gillon, 2000).

For choosing short-term speech goals, I like Tyler's first two principles of goal selection: 1) choose error patterns that have a major impact on the system in terms of severity and intelligibility, and 2) choose target sounds that have an impact on these error patterns and/or expand the inventory (see Chapter 6). Using these principles, I will almost always choose to target /s/ and/or /z/ because of the significant function these sounds have in morphosyntax. I have no problem targeting nonstimulable sounds or using the principle of maximum contrast (see Williams, Chapter 9); I would also target phonotactic structures and other aspects of speech as needed. In keeping with primary principle of keeping the long-term goal in mind, I would target these sounds or structures in different language levels and in varying communicative contexts. I would also never use a vertical goal attack strategy, the traditional Van Riper approach, or any other approach for which improved communication is not a short-term as well as a long-term goal.

FUTURE DIRECTIONS

One of my favorite exercises is to have students pretend that they are able to peer into the future 10, 20, or 30 years from now. The basic question I want them to answer is what has changed and what has not changed about how we assess, diagnose, classify, and treat children with speech sound disorders. I also ask them whether the prevalence of speech sound disorders has changed, whether a phenotypic marker for DAS has been found, whether the benefits of oral-motor therapy are still being debated, and what new technologies have been developed for assessment and treatment. I am not particularly good at predicting the future, so I am very interested in how knowledgeable students will answer these questions. Unfortunately, I haven't asked any of these questions to students for a while, so I have to find that crystal ball that's collecting dust in my file cabinet and see if there is anything in it.

Well, the good news is that I found the crystal ball, but the bad news is that it doesn't work. Like most crystal balls, mine is not made of crystal and even when I squint I don't see the future; all I see is the past. But I heard this saying once: "Today is yesterday's tomorrow," which suggests that one way to think about the future is to look back in order to look forward. In other words, the changes that have occurred in how children with speech sound disorders are diagnosed, assessed, and treated should provide some guideposts for the changes we expect to occur in the next several decades. So, what does the past tell us about the future?

Since 1975, there have been changes in almost every aspect of how speech sound disorders are diagnosed, assessed, and treated. In 1976, David Ingram's (1976) seminal book on phonological disabilities in children was published. Ingram introduced the notion of phonological disorders and error patterns/processes to our field and, more generally, raised questions about the language basis of speech sound disorders. I entered the profession in 1974, so I have witnessed the significant changes that have occurred in this disorder area. One area, however, that has seen little change is the actual procedures used to facilitate speech sound production. In fact, these procedures have not changed much in the past 50 years. Another area that has not changed is the importance of stimulability testing. My first class in articulation disorders was with Bob Milisen, the person who first wrote about stimulability testing in 1954.

If we look at the 20-year span since 1985, the pattern of change looks very similar. In 1985, many programs were still teaching courses in articulation disorders, and the use of phonological assessments was still new for many clinicians. For example, at about this time when I was at the University of Memphis, we changed the title of the course "Articulation Disorders" to "Phonological Disorders." This change eventually led to the hiring of a phonologist (Karen) to teach the class. In some cases, the initial excitement and appeal of phonology made some clinicians reluctant to use the traditional motor approaches and techniques they had been using in the past because children were viewed as having a language-based disorder rather than an articulation (motor) problem.

The past 10 years have seen fewer changes, in part because of the shorter time span, but also because scientific consensus is gradually occurring in many areas with this population of children. It is not that we know everything there is to know about speech sound disorders, but the research conducted in the past 30 years has answered many questions about the nature of speech sound disorders and how best to assess and treat children with these disorders. The interesting questions being asked today involve trying to identify diagnostic and phenotype markers for genetically transmitted speech delays (e.g., Shriberg et al., in press).

What has occurred from the early 1990s to the present is that the pendulum seems to have swung back to the motor side after spending 10–15 years on the side of language-based phonology. This is seen in the heightened interest in oral-motor approaches and the increasing number of children diagnosed with DAS. Since the mid-1990s, there has also been increasing awareness of the link between speech sound disorders and subsequent reading difficulties. Targeting early literacy skills such as phonological awareness is now seen as an important treatment goal for this population of children (Gillon, 2000; Justice & Schuele, 2004).

So what does the future hold? I read in the New York Times recently that scientists in Boulder, Colorado, and Innsbruck, Austria, teleported an atom (Chang, 2004). This does not mean that we will ever be teleporting real objects, but it does mean that the development of a quantum computer that uses teleportation to move results of a calculation from one part of the computer to another is possible. What are the possibilities for children with speech sound disorders? Can these disorders ever be eliminated with some future version of genetic engineering? Maybe, but probably not within the next 30 years. Is it possible that the future will see the development of a more effective treatment approach? If the past is a guide to the future, the answer to this question is "no." There does not appear to be any technological advance in the foreseeable future that will speed speech normalization. Visi-Pitch–like feedback systems may become a part of the treatment arsenal. It is possible to envision hand-held computers or phones that provide visual feedback for speech productions. This technology could clearly help older children and adults to modify speech errors or dialectal speech patterns, but I cannot imagine it aiding a 3- to 5-year-old child with a severe speech delay.

If the future mirrors the past, the most significant changes in the next 20–30 years will be in how we diagnose and assess children with speech sound disorders. It is not unthinkable to imagine that by 2025, we will have technology that will be able to record child speech and other developmental information and immediately provide a detailed speech analysis, diagnosis, short- and long-term goals, preferred treatment approach, expected time for speech normalization, and risk of subsequent reading problems. The data used to generate this information will be based on the existing knowledge base and the research that will be conducted in the next 10–30 years.

There is no doubt that some of the future will mirror the past, but the past also shows us that there are always unforeseen developments. Was there anyone in 1975 who envisioned the scope of the Internet and World Wide Web or wireless technology? Just because speech modification techniques have not changed much in the past 50 years does not mean there will not be some unforeseen change in the next 20–30 years. Perhaps you see something in your crystal ball that I don't see in mine. I hope so, for today's visions are tomorrow's reality.

REFERENCES

Bauman-Waengler, J. (2004). *Articulatory and phonological impairments: A clinical focus* (2nd ed.). Boston: Allyn & Bacon.

Bernthal, J., & Bankson, N. (2004). *Articulation and phonological disorders* (5th ed.). Boston: Allyn & Bacon.

Bird, J., Bishop, D., & Freeman, N. (1995). Phonological awareness and literacy development in children with excessive phonological impairments. *Journal of Speech and Hearing Research, 38,* 446–462.

Camarata, S. (1993). The application of naturalistic conversation training to speech production in children with specific disabilities. *Journal of Applied Behavioral Analysis, 26,* 173–182.

Campbell, T. (1999). Functional treatment outcomes in young children with motor speech disorders. In A. Caruso & E. Strand (Eds.), *Assessment procedures for treatment planning in children with phonologic and motor speech disorders* (pp. 385–396). New York: Thieme.

Chang, K. (2004). Scientists teleport not Kirk, but an atom. *The New York Times.* Retrieved June 17, 2004, from http://www.nytimes.com

Edwards, H., Fourakis, M., Beckman, M., & Fox, R. (1999). Characterizing knowledge deficits in phonological disorders. *Journal of Speech, Language, and Hearing Research, 42,* 169–186.

Gillon, G. (2000). The efficacy of phonological awareness intervention for children with spoken language impairment. *Language, Speech, and Hearing Services in Schools, 31,* 126–141.

Hodson, B., & Paden, E. (1991). *Targeting intelligible speech: A phonological approach to remediation* (2nd ed.). San Diego: College-Hill Press.

Hoffman, P., & Norris, J. (2002). Phonological assessment as an integral part of language assessment. *American Journal of Speech-Language Pathology, 11,* 230–246.

Ingram, D. (1976). *Phonological disability in children.* New York: Elsevier.

Ingram, D., & Ingram, K. (2001). A whole-word approach to phonological analysis and intervention. *Language, Speech, and Hearing Services in Schools, 32,* 271–283.

Justice, L., & Schuele, M. (2004). Phonological awareness: Description, assessment, and intervention. In J. Bernthal & N. Bankston (Eds.), *Articulation and phonological disorders* (5th ed., pp. 376–407). Boston: Allyn & Bacon.

Kamhi, A. (1994). Toward a theory of clinical expertise in speech-language pathology. *Language, Speech, and Hearing Services in Schools, 25,* 115–119.

Kamhi, A. (2000). Practice makes perfect: The incompatibility of practicing speech and meaningful communication. *Language, Speech, and Hearing Services in Schools, 31,* 182–186.

Kamhi, A. (2003, November). *How to decide which speech treatment approach to use.* Mini-seminar presented at the annual convention of the American Speech-Language-Hearing Association, Chicago.

Kamhi, A. (2004). A meme's eye view of speech-language pathology. *Language, Speech, and Hearing Services in Schools, 35,* 105–111.

Locke, J. (1980). Mechanisms of phonological development in children: Maintenance, learning, and loss. *Papers from the Sixteenth Regional Meeting of the Chicago Linguistic Society.* Chicago: Chicago Linguistic Society.

Locke, J. (1983). *Phonological acquisition and change.* New York: Academic Press.

Miccio, A.W., & Ingrisano, D. (2000). The acquisition of fricatives and affricates: Evidence from a disordered phonological system. *American Journal of Speech-Language Pathology, 9,* 214–229.

Milisen, R. (1954). The disorder of articulation: A systematic clinical and experimental approach. *Journal of Speech and Hearing Disorders, Monograph Supplement 4.*

Shriberg, L. (1997). Developmental phonological disorders: One or many. In B. Hodson & M. Edwards (Eds.), *Perspectives in applied phonology* (pp. 105–127). Gaithersburg, MD: Aspen Publishers.

Shriberg, L., Aram, D., & Kwiatkowski, J. (1997). Developmental apraxia of speech I: Descriptive and theoretical perspectives. *Journal of Speech, Language, and Hearing Research, 40,* 273–285.

Shriberg, L., Lewis, B., Tomblin, B., McSweeny, J., Karlsson, H., & Sheer, A. (in press). Toward diagnostic and phenotype markers for genetically transmitted speech delay. *Journal of Speech, Language, and Hearing Research.*

Stanovich, K. (2000). *Progress in understanding reading: Scientific foundations and new frontiers.* New York: Guilford.

Torgesen, J., & Bryant, B. (1994). *Test of Phonological Awareness.* Austin, TX: PRO-ED.

Van Riper, C. (1978). *Speech correction: Principles and methods* (6th ed.). Englewood Cliffs, NJ: Prentice Hall.

Velleman, S., & Vihman, M. (2002). Whole-word phonology and templates: Trap, bootstrap, or some of each? *Language, Speech, and Hearing Services in Schools, 33,* 9–24.

Wagner, R., Torgesen, J., & Rashotte, C. (1999). *Comprehensive Test of Phonological Processing.* Austin, TX: PRO-ED.

Williams, A.L. (2000). Multiple oppositions: Theoretical foundations for an alternative contrastive intervention approach. *American Journal of Speech-Language Pathology, 9,* 282–288.

Index

Page references followed by *t* or *f* indicate tables or figures, respectively.